D1472896

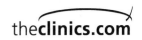

# MEDICAL CLINICS
## OF NORTH AMERICA

Allergy

GUEST EDITOR
Anthony Montanaro, MD

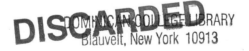

DISCARDED

DOMINICAN COLLEGE LIBRARY
Blauvelt, New York 10913

January 2006 • Volume 90 • Number 1

**SAUNDERS**

An Imprint of Elsevier, Inc.
PHILADELPHIA  LONDON  TORONTO  MONTREAL  SYDNEY  TOKYO

130005

## W.B. SAUNDERS COMPANY
*A Division of Elsevier Inc.*

1600 John F. Kennedy Boulevard • Suite 1800 • Philadelphia, Pennsylvania 19103-2899

http://www.theclinics.com

**MEDICAL CLINICS OF NORTH AMERICA**  Volume 90, Number
January 2006  ISSN 0025-71.
Editor: Rachel Glover  ISBN 1-4160-3442

Copyright © 2005 Elsevier Inc. All rights reserved. No part of this publication may be reproduced transmitted in any form or by any means, electronic or mechanical, including photocopy, recording, any information retrieval system, without written permission from the publisher.

Single photocopies of single articles may be made for personal use as allowed by national copyright law Permission of the publisher and payment of a fee is required for all other photocopying, including multip or systematic copying, copying for advertising or promotional purposes, resale, and all forms of docume delivery. Special rates are available for educational institutions that wish to make photocopies for non-pro educational classroom use. Permissions may be sought directly from Elsevier's Rights Department in Phil delphia, PA, USA at Tel.: (+1) 215-239-3804; Fax: (+1) 215-239-3805; E-mail: healthpermissions@elsevier.cor Requests may also be completed on-line via the Elsevier homepage (http://www.elsevier.com/locate permissions). In the USA, users may clear permissions and make payments through the Copyright Clearan Center, Inc., 222 Rosewood Drive, Danvers, MA 01923, USA; Tel.: (+1) 978-750-8400; Fax: (+1) 978-750-474 and in the UK through the Copyright Licensing Agency Rapid Clearance Service (CLARCS), 90 Tottenha Court Road, London W1P 0LP, UK; Tel.: (+44) 171-436-5931; Fax: (+44) 171-436-3986. Other countries m have a local reprographic rights agency for payments.

The ideas and opinions expressed in *Medical Clinics of North America* do not necessarily reflect those of t Publisher. The Publisher does not assume any responsibility for any injury and/or damage to persons property arising out of or related to any use of the material contained in this periodical. The reader is a vised to check the appropriate medical literature and the product information currently provided by t manufacturer of each drug to be administered to verify the dosage, the method and duration of admini tration, or contraindications. It is the responsibility of the treating physician or other health care profe sional, relying on independent experience and knowledge of the patient, to determine drug dosages ar the best treatment for the patient. Mention of any product in this issue should not be construed as endors ment by the contributors, editors, or the Publisher of the product or manufacturers' claims.

*Medical Clinics of North America* (ISSN 0025-7125) is published bimonthly by Elsevier. Corporate and editori offices: 1600 John F. Kennedy Boulevard, Suite 1800, Philadelphia, PA 19103-2899. Accounting and circulatio offices: 6277 Sea Harbor Drive, Orlando, FL 32887-4800. Periodicals postage paid at Orlando, FL 32862, ar additional mailing offices. Subscription prices are USD 145 per year for US individuals, USD 260 per year f US institutions, USD 75 per year for US students, USD 185 per year for Canadian individuals, USD 330 p year for Canadian institutions, USD 210 per year for international individuals, USD 330 per year for inte national institutions and USD 110 per year for Canadian and foreign students/residents. To receiv student/resident rate, orders must be accompanied by name of affiliated institution, date of term, and the si *nature* of program/residency coordinator on institution letterhead. Orders will be billed at individual rate un proof of status is received. Foreign air speed delivery is included in all *Clinics* subscription prices. All prices a subject to change without notice. POSTMASTER: Send address changes to *Medical Clinics of North Americ* W.B. Saunders Company, Periodicals Fulfillment, Orlando, FL 32887-4800. **Customer Service: 1-800-65 2452 (US). From outside of the USA, call (+1) 407-345-1000. E-mail: hhspcs@harcourt.com.**

*Reprints.* For copies of 100 or more, of articles in this publication, please contact the Commercial Reprin Department, Elsevier Inc., 360 Park Avenue South, New York, New York 10010-1710. Tel.: (+1) (212) 63 3813; Fax: (+1) (212) 462-1935; E-mail: reprints@elsevier.com.

*Medical Clinics of North America* is also published in Spanish by McGraw-Hill Interamericana Editores S. A P.O. Box 5-237, 06500 Mexico, D.F., Mexico.

*Medical Clinics of North America* is covered in *Index Medicus, Current Contents, ASCA, Excerpta Medic Science Citation Index,* and *ISI/BIOMED.*

Printed in the United States of America.

## GOAL STATEMENT
The goal of *Medical Clinics of North America* is to keep practicing physicians up to date with current clinical practice by providing timely articles reviewing the state of the art in patient care.

## ACCREDITATION
The *Medical Clinics of North America* is planned and implemented in accordance with the Essential Areas and Policies of the Accreditation Council for Continuing Medical Education (ACCME) through the joint sponsorship of the University of Virginia School of Medicine and Elsevier. The University of Virginia School of Medicine is accredited by the ACCME to provide continuing medical education for physicians.

The University of Virginia School of Medicine designates this educational activity for a maximum of 90 category 1 credits per year, 15 category 1 credits per issue, toward the AMA Physician's Recognition Award. Each physician should claim only those credits that he/she actually spent in the activity.

The American Medical Association has determined that physicians not licensed in the US who participate in this CME activity are eligible for AMA PRA category 1 credit.

Category 1 credit can be earned by reading the text material, taking the CME examination online at *http://www.theclinics.com/home/cme*, and completing the evaluation. After taking the test, you will be required to review any and all incorrect answers. Following completion of the test and evaluation, your credit will be awarded and you may print your certificate.

## FACULTY DISCLOSURE/CONFLICT OF INTEREST
The University of Virginia School of Medicine, as an ACCME accredited provider, endorses and strives to comply with the Accreditation Council for Continuing Medical Education (ACCME) Standards of Commercial Support, Commonwealth of Virginia statutes, University of Virginia policies and procedures, and associated federal and private regulations and guidelines on the need for disclosure and monitoring of proprietary and financial interests that may affect the scientific integrity and balance of content delivered in continuing medical education activities under our auspices.

The University of Virginia School of Medicine requires that all CME activities accredited through this institution be developed independently and be scientifically rigorous, balanced and objective in the presentation/discussion of its content, theories and practices.

All authors/editors participating in an accredited CME activity are expected to disclose to the readers relevant financial relationships with commercial entities occurring within the past 12 months (such as grants or research support, employee, consultant, stock holder, member of speakers bureau, etc.). The University of Virginia School of Medicine will employ appropriate mechanisms to resolve potential conflicts of interest to maintain the standards of fair and balanced education to the reader. Questions about specific strategies can be directed to the Office of Continuing Medical Education, University of Virginia School of Medicine, Charlottesville, Virginia.

*The authors/editors listed below have identified no professional or financial affiliations for themselves or their spouse/partner:*
Larry Borish, MD; Rachel Glover, Acquisitions Editor; Jon M. Hanifin, MD; Barry J. Mark, MD; Sameer K. Mathur, MD, PhD; Anna Nowak-Wegrzyn, MD; Hugh A. Sampson, MD; Eric L. Simpson, MD; Raymond G. Slavin, MD; and John W. Steinke, PhD.

*The authors/editors listed below identified the following professional or financial affiliations for themselves or their spouse/partner:*
**Leonard Bielory, MD** is a consultant for Alcon, Inspite, Medpointe, and Allergan in the area of ocular allergy.
**William W. Busse, MD** is an independent contractor and on the speakers's bureau for GlaxoSmithKline and Aventis; is an independent contractor and consultant for Fuijisawa, Dynavax, Hoffman-LaRoche, and Wyeth; is an independent contractor for Pfizer; a consultant for Bristol-Myers Squibb; and, is on the speakers' bureau for Merck.
**Donald A. Dibbern Jr., MD, FAAAAI** is on the speakers' bureau for Pfizer.
**David F. Graft, MD** is a consultant and on the speakers' bureau for Sanofi Aventis and Schering Plough, and is a consultant for Merck and GlaxoSmithKline.
**Alexander N. Greiner, MD** is on the speakers' bureau for Pfizer, Kos, Aventis, and MedPointe.
**Phillip Lieberman, MD** is a consultant and on the speakers' bureau for Dey and Verus.
**Anthony Montanaro, MD** is on the speakers' bureau for Aventis, GlaxoSMithKline, Merck, and Schering.
**Roland Solensky, MD** is on the speaker's bureau for Pfizer.
**Steven A. Tilles, MD** has grant and research support from Through A.S.T.H.M.A., Inc. research organization: Abbott, Altana, Amgen, Astellas, AstraZeneca, Allergy Therapeutics, Dey Labs, Genentech, GlaxoSmithKline, Janssen, Merck, Novartis, Pfizer, Sanofi-Aventis, Sepracor, UCB Pharma, National Heart, Lung and Blood Institute, MedPointe Pharmaceuticals, Medtronic Emergency Response Systems, Pharmaxis, CompleWare; is a consultant to Genentech, Janssen Pharmaceutica, Sanofi-Aventis, Novartis, Arriva Pharmaceuticals, and PDL; is on the speakers' bureau and has received honoraria from Glaxo Welcome, Pfizer/UCB Pharma, Aventis, Genentech, Schering.

*Disclosure of Discussion of non-FDA approved uses for pharmaceutical products and/or medical devices:*
The University of Virginia School of Medicine, as an ACCME provider, requires that all faculty presenters identify and disclose any "off label" uses for pharmaceutical and medical device products. The University of Virginia School of Medicine recommends that each physician fully review all the available data on new products or procedures prior to instituting them with patients.

## TO ENROLL
To enroll in the Medical Clinics of North America Continuing Medical Education program, call customer service at 1-800-654-2452 or visit us online at *http://www.theclinics.com/home/cme*. The CME program is available to subscribers for an additional fee of USD 205.

# FORTHCOMING ISSUES

# RECENT ISSUES

---

## THE CLINICS ARE NOW AVAILABLE ONLINE!

Access your subscription at:
http://www.theclinics.com

# GUEST EDITOR

**ANTHONY MONTANARO, MD,** Professor (Medicine); and Head, Division of Allergy and Clinical Immunology, Oregon Health and Science University, Portland, Oregon

# CONTRIBUTORS

**LEONARD BIELORY, MD,** Professor (Medicine, Pediatrics, and Ophthalmology); Director, Clinical Research and Development; Director, Division of Allergy, Immunology, and Rheumatology; and Co-Director, Immuno-Opthalmological Service, New Jersey Medical School, University of Medicine and Dentistry of New Jersey, Newark, New Jersey

**LARRY BORISH, MD,** Professor (Medicine), Asthma and Allergic Disease Center, Beirne Carter Center for Immunology Research, University of Virginia Health Systems, Charlottesville, Virginia

**WILLIAM W. BUSSE, MD,** Professor, Section of Allergy, Pulmonary, and Critical Care, Department of Medicine, University of Wisconsin Medical School, Madison, Wisconsin

**DONALD A. DIBBERN, JR, MD, FAAAAI,** Adjunct Assistant Professor (Medicine and Dermatology), Division of Allergy and Clinical Immunology, Oregon Health and Sciences University, Portland, Oregon

**DAVID F. GRAFT, MD,** Chairman, Asthma and Allergic Diseases, Park Nicollet Clinic; and Adjunct Professor, Department of Pediatrics, University of Minnesota Medical School, Minneapolis, Minnesota

**ALEXANDER N. GREINER, MD,** Assistant Clinical Professor, University of California at San Diego; and Allergy and Asthma Medical Group and Research Center, San Diego, California

**JON M. HANIFIN, MD,** Professor, Department of Dermatology, Oregon Health and Science University, Portland, Oregon

**PHILLIP LIEBERMAN, MD,** Clinical Professor (Medicine and Pediatrics), Division of Allergy and Immunology, Departments of Medicine and Pediatrics, University of Tennessee College of Medicine, Memphis, Tennessee

**BARRY J. MARK, MD,** Clinical Fellow, Division of Allergy and Immunology, Saint Louis University School of Medicine, St. Louis, Missouri

**SAMEER K. MATHUR, MD, PhD,** Clinical Instructor, Section of Allergy, Pulmonary, and Critical Care, Department of Medicine, University of Wisconsin Medical School, Madison, Wisconsin

**ANTHONY MONTANARO, MD,** Professor (Medicine); and Head, Division of Allergy and Clinical Immunology, Oregon Health and Science University, Portland, Oregon

**ANNA NOWAK-WEGRZYN, MD,** Assistant Professor (Pediatrics), Division of Allergy and Immunology, Department of Pediatrics, Mount Sinai School of Medicine; and Jaffe Food Allergy Institute, New York, New York

**HUGH A. SAMPSON, MD,** Professor (Pediatrics and Immunobiology), Division of Allergy and Immunology, Department of Pediatrics, Mount Sinai School of Medicine; and Jaffe Food Allergy Institute, New York, New York

**ERIC L. SIMPSON, MD,** Assistant Professor, Department of Dermatology, Oregon Health and Science University, Portland, Oregon

**RAYMOND G. SLAVIN, MD,** Director, Division of Allergy and Immunology, Saint Louis University School of Medicine, St. Louis, Missouri

**ROLAND SOLENSKY, MD,** Division of Allergy and Immunology, The Corvallis Clinic, Corvallis, Oregon

**JOHN W. STEINKE, PhD,** Assistant Professor (Medicine), Asthma and Allergic Disease Center, Beirne Carter Center for Immunology Research, University of Virginia Health Systems, Charlottesville, Virginia

**STEPHEN A. TILLES, MD,** Clinical Assistant Professor (Medicine), Department of Medicine, University of Washington School of Medicine, Seattle, Washington

CONTRIBUTORS

# CONTENTS

measures and array of medications, both those currently available and on the horizon, provide an armamentarium for effective diagnosis, management, and monitoring of asthma. In coming years, it is expected that additional testing modalities will be available for more precise monitoring of asthma control, and an increased understanding of pharmacogenetics will enable the tailoring of asthma medications to specific patients, providing customized therapy to maximize asthma control.

Asthma is a common syndrome that affects approximately 5% of the adult population in the United States. This article focuses on the differential diagnosis of adult asthma, including a discussion of reasonable clinical approaches to determining the correct diagnosis. Chronic obstructive pulmonary disease and vocal cord dysfunction are discussed in the most detail because these are more likely to be mistaken for asthma in clinical practice. Less common asthma masqueraders are then discussed, including those that also may confound or aggravate asthma.

Anaphylaxis is an acute multisystem allergic reaction that is potentially fatal. Anaphylactic episodes are most commonly caused by foods or drugs, but in many instances have no known cause. Each physician should be equipped in office for therapy of the acute event. The drug of choice, which should be administered immediately, is epinephrine. Although there is some debate as to the preferred injection site, it is clear that of sites studied to date, injection in the lateral thigh (vastus lateralis) produces the most rapid rise in serum level. Any patient predisposed to anaphylactic episodes should wear identifying medical jewelry and avoid, whenever possible, drugs that could worsen an event or complicate its therapy.

Over the past 20 years, food allergy has emerged as an important clinical problem in Westernized countries. Not only has food allergy prevalence almost doubled but its severity and scope have increased. Consequently, research focusing on characterization, mapping, and cloning of food allergens, as well as on deciphering the nature of immune responses to food allergens and the mechanisms of oral tolerance, has blossomed. It is hoped that this research will lead to the development of therapeutic modalities for food allergy in the near future. This article discusses the pathomechanism of food allergic reactions, classification and manifestations of clinical food allergic disorders, and an approach to diagnosis and management.

with an autoimmune etiology. Although some progress has been made at improving symptomatic control of urticaria, further research and discovery are necessary before there is an effective impact on the underlying course and natural history of this condition.

ELSEVIER
SAUNDERS

Med Clin N Am 90 (2006) xi–xiii

THE MEDICAL
CLINICS
OF NORTH AMERICA

Preface

# Allergy

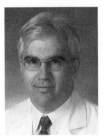

Anthony Montanaro, MD
*Guest Editor*

Allergic disease remains one of the greatest challenges in clinical medicine. In this issue we explore some of these challenges and attempt to highlight the new developments in the diagnosis and management of these disorders. We have assembled some of the leading experts in the field of allergy and immunology, who have authored scholarly reviews in their areas of expertise.

I invite the reader to consider the background of the epidemic of allergic disease. This epidemic appears to be a phenomenon of Western civilization. The hypotheses that underlie this phenomenon are explored in the article on the genetics of allergic disease. Although it is unlikely that a single atopic genotype exists, there appear to be multiple candidate genes that provide the genetic basis for multiple atopic phenotypes.

Clearly, the most common phenotype of atopy is expressed clinically as allergic rhinitis. As Dr. Greiner points out in his article, allergic rhinitis is not only the most common allergic disease but also the most common respiratory disorder. Dr. Greiner further indicates the substantial direct and indirect costs, as well as the significant comorbidities, that are associated with this common illness. A comprehensive diagnostic and therapeutic approach to this condition is highlighted, encompassing education, environmental controls, pharmacotherapy, and allergen immunotherapy.

Asthma is one of the most important challenges in clinical medicine, accounting for significant morbidity and mortality and tremendous direct and indirect cost to society. No specialists in this field have more expertise than Dr. Busse and his colleagues at the University of Wisconsin. In their article, Drs. Busse and Mathur review the pathophysiology and the epidemiology of

0025-7125/06/$ - see front matter © 2005 Elsevier Inc. All rights reserved.
doi:10.1016/j.mcna.2005.09.001          *medical.theclinics.com*

asthma. They provide an up-to-date treatise on diagnosis, as well as guide-line-directed treatment options.

Dr. Stephen Tilles provides further expert analysis of the differential diagnosis of asthma. Because this condition is so common, there are significant problems with misdiagnoses and underdiagnoses of reversible airway obstruction. Dr. Tilles shares his expertise in the challenging area of asthma masqueraders, with a focus on vocal cord dysfunction, an area in which he has greatly added to our understanding. In addition, Dr. Tilles expands the differential diagnosis by highlighting the features distinguishing asthma from many common conditions, including chronic obstructive pulmonary disease and gastroesophageal reflux.

Dr. Philip Lieberman has spent much of his distinguished career in the clinical study of anaphylaxis. In his article on anaphylaxis, Dr. Lieberman shares his wealth of experience and his mastery of the literature in this important area. I suspect that no condition in clinical medicine instills more fear in the hearts of patients and their care providers than this one. Dr. Lieberman presents a concise and learned approach to anaphylaxis that can save lives and minimize patients' appropriate apprehension regarding this life-threatening condition.

Adverse reactions to foods are among the most difficult and common clinical problems in medicine. Drs. Nowak-Wegrzyn and Sampson present a diagnostic approach to this challenge in children and adults. Their experiences at the Jaffe Food Allergy Institute at the Mount Sinai School of Medicine provide the foundation for much of the clinical research being published in this area. They help sort through the differential diagnosis of food-related disorders based on age and pathologic mechanisms. Non–IgE-mediated as well as IgE-mediated food allergies are detailed. The superb figures in their article should provide a useful reference source for any clinician.

Dr. Bielory is an internationally highly regarded expert in the area of ocular allergy. In his article, Dr. Bielory reviews clinically relevant pathophysiology and details the important aspects of the differential diagnosis of ocular allergy, including the emerging area of dry eye syndrome. He further reviews newer treatment options for ocular allergy and describes a rational, cost-effective approach to treatment, including the benefits of immunotherapy.

Drs. Simpson and Hanifin at the Oregon Health and Science University (OHSU) review the challenges of atopic dermatitis. Dr. Hanifin and his colleagues at OHSU are regarded as leading experts in this important clinical area and have initiated many exciting new scientific advances in the field of atopic dermatitis. The authors summarize differential diagnosis, relevant clinical findings, and updated treatment regimens. They include a discussion of the controversy regarding the recently released black box warnings on nonsteroidal topical immunomodulatory agents that places this issue in proper perspective.

Dr. Raymond Slavin at Washington University School of Medicine is one of the most respected experts in the field of allergy. Many specialists and generalists have benefited over the years from his expertise in the difficult area of contact dermatitis. In their article on contact dermatitis, Drs. Mark and Slavin review the clinical features and underlying immunologic basis of this condition. They help to distinguish specific contact allergic dermatitis from contact irritant dermatitis and highlight the importance of identifying the offending agents. Historical clues in and outside the workplace that can aid in the identification of these agents are presented. Practical management issues are reviewed, including caveats for the practitioner who may encounter this problem.

Dr. Donald Dibbern shares his wealth of clinical experience as the Director of the OHSU Multidisciplinary Urticaria Clinic. He is able to summarize aspects of clinical presentation and evaluation that enable the clinician to undertake a pragmatic approach to perhaps the most frustrating allergic problem for patient and care provider alike. Recent advances, such as those in the area of autoimmune urticaria, are discussed. The evidence for the use of traditional as well as newer and more aggressive therapeutic options is detailed.

The challenge of stinging insect venom sensitivity is detailed in an outstanding review by Dr. David Graft. The importance of identifying appropriate patients for venom-specific immunotherapy is reviewed. The conundrum of the history-positive, skin test– negative patient is addressed, and recommendations for evaluating these patients are presented. Clinicians will be more effective when they can present patients with a therapeutic option that is more than 95% effective in preventing a potentially life-threatening event.

Dr. Solensky has reviewed the clinical challenge of drug hypersensitivity. Dr. Solensky and colleagues at Southwestern Medical School have been highly regarded leaders in this area and have contributed significantly to the drug allergy literature. In Dr. Solensky's article, he has addressed the value of and indications for skin testing in drug allergy. He addresses the confusing area of cephalosporin cross-reactivity and makes specific recommendations for evaluating patients with this clinical dilemma.

I hope that you enjoy reading this issue. The authors have assembled the latest findings in this challenging area of medicine. This compendium of updates should provide the clinical practitioner with a valuable resource for problems that are encountered on a daily basis. I have been privileged to work with such a distinguished group of authors. I hope you learn as much as I have in preparing this issue.

Anthony Montanaro, MD
*Division of Allergy and Clinical Immunology*
*Oregon Health and Science University*
*3181 SW Sam Jackson Park Road, OP34*
*Portland, OR 97201-3098, USA*

*E-mail address:* montanar@ohsu.edu

THE MEDICAL
CLINICS
OF NORTH AMERICA

ELSEVIER
SAUNDERS

Med Clin N Am 90 (2006) 1–15

# Genetics of Allergic Disease

John W. Steinke, PhD, Larry Borish, MD*

Asthma and Allergic Disease Center, Beirne Carter Center for Immunology Research,
University of Virginia Health Systems, Charlottesville, VA, USA

The understanding that genetics play a role in allergic disease and asthma has been recognized for more than 100 years. This genetic component was suggested through observations that allergic subjects had a significantly higher incidence of family histories of disease as compared with controls [1,2]. Follow-up studies have shown that if one parent has allergies, a child has a 33% chance of developing allergies and if both parents are allergic that number jumps to a 70% chance. The link to asthma is not quite as strong, because a child only has a 15% chance of developing asthma if one parent has the disease. A dominant or recessive model of inheritance for atopy or asthma has not been supported in association studies, which led to a period of time where the idea of inheritance of atopy was in question. Eventually, it was recognized that allergies and asthma represent complex genetic disorders, defined as disorders that have numerous contributing genes, each having variable degrees of involvement in any given individual. In addition to specific genes, environmental exposures (including allergen exposure, secondhand cigarette smoke, pollutants), low birth weight, infectious agents, and numerous other factors have been recognized to contribute to the development of allergies and asthma through their ability to influence gene expression. The results of twin studies suggest that approximately 50% of the risk for developing asthma is related to genetic factors with an equivalent risk associated with environment [3]. This article covers three areas involved in the genetics of allergic disease: (1) the association studies performed in allergy and asthma, (2) functional genomics of candidate genes, and (3) pharmacogenetics.

* Corresponding author. Asthma and Allergic Disease Center, Beirne Carter Center for Immunology Research, University of Virginia Health Systems, 409 Lane Road, PO Box 801355, Charlottesville, VA 22908–1355.

E-mail address: lb4m@virginia.edu (L. Borish).

0025-7125/06/$ - see front matter © 2005 Elsevier Inc. All rights reserved.
doi:10.1016/j.mcna.2005.08.005
medical.theclinics.com

## Genome-wide screens, association studies, and candidate genes

One approach to identifying disease-causing genes involves scanning the entire genome with a technique termed "positional cloning." This technique is based on the presence of highly polymorphic genetic markers whose position on a chromosome is known. Markers close to the disease gene are statistically coinherited with the disease when multiple families are analyzed. Typically, these approaches localize a marker to within approximately $10^6$ DNA base pairs of the actual gene. Identification of such a closely linked marker is followed by a technique termed "chromosomal walking" until the mutant gene is found. This process requires an enormous amount of work, even using today's molecular biology techniques. Since completion of the human genome project, the typical approach has been to access the map of the human genome and obtain a list of the genes localized to the chromosomal region where a linkage marker has been identified. It is then possible to determine whether mutations either in one of these genes or in adjacent regions contribute to the development of allergies and asthma. Obvious candidate genes can often be identified within a linkage region; however, the function of most of the genes identified through the human genome project is not known. It is likely that these unknown genes may provide insight into the asthmatic and atopic disease processes, because they focus attention on pathways not previously implicated in disease progression.

Advances in the past 15 years have opened the door to positional cloning using linkage studies within families as a means of identifying markers that may be linked to allergies and asthma. Several problems have limited the value of these studies. These include the confounding influences of genetic heterogeneity (mutations in different genes that result in the same phenotype) and the incomplete penetrance of genetic phenotypes that reflects the importance of both gene-environment and gene-gene interactions. Examples of gene-environment interactions include the requirement for exposures to cigarette smoke, endotoxin, diet, viral infections, or the presence and dose of specific aeroallergens, before certain genotypes manifest themselves. For example, links have been demonstrated to genes within chromosomes 1p, 5q, and 9q only when tobacco smoke is included as a risk factor for asthma [4]. Similarly, genetic mutations involving CD14 or toll-like receptors are more likely to manifest as asthma when endotoxin is prevalent in the environment. Other specific genetic variants may only achieve penetrance when allowed to synergize with mutations in related genes. For example, a gene-gene interaction has been shown between an allele at position −1112 of the interleukin (IL)-13 gene and an allele at position 478 of the IL-4 receptor α gene, a component of the IL-13 receptor. Individuals with both affected genes had a fivefold greater risk for the development of asthma as compared with individuals with nonrisk genotypes [5].

Positional cloning studies optimally require unambiguous phenotypes. The absence of an exact definition of asthma, atopic dermatitis, or other atopic diseases has contributed, however, to the lack of replication observed in numerous linkage studies. A more useful, but still problematic, approach has been to perform linkages to intermediate phenotypes that are more easily quantified. A few examples of intermediate phenotypes include bronchial hyperresponsiveness, skin test reactivity to inhalant allergens, and total and specific IgE levels. The inability to phenotype family members unambiguously and the lack of a general consensus on how these available measures should be performed and interpreted has contributed to the current confusion. Many genome-wide searches have also been inconclusive because of their being underpowered with regards to the numbers of families used in the genetic analysis. The genetic component of asthma and allergies represents the cumulative influence of many genes. As a result, thousands of families need to be studied to draw conclusive evidence for a role for a given genetic marker in complex genetic disorders. This represents a daunting task. Nonetheless, over the past decade, more than 18 genome-wide screens using a variety of intermediate phenotypes have been published [6–8]. One of the earliest genome-wide searches for asthma genes was performed by Cookson's group at Oxford. Using the technology available at the time, these investigators performed linkage analyses on a very limited number of polymorphic DNA markers to allergen-specific IgE and high total serum IgE. Their analysis found a linkage to chromosome 11q when linked to maternal (but not paternal) phenotype [9]. Analysis of 11q demonstrated that this marker mapped close to the gene for the β chain of the high-affinity IgE receptor. Although the α and γ chains of the high-affinity IgE receptor are sufficient for sending signals to the cell for activation, the β chain acts as an amplification mechanism for this signaling pathway and permits mast cell activation in the presence of fewer cross-linked IgE molecules. These authors have suggested that base exchanges in the cytoplasmic region of the β-chain may be the disease-causing mutations. As has been typical of many genetic studies, significance of this linkage to chromosome 11 has been controversial insofar as several other groups were not able to confirm this linkage [10–12].

Several other extensive genome-wide searches have now been reported [6,7,13]. The National Heart, Lung, and Blood Institute funded a multicenter Collaborative Study on the Genetics of Asthma. Their initial genome screen involved three racial groups (African-Americans, whites, and Hispanics) [13], and more recently this group has reported information on individuals of Hutterite ancestry [7]. Together, these studies uncovered approximately 15 separate promising linkages, including several in previously unsuspected regions of the human genome. Several of these linkages have been confirmed by competing investigators in separate populations (Table 1). These include a locus on chromosome 2 near the IL-1 cluster that includes the genes for CD28 and CTLA-4 and the major histocompatibility complex on chromosome 6. Not surprisingly, the chromosome 5 cytokine gene cluster that includes the genes for IL-3, IL-4, IL-5, IL-9, IL-13, granulocyte-macrophage

Table 1
Linkages to asthma and allergy

| Chromosome | Candidate genes |
|---|---|
| 1p | IL-12 receptor, JAK1, PAF receptor, endothelin 2 |
| 2q | IL-1, IL-1Ra, ICOS, CTLA-4, CD28 |
| 3p24 | bcl-6 (stat-6 binding inhibition), CCR4 |
| 5q23–q25 | IL-3, IL-4, IL-5, IL-9, IL-13, GM-CSF, leukotriene $C_4$ synthase, macrophage-CSF receptor, β2-AR, GR, TIM-1, TIM-3, CD14, SPINK5 |
| 6p21–p23 | MHC, TNFs, transporters involved in antigen processing and presentation (TAP-1 and -2), LMP particles |
| 7q11–q14 | T-cell receptor γ chain, IL-6 |
| 10q | 5-LO |
| 11q13 | High-affinity IgE receptor (Fc∈RI), β chain, Clara cell protein 16, FGF-3 |
| 12q14–q24 | IFN-γ, IL-22, SCF, nitric oxide synthetase (constitutive), NF-YB (transcription factor for HLA genes), ILGF-1, leukotrien $A_4$ hydrolase, Stat 6 (IL-4 stat) |
| 13q21–q24 | Cysteinyl leukotriene 2 receptor |
| 14q11–q13 | T-cell receptor (α/δ chains) |
| 16p11–p12 | NF-κB, MCC |
| 17p12–p17 | IL-4 receptor |
| 17q | CCL5 (RANTES) |
| 19q13 | CD22, TGF-β1 |
| 20p13 | ADAM33 |
| Xq13 | IL-13 receptor, common γ chain |
| Xp | MAOB |
| Y | IL-9 receptor |

*Abbreviations:* AR, adrenergic receptor; FGF, fibroblast growth factor; GM-CSF, granulo-cyte-macrophage colony–stimulating factor; GR, glucocorticosteriod receptor; IFN, interferorn; IL, interleukin; ILGF, insulin-like growth factor; LMP, large multicatalytic protelytic; LO, lipoxygenase; MHC, major histocompatibility complex; NF, nuclear factor; SCF, stem cell factor; TNF, tumor necrosis factor.

colony–stimulating factor, and leukotriene C4 synthase ($LTC_4S$) has been linked to allergies and asthma. Genome-wide searches have also supported presence of potential allergy and asthma genes on chromosome 12 in association with interferon-γ and stat-6. It is likely that many of the reported sites of asthma susceptibility genes will ultimately fail to be confirmed in other studies. Similarly, it would not be surprising if other asthma susceptibility genes are identified as mapping techniques and understanding of the disease improves. The application of positional cloning to the identification of genes in complex genetic disorders has been disappointing and this disappointment has led to greater attention to detection of polymorphisms in candidate genes.

The understanding that whole genome screens are difficult to interpret and may not be the best way to analyze the genetics of a complex disease, such as asthma and atopy, has led to use of candidate gene studies. Candidate genes include the numerous biochemical products that are known to be abnormally regulated or otherwise function inappropriately that lead to allergies and asthma or influence the severity of disease (Table 2). Candidate gene studies are performed by aggressively studying a narrow region of the genome with numerous polymorphic markers, which saturate the region of interest in a fashion that is not practical with a genome-wide scan [14]. Several statistical techniques are used in these candidate gene approaches. In association studies, a particular gene thought to have pathologic consequences is examined for its variance in predicted frequency in populations with and without the suspected disease. This approach can confirm candidates as being important to the genetics of atopy and asthma, but ignores the contributions of other unknown and unbiased loci that may be important. A tool that has been used to enhance the power of association studies and maintain some of the power of linkage studies has been to perform transmission disequilibrium testing. This involves assessing the frequency with which a potential disease-causing allele is transmitted to an affected offspring from either parent [15,16].

A recent study has demonstrated the use of positional cloning techniques when combined with candidate gene analyses to identify asthma and allergy genes. A genome-wide scan performed on 460 families identified a relatively

Table 2
Candidate genes of atopy and allergy

| Type | Examples |
| --- | --- |
| *Cytokines influencing allergic phenotype* | |
| Eosinophil growth-, activation-, and apoptosis-inhibiting factors | IL-5, IL-3, GM-CSF, CCL11, CCL5 |
| Mast-cell growth factors | IL-3, IL-9, IL-10, NGF, SCF, TGF-β |
| Histamine-releasing factors | CCL2 (MCP-1), CCL7 (MCP-3), CCL5 |
| IgE isotype switch factors | IL-4, IL-13 |
| Inhibition of IgE isotype switch | IFN-γ, IL-12, IL-18, IL-23 |
| Lipoxygenase pathway metabolism | 5-LO, 5-LO–activating peptide, leukotriene $C_4$ synthase |
| Proinflammatory cytokines | IL-1α, IL-1β, TNF-α, IL-6 |
| Anti-inflammatory cytokines | TNF-β, IL-10, IL-1Ra |
| | |
| *Receptors* | |
| Antigen receptors | T-cell receptors (α/β, γ/δ), B-cell receptor (IG, κ/λ light chain) |
| IgE | FcεRI β chain, FcεRII (CD23) |
| Cytokine gene receptors | IFN-γR β chain, M-CSF receptor, IL-1R, IL-4R, IL-9R, TNF receptors |
| Adhesion molecules | VLA-4, VCAM-1, ICAM-1, LFA-1 |
| Corticosteroid receptor | Grl-hsp90 |
| Neurogenic receptors | β2-Adrenergic, cholinergic receptors |
| | |
| *Nuclear transcription factors* | AP-1, NFIL-2, Oct-1, Stat-1/2, GATA3, Tbet, NF-κB, IκB, NFAT, Stat-4, Stat-6, bcl-6 |

*Abbreviations:* GM-CSF, granulocyte-macrophage colony–stimulating factor; ICAM, intercellular adhesion molecule; IFN, interferorn; IL, interleukin; LFA, lymphocyte function-associated antigen; MCP, monocyte chemotactic protein; NF, nuclear factor; SCF, stem cell factor; TNF, tumor necrosis factor; VCAM, vascular cell adhesion molecule; VLA, very late antigen.

strong linkage of asthma and bronchial hyperresponsiveness to markers on chromosome 20p13. A subsequent survey of 135 polymorphisms in 23 genes within this region identified the ADAM33 gene as being significantly associated with asthma using both association and transmission disequilibrium analyses [17]. This linkage has been confirmed in two separate genome screens in United Kingdom and United States outbred populations [18,19] and a polymorphism within the gene has been associated specifically with an accelerated decline in lung function [20]. ADAM33 is a protease with multiple isoforms that is active at the cell surface and is part of the matrix metalloproteinase family. Its role in asthma is speculative but expression of this protein on airway fibroblasts, myofibroblasts, and smooth muscle cells may alter the response of lymphocytes and inflammatory cells by proteolytic release of cytokines and chemokines from precursor molecules that influence cell migration. It also might alter growth factor expression and remodeling responses in the basement membrane to damaged epithelium and smooth muscle of the airway [21].

## Functional genomics

It is thought that most genetic variants that contribute to complex genetic disorders probably represent the contribution of base exchange mutations in individual DNA bases, termed "single nucleotide polymorphisms" (SNPs). SNPs occur in approximately 1 in 1000 base pairs throughout human genomic DNA. Because there are 4.2 billion bases within the human genome, this suggests that there are at least 4 million SNPs that contribute to all individual characteristics including height, weight, personality, eye color, hair color, and so forth. Other genetic mechanisms may also play a role including deletions and transpositions. Once a region has been identified through a genome-wide search or an association study, the role of a particular polymorphism needs to be confirmed in a functional study. Often most of the polymorphisms are silent, having no effect on either gene structure or gene expression, and any observed linkages are caused by other polymorphisms in the same or nearby gene. A large interest has been focused on the contributions of SNPs in the coding sequence of genes that have the potential to impact protein structure. SNPs that occur in gene promoters, enhancers, or in sequences that influence chromatin structure or RNA stability, however, may modify gene expression and thereby also have important genetic effects. In this section, several examples are given in which a polymorphism identified in an association study was subsequently confirmed to have a functional effect.

### Interleukin-10

IL-10 is a cytokine that displays pleiotropic effects in immunoregulation and inflammation. IL-10 inhibits Th1 production of interferon-γ and expression of IL-4 and IL-5 by Th2 lymphocytes. Monocytes are the major source for human IL-10. Other sources include T regulatory cells, cytotoxic T cells, B lymphocytes, myeloid dendritic cells, and mast cells. In addition to its effects on Th1 and Th2 cytokine production, IL-10 inhibits production of cytokines from mononuclear phagocytes. IL-10 also inhibits monocyte major histocompatibility complex class II, B7.1–B7.2 (CD80–CD88) expression, and accessory cell functions. Expression of IL-10 by antigen-presenting cells represents an established pathway for induction of tolerance to allergens. Support for a modulating role for IL-10 in human allergic diseases is derived from observations that IL-10 inhibits eosinophil survival, inhibits IgE synthesis, and enhances IgG4 synthesis [22]. The present authors described a C→A exchange in the IL-10 promoter located 571 base pairs upstream from the transcription start site, which is located between putative consensus binding sequences for Sp1 and ets family proteins [23]. This polymorphism was associated with elevated total serum IgE in subjects heterozygotic or homozygotic for this base exchange. In a study of white families, the polymorphism was confirmed as an asthma-associated gene associated with an increase in eosinophil cell counts [24]. In vitro and in vivo binding assays demonstrated that the transcription factors Sp1 and Sp3 bound to a sequence immediately upstream of the polymorphism. Experiments designed to address the functionality of the Sp1 site and the −571 base exchange were performed in B cells and demonstrated that the Sp1 site was a transcriptional repressor of the IL-10 gene. Changing the promoter from C-containing to A-containing resulted in an increase in transcription [25]. The present authors' results are different from others that have shown, in response to lipopolysaccharide stimulation of monocytes, the A at position −571 results in lower promoter activity [26]. This most likely reflects differences in cell-type expression of IL-10 and points to the need to examine the functionality of base exchanges in multiple cell types with a variety of stimuli.

## CD14

CD14 is a receptor that has specificity for lipopolysaccharides and other bacterial wall-derived components that is constitutively expressed on the surface of monocytes, macrophages, and neutrophils. CD14 can exist as a soluble receptor by way of direct secretion or by enzymatic cleavage of the membrane anchored CD14. Engagement of CD14 is associated with strong IL-12 responses in antigen-presenting cells and is a necessary signal in the formation of Th1 cells from naïve T cells [27]. It is thought that changes in CD14 levels could change the ratio of Th1- to Th2-type cells and alter IgE levels. A C→T transition at position −159 of the CD14 promoter in relation to the transcription start site was found. Individuals homozygous for the T allele were found to have higher sCD14 in the serum and lower total IgE levels in skin test–positive children [28]. The functional role of this polymorphism was then investigated. Members of the Sp transcription factor family bound to the promoter and the affinity of binding was lower for promoters containing the T allele. Using reporter assays, it was found that transcription from promoters containing the T allele was higher than constructs containing the C allele, and that was dependent on the ratio of Sp3 to Sp1 and Sp2 [29].

## CCL5

CCL5 (RANTES) is a C-C chemokine that acting in synergy with IL-5 is one of the most important eosinophil chemoattractants in allergic inflammation. Other cells including lymphocytes, monocytes, and basophils can migrate in response to CCL5 secretion. CCL5 is expressed in activated T lymphocytes, airway and renal epithelial cells, platelets, and fibroblasts [22]. Several genetic studies have implicated two regions of the CCL5 promoter as associating with disease: a G→A exchange at −403 and a C→G exchange at −28 in relation to the transcription start site. In white populations, the −403 A allele seems to be associated with an increased risk of atopy and airway obstruction [30,31]. Functional studies of this site demonstrated that the presence of the A allele creates a GATA transcription factor binding site that results in an eightfold increase in basal promoter activity [32]. In contrast to the results of the studies in the white populations, studies in several Asian populations have failed to demonstrate an association with the −403 polymorphism, but have observed associations with the −28 C→G polymorphism and asthma [33,34]. The polymorphism is located adjacent to a NF-κB binding site and in vitro reporter assays have shown that the G allele results in a twofold activation of transcription [35]. Mononuclear cells isolated from patients with the −28 C/G alleles confirmed that when stimulated, cells from carriers of the G allele secreted more CCL5 protein than cells from carriers of the C allele [33]. These studies point to the possibility that certain polymorphisms in a gene might be important in one population, but that other polymorphisms might play a bigger role in other populations. This points to the need to repeat the association studies in multiple ethnically diverse populations.

## Interleukin-13

The IL-13 locus has been one of the most-cited candidate genes in association with asthma and atopy, with more than 70 reported SNPs in the gene and promoter region [36]. IL-13 is homologous to IL-4 and shares many of the same biologic activities on mononuclear phagocytic cells, endothelial cells, epithelial cells, and B cells, but because of differential expression of the IL-13 receptors, IL-13 has unique properties distinct from IL-4. Like IL-4, IL-13 can induce the IgE isotype switch and vascular cell adhesion molecular−1 expression. IL-13 has been shown to induce eosinophilic inflammation, and may be uniquely important in inducing mucus cell hypersecretion, airway fibrosis, and airway hyperreactivity [22]. Two SNPs have consistently shown associations with disease in multiple studies: a $C \rightarrow T$ exchange at position $-1112$ of the promoter and a $G \rightarrow A$ at position $+2044$ of the gene. In a Dutch family study, the $-1112T$ allele was associated with asthma, bronchial hyperresponsiveness, and skin-test reactivity [37]. Functional studies demonstrated that the C allele at $-1112$ displayed 30% higher transcriptional activity as compared with the T allele. When examined on the molecular level, it was found that the T allele created an Oct-1 transcription factor binding site that may function as a repressor by preventing binding of the transcription activator STAT1 to a site just upstream of the polymorphism [38]. Several studies have shown an association of the $+2044A$ allele and increased IgE levels [39,40]. The polymorphism results in a nonconservative replacement of the basic amino acid arginine (Arg)130 with a neutral amino acid glutamine (Gln) in the IL-13 protein. Using recombinant proteins, the two forms of the IL-13 protein did not differ in binding affinity to the IL-13Rα1 type receptor, but the Gln130 protein bound to the IL-13Rα2 with lower affinity and was more stable in the extracellular environment [41]. The increased stability may result in higher levels of circulating IL-13 levels in individuals with the Gln130 protein, leading to the observed associations of IL-13 and asthma and atopy.

### Haplotype analysis and phylogenetic shadowing

One problem facing the study of functional genomics is determining which SNPs are likely to be involved in disease processes and which ones serve as markers of disease because of linkage disequilibrium. More than 70 SNPs have been reported for the IL-13 gene, but only two of these have been analyzed further in epidemiologic and functional studies [36]. Two approaches are used to address this problem: haplotype analysis and phylogenetic shadowing. Individual SNPs do not segregate randomly, but usually are present on a chromosome with other specific SNPs. This combination of SNPs on a chromosome that is inherited together is termed a "haplotype." Rather than looking at each SNP individually for association with disease, the haplotype is examined instead. This approach strengthens the identification of that region on the chromosome as containing the disease-causing gene, but does not help determine which SNP is functionally important. A new approach termed "phylogenetic shadowing" has the promise of taking some of the guesswork out of identifying important polymorphisms. This process makes comparisons of sequences from many closely related primate species taking into account the phylogenetic relationships of the species being compared. Coding exons and important regulatory elements tend to be highly conserved, so if the sequence has little variation across many species it is likely to be important, whereas sequences with high variability are less likely to be important [42]. Extending this analogy to SNPs, if a SNP falls in a highly conserved area, this is a good candidate for further functional studies. If the polymorphism is in a nonconserved or variable region, then there is a decreased likelihood that the change has a functional effect.

## Pharmacogenetics

Pharmacogenetics is defined as the study of variation in drug response in different individuals caused in part by their genetic composition. Genetic variations in drug target genes can be used to predict clinical responsiveness to treatment and represents the first area where genetic information concerning allergic response will be used in the clinical setting. An early study by Malmstrom and coworkers [43] examined the response of individuals with asthma to the inhaled corticosteroid beclomethasone or the leukotriene modifier montelukast. This study demonstrated that there was a wide spectrum of interindividual responses to each drug as measured by changes in forced expiratory volume in 1 second ($FEV_1$) from baseline. Of the patients receiving beclomethasone, 22% failed to show improvement in $FEV_1$, whereas 34% receiving montelukast failed to show improvements in $FEV_1$ [43]. Recently, new data have shed some light on the variable response to inhaled corticosteroids observed in some patients. In three independent asthmatic clinical trial populations, variation in the corticotropin-releasing hormone receptor 1 (CRHR1) gene was associated with increased response to inhaled corticosteroids [44]. Individuals homozygous for the variation displayed a doubling to quadrupling of lung function following treatment with corticosteroids as compared with individuals without the variation.

Polymorphisms have been reported in the promoters of the 5-lipoxygenase (5-LO) and $LTC_4S$ genes that are involved in arachidonic acid metabolism and cysteinyl leukotriene production. Abnormalities in the transcriptional regulation of these genes may be important in producing the aspirin-sensitive phenotype and may identify individuals who are more responsive to leukotriene modifiers. Base exchanges in the 5-LO promoter alter the number of binding sites for the transcription factors Sp1 and Egr-1 [45,46]. The most common allele in the 5-LO promoter consists of five tandem Sp1-binding motifs with variants having deletions or additions to the number of Sp1-binding motifs. Reporter gene assays have demonstrated that a promoter with five repeats is the most active [45]. Their role in inducing aspirin sensitivity remains speculative; however, these alternative genotypes can influence responsiveness to a leukotriene modifier. In a controlled trial of the 5-LO inhibitor zileuton, patients with at least one allele containing five Sp1-binding motifs had an 18.8% improvement in $FEV_1$ compared with a 1.1% decline in $FEV_1$ in individuals in whom neither allele contained the five repeats [47]. Even though there is a functional effect of polymorphisms in the 5-LO promoter and these result in changes in clinical responsiveness to a leukotriene modifier, the polymorphisms are only present in 5% of asthmatic patients and can only account for a small proportion of the variability in response to leukotriene modifier therapy. Mutations with the $LTC_4S$ gene (an $A \rightarrow C$ transversion at position $-444$), coded for in the cytokine gene cluster complex on 5q, link to aspirin-sensitive asthma. Unlike the 5-LO polymorphisms, the $LTC_4S$ C allele is found at frequency of 23% in a normal population with a frequency up to 44% in an aspirin-intolerant population [48]. Sampson and coworkers [49] demonstrated that stimulated eosinophils from carriers of the C allele produced almost three times the levels of $LTC_4$ as compared with eosinophils from individuals without the C allele. Carriers of the C allele have decreased basal $FEV_1$ levels and using the transmission disequilibrium test, an association between the C allele and bronchial hyperreactivity to methacholine was observed [50]. It might be expected that carriers of the C allele are good responders to leukotriene modifier therapy. Support for this idea came from a small study in which asthmatic patients were given zafirlukast for 2 weeks. Those who had a C allele displayed a 9% improvement in $FEV_1$, whereas those without a C allele had a 12% decrease in $FEV_1$ [49]. This was a small study and needs to be repeated.

Similar findings have been related to the response of airways to β-agonists. Four structural genetic variations within the β2-adrenergic receptor gene, which is also coded within the 5q31 complex, have been identified [51]. Although none of these amino acid substitutions have been conclusively linked to the presence of asthma, they have been associated with response to β-agonists. Retrospective studies have suggested that the presence of glycine (caused by an $A \rightarrow G$ base exchange at nucleic acid position 46 of the gene) at amino acid residue 16 is associated with the presence of corticosteroid-dependence, nocturnal symptoms, and loss of bronchodilator responsiveness with long-term administration of albuterol [52]. In a recent prospective study, individuals homozygous for arginine rather than homozygous for glycine at amino acid 16 had lower peak expiratory flow rates and lower $FEV_1$ when treated with albuterol [53]. It should be noted that in the African-American population, there is an increase in the number of individuals homozygous for arginine at amino acid 16 and this may explain the reported increased morbidity associated with long-term administration of β-agonists in this population [54]. These results suggest that individuals homozygous for arginine at amino acid 16 should avoid regular bronchodilator treatments using albuterol or long-acting β-agonists.

## Genes and the environment

The increase in asthma that has been observed over the past 20 to 30 years has been attributed in part to what is termed the "hygiene hypothesis." This states that the reduced exposure to childhood infections, or other immune stimuli, such as farming and endotoxin exposure, may explain the increased prevalence of allergic diseases in industrialized countries [55]. Although not likely to be the sole explanation for the increase in asthma prevalence, it leads to the question of whether changes in the environment imposed on genetic background may have led to the increase in asthma and allergies. One component of the hygiene hypothesis is that decreased endotoxin exposure and reduced innate immune responses drive the increased sensitivity to allergens. Endotoxin functions through engagement of the toll-like receptor (TLR) 4 and the costimulatory molecule CD14. Polymorphisms have been found in the CD14 gene that lead to a functional change in the expression of the gene [28], and recently, associations of polymorphisms and asthma have been noted in the TLR4 gene that alter response to endotoxin [56]. It is likely that influences of these functional genetic polymorphisms on disease development are only observed in individuals whose environment produces significant endotoxin exposures. Studies have not yet been performed addressing the direct environmental influence on phenotype expression in response to these polymorphisms. Presence in the environment of ligands interacting through other TLRs (including TLR 2, 3, 7, and 9) are similarly also likely to determine a role for polymorphisms in these receptors in causing (or protecting against) allergic sensitization. Supporting this is the finding that TLR2 has been identified as a major asthma gene in children of European farmers [57]. TLR2 is a ligand for peptidoglycans and lipoproteins. Associations of SNPs in this receptor are not observed in nonfarmers because presumably they do not have the same level of exposures. As industrialization has increased, exposure and infections caused by helminths, tuberculosis, and others have decreased. Another example of a major environmental change that has occurred and might influence expression of genetic polymorphisms is the increase in airborne diesel particulate matter caused by motorized vehicles. Although likely to alter many pathways, one recent study has shown that a variant of the glutathione-S-transferase gene modifies the adjuvant effect of diesel particles on allergic inflammation [58]. Glutathione-S-transferase can metabolize reactive oxygen species and detoxify xenobiotics present in diesel exhaust particles. Mutations in glutathione-S-transferase that inhibit this function could lead to increased inflammation and response to benign substances, such as aeroallergens. These effects are only observed, however, in areas where concentrations of airborne diesel particulate matter are high, such as in large cities. Because of the complexity of response to diesel particles, this represents an area where a strong gene-environment interaction should be observed.

**Summary**

Currently, more than 20.3 million Americans report having asthma and an even greater number suffer from allergies. The cost for treatment of these diseases in the United States is greater than $8 billion with more than 40% of this total representing drug expenditure [59]. An intense effort has been made to understand the genetic components of asthma and allergies and how the identified genetic differences influence disease progression and response to drugs. In the future, it will be possible in the clinical setting to analyze a patient's genetic repertoire. From this information, the physician will gain insight into the genes involved in producing that subject's allergic and asthmatic phenotype; understand the natural history of that patient's disease; and predict responses (positive and negative) to pharmacologic agents. The end result will be the ability to tailor a specific treatment regime for each patient and reduce the overall cost of health care related to allergies and asthma.

## References

[1] Cooke RA, van der Veer A. Human sensitization. J Immunol 1916;1:201–5.
[2] Coca AF, Cooke RA. On the classification of the phenomenon of hypersensitiveness. J Immunol 1923;8:163–82.
[3] Hopp RJ, Bewtra AK, Watt GD, et al. Genetic analysis of allergic disease in twins. J Allergy Clin Immunol 1984;732:265–70.
[4] Colilla S, Nicolae D, Pluzhnikov A, et al. Evidence for gene-environment interactions in a linkage study of asthma and smoking exposure. J Allergy Clin Immunol 2003;111:840–6.
[5] Howard TD, Koppelman GH, Xu J, et al. Gene-gene interaction in asthma: *IL4RA* and *IL13* in a Dutch population with asthma. Am J Hum Genet 2003;70:230–6.
[6] Daniels SE, Bhattacharrya S, James A, et al. A genome-wide search for quantitative trait loci underlying asthma. Nature 1996;383:247–50.
[7] Ober C, Cox NJ, Abney M, et al. Genome-wide search for asthma susceptibility loci in a founder population. The Collaborative Study on the Genetics of Asthma. Hum Mol Genet 1998;7:1393–8.
[8] Wjst M, Fischer G, Immervoll T, et al. A genome-wide search for linkage to asthma. German Asthma Genetics Group. Genomics 1999;58:1–8.
[9] Moffatt MF, Sharp PA, Faux JA, et al. factors confounding genetic linkage between atopy and chromosome 11q. Clin Exp Allergy 1992;22:1046–51.
[10] Lympany P, Welsh K, MacCochrane G, et al. Genetic analysis using DNA polymorphism of the linkage between chromosome 11q13 and atopy and bronchial hyperresponsiveness to methacholine. J Allergy Clin Immunol 1992;89:619–28.
[11] Hizawa N, Yamaguchi E, Ohe M, et al. Lack of linkage between atopy and locus 11q13. Clin Exp Allergy 1992;22:1065–9.
[12] Rich SS, Roitman-Johnson B, Greenberg B, et al. Genetic analysis of atopy in three large kindreds: no evidence of linkage to D11S97. Clin Exp Allergy 1992;22:1070–6.
[13] (CSGA) CSotGoA. A genome-wide search for asthma susceptibility loci in ethnically diverse populations. Nat Genet 1997;15:389–92.
[14] Thomas NS, Wilkinson J, Holgate ST. The candidate region approach to the genetics of asthma and allergy. Am J Respir Crit Care Med 1997;156:S144–51.
[15] Risch NJ. Searching for genetic determinants in the new millennium. Nature 2000;405: 847–56.
[16] Gabriel SB, Schaffner SF, Nguyen H, et al. The structure of haplotype blocks in the human genome. Science 2002;296:2225–9.
[17] Van Eerdewegh P, Little RD, Dupuis J, et al. Association of the ADAM33 gene with asthma and bronchial hyperresponsiveness. Nature 2002;418:426–30.
[18] Howard TD, Postma DS, Jongepier H, et al. Association of a disintegrin and metalloprotease 33 (ADAM33) gene with asthma in ethnically diverse populations. J Allergy Clin Immunol 2003;112:717–22.

[19] Werner M, Herbon N, Gohlke H, et al. Asthma is associated with single-nucleotide polymorphisms in ADAM33. Clin Exp Allergy 2004;34:26–31.

[20] Jongepier H, Boezen HM, Dijkstra A, et al. Polymorphisms of the ADAM33 gene are associated with accelerated lung function decline in asthma. Clin Exp Allergy 2004;34: 757–60.

[21] Holgate ST, Davies DE, Rorke S, et al. Identification and possible functions of ADAM33 as an asthma susceptibility gene. Clin Exp All Rev 2004;4:49–55.

[22] Borish L, Steinke JW. Cytokines and chemokines. J Allergy Clin Immunol 2003;111: S460–75.

[23] Hobbs K, Negri J, Klinnert M, et al. Interleukin-10 and transforming growth factor-beta promoter polymorphisms in allergies and asthma. Am J Respir Crit Care Med 1998;158: 1958–62.

[24] Immervoll T, Loesgen S, Dutsch G, et al. Fine mapping and single nucleotide polymorphism association results of candidate genes for asthma and related phenotypes. Hum Mutat 2001; 18:327–36.

[25] Steinke JW, Barekzi E, Hagman J, et al. Functional analysis of -571 IL-10 promoter polymorphism reveals a repressor element controlled by Sp1. J Immunol 2004;173:3215–22.

[26] Crawley E, Kay R, Sillibourne J, et al. Polymorphic haplotypes of the interluekin-10 5′ flanking region determine variable interleukin-10 transcription and are associated with particular phenotypes of juvenile rheumatoid arthritis. Arthritis Rheum 1999;42:1101–8.

[27] Ulevitch RJ, Tobias PS. Receptor-dependent mechanisms of cell stimulation by bacterial endotoxin. Annu Rev Immunol 1995;13:437–57.

[28] Baldini M, Lohman IC, Halonen M, et al. A polymorphism in the 5′ flanking region of the CD14 gene is associated with circulating soluble CD14 levels and with total serum immunoglobulin E. Am J Respir Cell Mol Biol 1999;20:976–83.

[29] LeVan TD, Bloom JW, Bailey TJ, et al. A common single nucleotide polymorphism in the CD14 promoter decreases the affinity of Sp protein binding and enhances transcriptional activity. J Immunol 2001;167:5838–44.

[30] Al-Abdulhadi SA, Helms PJ, Main M, et al. Preferential transmission and association of the −403 G→A promoter RANTES polymorphism with atopic asthma. Genes Immun 2005; 6(1):24–30.

[31] Fryer AA, Spiteri MA, Bianco A, et al. The -403 G→A promoter polymorphism in the RANTES gene is associated with atopy and asthma. Genes Immun 2000;1:509–14.

[32] Nickel RG, Casolaro V, Wahn U, et al. Atopic dermatitis is associated with a functional mutation in the promoter of the C–C chemokine RANTES. J Immunol 2000;164:1612–6.

[33] Hizawa N, Yamaguchi E, Konno S, et al. A functional polymorphism in the RANTES gene promoter is associated with the development of late-onset asthma. Am J Respir Crit Care Med 2002;166:686–90.

[34] Yao T-C, Kuo M-L, See L-C, et al. The RANTES promoter polymorphism: a genetic risk factor for near-fatal asthma in Chinese children. J Allergy Clin Immunol 2003;111:1285–92.

[35] Liu H, Chao D, Nakayama EE, et al. Polymorphism in RANTES chemokine promoter affects HIV-1 disease progression. Proc Natl Acad Sci U S A 1999;96:4581–5.

[36] Vercelli D. Genetics of IL-13 and functional relevance of IL-13 variants. Curr Opin Allergy Clin Immunol 2002;2:389–93.

[37] Howard TD, Whittaker PA, Zaiman AL, et al. Identification and association of polymorphisms in the interleukin-13 gene with asthma and atopy in a Dutch population. Am J Respir Cell Mol Biol 2001;25:377–84.

[38] Cameron L, Kabesch M, Vercelli D. The single nucleotide polymorphism -1112C/T attenuates IL-13 transcription and creates an Oct-1 binding site that interferes with Stat-1 dependent promoter activation. J Allergy Clin Immunol 2002;109:S255.

[39] Taussig LM, Wright AL, Morgan WJ, et al. The Tucson Children's Respiratory Study. I. Design and implementation of a prospective study of acute and chronic respiratory illness in children. Am J Epidemiol 1989;129:1219–31.

[40] von Mutius E, Weiland SK, Fritzsch C, et al. Increasing prevalence of hay fever and atopy among children in Leipzig, East Germany. Lancet 1998;351:862–86.

[41] Arima K, Umeshita-Suyama R, Sakata Y, et al. Upregulation of IL-13 concentration in vivo by the IL-13 variant associated with bronchial asthma. J Allergy Clin Immunol 2002;109: 980–7.

[42] Gibbs RA, Nelson DL. Primate shadow play. Science 2003;299:1331–3.

[43] Malmstrom K, Rodriguez-Gomez G, Guerra J, et al. Oral montelukast, inhaled beclomethasone, and placebo for chronic asthma. Ann Intern Med 1999;130:487–95.

[44] Tantisira KG, Lake S, Silverman ES, et al. Corticosteroid pharmacogenetics: association of sequence variants in CRHR1 with improved lung function in asthmatics treated with inhaled corticosteroids. Hum Mol Genet 2004;13:1353–9.

[45] In KH, Asano K, Beier D, et al. Naturally occurring mutations in the human 5-lipoxygenase gene promoter that modify transcription factor binding and reporter gene transcription. J Clin Invest 1997;99:1130–7.

[46] Silverman ES, Du J, De Sanctis GT, et al. Egr-1 and Sp1 interact functionally with the 5-lipoxygenase promoter and its naturally occurring mutants. Am J Respir Cell Mol Biol 1998; 19:316–23.

[47] Drazen JM, Yandava CN, Dube L, et al. Pharmacogenetic association between ALOX5 promoter genotype and the response to anti-asthma treatment. Nat Genet 1999;22:168–70.

[48] Sanak M, Simon H-U, Szczeklik A. Leukotriene C4 synthase promoter polymorphism and risk of aspirin-induced asthma. Lancet 1997;350:1599–600.

[49] Sampson AP, Siddiqui S, Buchanan D, et al. Variant LTC4 synthase allele modifies cysteinyl leukotriene synthesis in eosinophils and predicts clinical response to zafirlukast. Thorax 2000;55:S28–31.

[50] Sayers I, Barton S, Rorke S, et al. Allelic association and functional studies of promoter polymorphism in the leukotriene C4 synthase gene (LTC4S) in asthma. Thorax 2004;58: 417–24.

[51] Reihsaus E, Innis M, MacIntyre N, et al. Mutations in the gene encoding for the beta 2-adrenergic receptor in normal and asthmatic subjects. Am J Respir Cell Mol Biol 1993;8:334–9.

[52] Israel E, Drazen JM, Liggett SB, et al. The effect of polymorphisms of the β2-adrenergic receptor on the response to regular use of albuterol in asthma. Am J Respir Crit Care Med 2000;162:75–80.

[53] Israel E, Chinchilli VM, Ford JG, et al. Use of regularly scheduled albuterol in asthma: genotype-stratified, randomised, placebo-controlled cross-over trial. Lancet 2004;364:1464–6.

[54] Perera BJ. Salmeterol multicentre asthma research trial (SMART): interim analysis shows increased risk of asthma related deaths. Ceylon Med J 2003;48:99.

[55] Eder W, von Mutius E. Hygiene hypothesis and endotoxin: what is the evidence? Curr Opin Allergy Clin Immunol 2004;4:113–7.

[56] Fageras Bottcher M, Hmani-Aifa M, Lindstrom A, et al. A TLR4 polymorphism is associated with asthma and reduced lipopolysaccharide-induced interleukin-12(p70) responses in Swedish children. J Allergy Clin Immunol 2004;114:561–7.

[57] Eder W, Klimecki W, Yu L, et al. Toll-like receptor 2 as a major gene for asthma in children of European farmers. J Allergy Clin Immunol 2004;113:482–8.

[58] Gilliland FD, Li YF, Saxon A, et al. Effect of glutathione-S-transferase M1 and P1 genotypes on xenobiotic enhancement of allergic responses: randomised, placebo-controlled crossover study. Lancet 2004;363:119–25.

[59] Weiss KB, Sullivan SD. The health economics of asthma and rhinitis. I. Assessing the economic impact. J Allergy Clin Immunol 2001;107:3–8.

ELSEVIER
SAUNDERS

Med Clin N Am 90 (2006) 17–38

THE MEDICAL
CLINICS
OF NORTH AMERICA

# Allergic Rhinitis: Impact of the Disease and Considerations for Management

Alexander N. Greiner, MD[a,b,*]

[a]Allergy and Asthma Medical Group and Research Center, San Diego, CA, USA
[b]University of California at San Diego, San Diego, CA, USA

Allergic rhinitis (AR) is a common yet underappreciated inflammatory condition of the nasal mucosa characterized by pruritus, sneezing, rhinorrhea, and nasal congestion. It is mediated by an IgE-associated response to indoor and outdoor environmental allergens. AR affects a large portion of the United States population at all stages of life. Onset of symptoms after age 20 should raise the suspicion that nonallergic rhinitis (NAR) is the primary diagnosis or contributes significantly to the nasal symptoms due to AR. Epidemiologic relationships and basic science support the concept that AR is part of a systemic inflammatory process and hence is associated with other mucosal inflammatory conditions, such as asthma, rhinosinusitis, allergic conjunctivitis, and otitis media with effusion. It is now recognized that AR can affect quality of life to a similar degree with asthma. The Allergic Rhinitis and Its Impact on Asthma (ARIA) guidelines have provided a pragmatic, stepwise approach to treatment of AR. Allergen avoidance remains one of the guiding principles of treatment, although it may be difficult to implement. Although an ever-increasing armamentarium of pharmacotherapeutic agents is available to the clinician, intranasal corticosteroids remain the single most effective class of medications for treating AR. Immunotherapy (allergy vaccination) is the only treatment modality with the potential to modulate the immune system permanently, leading to long-lasting improvement. It is somewhat time-intensive and carries a small risk of serious adverse reactions. New specific immunomodulating biologic agents will most likely become available. However, their role in the treatment of AR may be dependent on their cost.

* Allergy and Asthma Medical Group and Research Center, APC, 9610 Granite Ridge Drive, Suite B, San Diego, CA 92123.
   E-mail address: greineran@yahoo.com

0025-7125/06/$ - see front matter © 2005 Elsevier Inc. All rights reserved.
doi:10.1016/j.mcna.2005.08.011                    *medical.theclinics.com*

## Classification

Traditionally, AR has been classified as seasonal or perennial, depending on whether an individual is sensitized to cyclic pollens or to year-round allergens, such as dust mites, pets, cockroaches, and molds. This classification scheme has proved to be artificial and often inconsistent, because, depending somewhat on the locale, allergic sensitization to multiple seasonal allergens may result in year-round disease. Conversely, allergic sensitization to perennial allergens, such as animal dander, may result in symptoms during only a limited period of time. Furthermore, molds, depending on the species and geographic area, may function as seasonal or perennial allergens. Nonetheless, throughout this article the older classification scheme is used along with the newer one, owing to the former's use in many research studies and regulatory approvals.

Recent global guidelines for classification and treatment of AR have led to the definitions of allergic nasal disease as intermittent or persistent and mild or moderate–severe [1]. Intermittent rhinitis is defined on the basis of symptoms that are present for fewer than 4 days per week or fewer than 4 weeks. When symptoms are present for more than the 4 days per week and are present for more than 4 weeks, the rhinitis is defined as persistent (Fig. 1). Mild symptoms do not affect sleep, impair participation in daily activities, sports, and leisure, or interfere with work or school and are not considered troublesome. Conversely, moderate–severe symptoms result in abnormal sleep, interfere with daily activities, sports, and leisure, impair work and school activities, and are considered troublesome. The diagnosis of AR may be made presumptively based on the symptoms and the history of allergen triggers. However, confirmation of the diagnosis requires documentation of specific IgE reactivity. Appropriate determination of allergen sensitivity by skin-prick testing or in vitro methods, such as the radioallergosorbent test (RAST) or ELISA, may not only help in diagnosing AR but

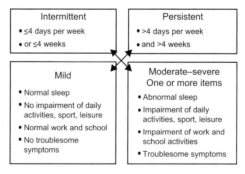

Fig. 1. Classification of allergic rhinitis according to ARIA. (*From* Bachert C, van Cauwenberge P, Khaltaev N; World Health Organization. Allergic rhinitis and its impact on asthma. In collaboration with the World Health Organization. Executive summary of the workshop report. Geneva, Switzerland, December 7–10, 1999. Allergy 2002;57:841–55; with permission.)

also provide information on how to intervene with specific environmental control measures. Specific IgE analysis by RAST or ELISA is slower and less cost-effective than skin-prick testing, but it is useful in patients who have dermatographism or for those who are unable to discontinue antihistamine therapy. Although current second- and third-generation RAST assays produce more quantifiable and reproducible measurements of IgE than ever before, skin testing remains a more sensitive tool and hence continues to be the gold standard for the detection of allergen-specific IgE [2].

**Epidemiology**

AR affects a large portion of the United States population at all stages of life, including infancy [3]. The prevalence of AR has been estimated to be between 15% and 20% [4], but physician-diagnosed AR in the pediatric age group has been reported in as many as 42% [5]. Older children have a higher prevalence of AR than younger ones, with a peak occurring in children aged 13 to 14. Approximately 80% of individuals diagnosed as having AR develop symptoms before the age of 20 [6]. Although boys are more likely than girls to be afflicted with AR, this tendency tends to reverse in puberty so that equal numbers are affected in adulthood. Onset of symptoms after age 20 should raise the suspicion that NAR is the primary diagnosis or at least contributes significantly to the rhinitis symptoms the patient experiences (mixed rhinitis). NAR is characterized by sporadic or persistent perennial symptoms not resulting from IgE-mediated immunopathologic events [7]. Many forms of NAR are noninflammatory in nature and thus are more appropriately termed rhinopathies. Allergic and nonallergic forms of rhinitis and other rhinopathies, as well as conditions that mimic AR, are listed in Box 1. These possibilities should be considered when patients present with nasal congestion, sneezing, itching of the nose, and anterior rhinorrhea or postnasal drainage.

**Atopy, risk factors, and comorbid disorders**

Atopy is the abnormal tendency to develop specific IgE in response to normally innocuous environmental allergens. Atopic diseases include allergic rhinoconjunctivitis, asthma, atopic dermatitis, and food allergies. Atopy has been linked to multiple genetic loci, including those on chromosomes 2, 5, 6, 7, 11, 13, 16, and 20 [8]. Therefore, a family history represents a major risk factor for AR. In one study, development of atopic disease in the absence of parental family history was only present in 13%, whereas, when one patient or sibling was atopic, the risk increased to 29%. When both parents were atopic, the risk for developing an atopic disorder was 47% in the next generation [9].

Other risk factors linked to the development of AR include higher socioeconomic status, ethnicity other than white, polluted environments, birth during a pollen season, lack of older siblings, late entry into daycare, heavy maternal smoking during the first year of life, exposure to indoor allergens such as

**Box 1. Differential diagnosis of rhinorrhea and nasal obstruction in children and adults**

*Allergic rhinitis*
- Seasonal
- Perennial
- Perennial with seasonal exacerbations
- Occupational (may also be nonallergic)

*Nonallergic rhinitis*
Mechanical obstruction/structural factors
- Septal deviation—may compound nasal obstruction for allergic rhinitis.
- Foreign body. Unilateral purulent nasal discharge is the usual manifestation of a foreign body and resolves after removal.
- Adenoidal hypertrophy—occurs mainly in children.
- Hypertrophic turbinates
- Nasal tumors (may be benign [eg, polyps] or malignant [eg, squamous cell carcinoma])
- Choanal atresia or stenosis. Bilateral choanal atresia must be diagnosed early in life, but unilateral choanal atresia or stenosis may go unnoticed for several years. Easily diagnosed by nasal endoscopy and axial CT of the midfacial skeleton.
Infectious rhinitis/rhinosinusitis
- Bacterial
- Viral
- Fungal
Perennial (vasomotor, idiopathic). Constant symptoms of profuse, clear rhinorrhea and nasal congestion without correlation to specific allergen exposure or signs of atopy. Often triggered by environmental triggers:
- Cold air–induced. Nasal congestion and rhinorrhea on exposure to cold, windy weather. Occurs in both allergic and nonallergic individuals.
- Odors
- Barometric pressure
Nonallergic rhinitis with eosinophilia syndrome. Most often seen in adults; characterized by eosinophilia on nasal smears with negative testing for specific allergens.

Reflex-induced
- Gustatory rhinitis: vagally mediated copious, watery rhinorrhea occurring immediately after food ingestion, particularly hot and spicy foods
- Chemical- or irritant-induced
- Postural reflexes: many different postural reflexes exist; a commonly encountered reflex involves ipsilateral nasal congestion when supine or prone with the head turned to one side.
- Nasal cycle: refers to the unilateral nasal congestion that cycles from one side to the other over time in normal individuals.

*Drug-induced rhinitis*
- Oral contraceptives
- Antihypertensives: hydralazine, β-adrenergic blockers
- Aspirin (ASA) and other nonsteroidal anti-inflammatory drugs (with or without the ASA triad/Samter's syndrome: rhinosinusitis, nasal polyps, asthma)
- Topical decongestants (rhinitis medicamentosa)

*Hormonally-induced rhinitis*
- Hypothyroidism
- Pregnancy
- Menstrual cycle
- Exercise
- Atrophic

*Granulomatous rhinitis*
- Sarcoidosis
- Wegener's granulomatosis

*Miscellaneous*
- Cerebrospinal rhinorrhea (usually presents with unilateral, clear rhinorrhea)

*Adapted from* Baroody FM, Naclerio RM. Allergic rhinitis. In: Rich RR, Fleisher TA, Shearer WT, editors. Clinical immunology: principles and practice. 2nd edition. London: Mosby; 2001. p. 48.7.

animal dander and dust mites, higher serum IgE levels ($> 100$ IU/mL before age 6), positive allergen skin-prick tests, and early introduction of foods or formula [1]. Increasing evidence suggests that early environmental exposure to various infectious agents, such as hepatitis A, mycobacterium, *Toxoplasma gondii*, and bacterial products derived from microbes such as lipopolysaccharide, protects against development of atopy [10,11]. These micro-organisms and microbial products, when encountered at the right time in the right amount, appear to stimulate innate immunity so as to bias the adaptive portion of the immune system toward development of a non-atopic phenotype.

It is increasingly understood that AR is part of a systemic inflammatory process rather than an isolated local disease. As such, it is closely linked to other inflammatory diseases affecting the respiratory mucous membranes, such as asthma, rhinosinusitis, otitis media with effusion, and allergic conjunctivitis. Epidemiologic evidence has repeatedly and consistently demonstrated the coexistence of rhinitis and asthma. Nasal symptoms have been noted in as many as 80% of the asthmatic population [12]. In subsets, such as allergic asthmatic adolescents, this link may be even stronger, with as many as 93% experiencing nasal symptoms. Conversely, asthma is present in as many as 22.5% of adults who have AR, versus 7.2% in the general population [13,14]. In children, the ratio of asthmatics with AR to asthmatics without AR is even higher [5].

This epidemiologic relationship has led to further analysis of the potential integration of the upper and lower airways. In one such study, segmental endobronchial allergen challenge led to the development of nasal and bronchial symptoms as well as to reductions in pulmonary and nasal function in the AR subjects but not in the healthy group [15]. By contrast, nasal allergen challenge in the AR subjects led to increased peripheral blood eosinophilia and increased nasal and bronchial airway inflammation through upregulation of adhesion molecules [16].

Considerable epidemiologic evidence also supports the linkage between sinus disease and AR. Studies have noted that 25% to 30% of patients who have acute sinusitis have AR, as do 40% to 67% of patients who have unilateral chronic sinusitis and as many as 80% of those who have chronic bilateral sinusitis. In acute rhinosinusitis, the putative mechanism by which AR predisposes to sinusitis is nasal inflammation that results in nasal congestion and obstruction of the ostia, which connect the sinuses to the nasal cavity. Decreased ventilation of the mucosa in the sinus cavity leads to ciliary dysfunction, transudation of fluids, and stagnation of mucus, thereby promoting the growth of bacterial pathogens. Chronic rhinosinusitis is an inflammatory disorder that has different phenotypes and is most likely due to multiple factors. The two most commonly recognized forms of chronic rhinosinusitis are characterized by either eosinophilic or neutrophilic infiltration. Some appear to share the same underlying immune mechanism as other atopic disorders, including AR. Although intriguing, the proposal that most chronic inflammatory sinus disease is driven by an abnormal response to inhaled ubiquitous fungal material [17] remains controversial.

Allergic conjunctivitis (AC) is characterized by ocular itching, swelling, and discharge that may be clear or resemble string-cheese. Eye symptoms are common in sufferers of AR, especially among those sensitized to pollen and animal dander. Although eye symptoms are often overlooked, at times they may over-shadow nasal symptoms and represent the chief reason patients present to the office. Although perennial AC is the second most common form of AC after seasonal conjunctivitis, one needs to pay special attention to two more severe forms of AC common to the atopic population: vernal and atopic keratoconjunctivitis [18]. These atopic eye diseases are potentially sight-threatening and should be managed in cooperation with an ophthalmologist.

Vernal keratoconjunctivitis is characterized by chronic inflammation of the conjunctivae. It presents most commonly in children and adolescents, more frequently in males, and usually resolves by early adulthood. The symptoms of vernal keratoconjunctivitis are severe itching, thick mucus, and photophobia. It may threaten sight if the corneal erosions occur. On examination, giant papillae may be noted on the tarsal conjunctive as well as the ropy mucoid discharge.

Atopic keratoconjunctivitis manifests as inflammatory changes of the conjunctivae and cornea and presents with eye itching, burning, tearing, and photophobia. Usually, affected individuals have concomitant eczema including the eyelids. On examination, the conjunctival lining of the eyelids, especially the lower ones, is usually red and swollen. Untreated, atopic keratoconjunctivitis can progress to ulceration, scarring, cataracts, keratoconus, and corneal vacularization. Secondary infections are not common.

## Quality of life

Until recently, study of AR and its treatment has focused on symptoms and symptom improvement rather than on how well-being or quality of life (QOL) is affected. It is now recognized that AR significantly affects QOL. Consequently, questionnaires have been devised and validated to determine the impact of AR on an individual's health. These health-related quality of life (HRQOL) instruments measure a series of variables. Although symptom severity is an important contributing factor in determining HRQOL, psychosocial factors, such as perceived control of disease, poor physical functioning, and greater psychologic distress, appear to explain a substantial amount of the variability in HRQOL among adults with rhinitis [19].

Using the short form–36 (SF-36) health survey, a generic instrument focusing on sleep, work and school performance, family functioning, and social relationships, investigators noted that perennial AR impaired the HRQOL to a similar degree to asthma, which has long been recognized to have a significant impact on QOL [20,21]. In a study of 850 young adults, subjects who had AR but not asthma (n = 240) were more likely than subjects who had neither asthma nor rhinitis (n = 349) to report problems with social activities, difficulties with daily activities as a result of emotional problems, and poorer mental well-being. Patients who had both asthma and AR (n = 76) experienced more physical limitations than patients with AR alone, but no difference was found between these two groups for questions related to social and mental health [22]. To improve understanding of the impact of rhinitis on work productivity, a random phone survey was conducted among adults, yielding 125 persons who had asthma (with or without concomitant rhinitis) and 175 persons who had rhinitis alone. Although asthmatics were less likely than those who had rhinitis to hold a job since their health problem began (88% versus 97%; $P = .002$), among those employed, decreased job effectiveness was more frequently reported in the rhinitis group (43 of 121; 36%) than in the asthmatic group (14 of 72; 19%; $P = .02$) [23].

## Treatment modalities

### Environmental control measures

The ARIA guidelines have provided a pragmatic, stepwise approach to treatment of AR (Fig. 2). As noted, the choice of the various modalities of treatment depends on the perceived severity of symptoms as well as on whether symptoms are persistent.

Allergen avoidance is one of the guiding principles of treatment. However, it often proves impractical and difficult to implement, and it may not be effective when used alone. Individuals sensitive to pollen may need to minimize time spent outdoors during times of high pollen count. Environmental measures to minimize indoor pollen exposure include keeping the windows of homes and cars closed and employing an air conditioner in the recycling/indoor mode.

For individuals allergic to dust mite, proposed measures include encasing mattresses, pillows and quilts or duvets in impermeable covers, as well as washing all bedding weekly in a hot cycle ($55°C–60°C$; $131°F–140°F$) to reduce dust mite allergen levels and live dust mites [1]. A recent study looking at the addition of impermeable bed covers in AR did not show any additional benefits over nonimpermeable covers [24]. High-efficiency particulate air (HEPA) filters can reduce allergen loads and may lead to symptom improvement in those with allergic sensitization to dust mite [25]. Although some acaricides, such as disodium octaborate tetrahydrate, can lower the number of live dust mites in carpets, it is unknown whether this effect translates into symptom mitigation [26]. House dust mites are sensitive to humidity, and hence growth should be suppressible with sufficient dehumidification. However, a recent randomized controlled trial in the United Kingdom showed that dehumidifiers did not have a major effect on house dust mite counts or allergen levels [27].

Individuals allergic to cats and dogs have few effective ways to reduce their exposure to pet allergens, short of ridding themselves of the animals. Although weekly washing can reduce allergens, clinical studies have not shown a clear benefit on rhinitis [28]. Similarly, HEPA filters did not lead to symptom improvement in cat-sensitized individuals with AR in a placebo-controlled study [29].

Cockroach infestation is associated with AR and asthma, especially in the inner city. Control measures are based on eliminating suitable environments

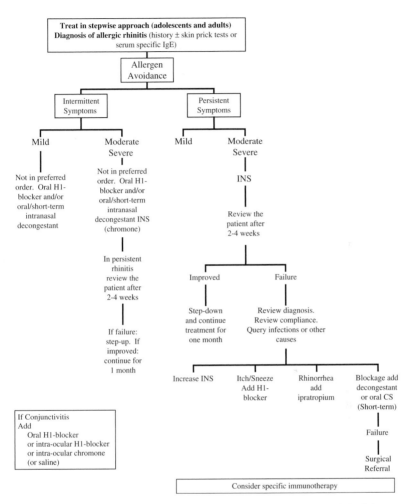

Fig. 2. Stepwise approach to treatment of allergic rhinitis. CS, corticosteroid; INS, intranasal corticosteroid. (*Adapted from* Bachert C, van Cauwenberge P, Khaltaev N; World Health Organization. Allergic rhinitis and its impact on asthma. In collaboration with the World Health Organization. Executive summary of the workshop report. Geneva, Switzerland, December 7–10, 1999. Allergy 2002;57:841–55; with permission.)

and restricting access by sealing, caulking, and controlling the food supply, as well as using chemical control and traps [1]. Although cockroach extermination by professionals may reduce allergen levels by 80% to 90%, no studies have evaluated the clinical significance of this reduction [30]. Reinfestation from adjacent apartments is a frequent problem, and thus extermination efforts will most likely need to be repeated and extended beyond the affected home.

Molds are ubiquitous both indoors and outdoors. Mold-allergic individuals should carefully inspect their homes for mold damage, paying especial attention to the more humid areas of the house. When indoor levels of a specific mold are significantly greater than outdoor levels, mold contamination is most likely present. Localized mold growth may be removed with a dilute bleach solution. More extensive mold damage may require more aggressive measures, such as replacing the affected surface. Controlled clinical studies showing that these measures effectively reduce suffering from rhinitis have not been undertaken.

## Overview of pharmacologic treatment

With mild intermittent AR, suggested initial pharmacologic therapy consists of an oral histamine-1 (H1)-blocker, an intranasal H1-blocker, or an oral decongestant. When intermittent disease is moderate or severe, intranasal corticosteroids provide an alternative to the aforementioned pharmacologic agents. Persistent mild AR is treated in the same manner as moderate or severe intermittent AR. When symptoms are persistent and moderate or severe, intranasal corticosteroids should be the first class of medications employed. Investigation into the presence of AC should also take place, because appropriate therapy with oral H1-blockers, intraocular H1-blockers, or intraocular chromomes will need to be integrated into a comprehensive therapeutic approach. With all grades of severity, appropriate follow-up should take place in a reasonable amount of time and therapy then stepped up or stepped down, as indicated.

### Intranasal corticosteroids

Intranasal corticosteroids (INS) represent the single most effective class of medications for AR and improve all nasal symptoms, including nasal congestion, rhinorrhea, itching, and sneezing. Most studies [31,32] but not all [33] have shown that treatment of rhinitis with INS also leads to decreased methacholine sensitivity of the lower airways, better asthma control [34], and fewer asthma-related emergency room visits [35]. The comprehensive clinical effects of INS are based on a broad mechanism of action. As glucocorticoids diffuse across the cell membrane, they bind to specific intracellular receptors, forming a complex that is then transported into the nucleus, where it binds to glucocorticoid response elements (GREs) [36]. As a result, transcription of GRE-associated genes is either downregulated or, less commonly, upregulated [37]. This effect leads to a reduction in inflammatory cells and their associated cytokines in the nasal mucosa.

Currently available INS in the United States include beclomethasone dipropionate, budesonide, flunisolide propionate, fluticasone, mometasone, and triamcinolone acetonide. Although INS may vary in their sensory attributes (eg, taste or smell) and thus in degree of patient acceptance and adherence, there do not appear to be any clear, clinically relevant differences in efficacy among them [38]. A list of currently available INS and their various attributes is presented in Table 1.

Table 1
Currently available intranasal corticosteriods

| Generic name (trade name) | Strength (µg/spray) | Daily dose (sprays per nostril) | | t½ (h) | Liquid type | Phenyl etoh/ fragrance | Volume (µL) | No. of sprays per bottle | Cost |
|---|---|---|---|---|---|---|---|---|---|
| | | Adult starting | Maintenance | | | | | | |
| Fluticasone (Flonase) | 50 | 2/nost | 1/nost | 7.8 | Susp | + | 95 | 120 | ++ |
| Triamcinolone (Nasacort AQ) | 55 | 2/nost | 2/nost | 3.1 | Susp | – | 130 | 120 | ++ |
| Flunisolide (Nasarel) | 29 | 2/nost | 1/nost | 1.8 | Sol | – | 120 | 200 | + |
| Mometasone (Nasonex) | 50 | 2/nost | 2/nost | 5.8 | Susp | – | 100 | 120 | ++ |
| Budesonide (Rhinocort Aqua) | 32 | 1/nost | 1/nost | 2–3 | Susp | – | 50 | 120 | ++ |

*Abbreviations:* nost, nostril; Susp, suspension; Sol, solution; +, moderate; ++, high.

Among the reported side effects are nasal burning and stinging, dryness, and epistaxis. These may occur in 5% to 10% of patients. Local atrophy, such as occurs with dermatologic high-potency corticosteroids, was not observed in two year-long studies with fluticasone propionate and mometasone furoate [39,40]. Local candidiasis, sometimes seen with inhaled corticosteroids, is rarely seen with nasal corticosteroids. In terms of systemic side effects, laboratory evaluations of the hypothalamic-pituitary-adrenal axis by multiple means have shown minimal or no suppression [41]. Osteocalcin, a marker of bone turnover, and eosinophilia were unaffected by a variety of INS when compared with placebo, suggesting that the systemic glucocorticoid burden was insignificant [42]. A recent case-control study showed no increased likelihood of bone fracture among octogenarians using INS, regardless of the dose [43].

## H1-antihistamines

Although many chemical mediators can induce one or more symptoms of AR, histamine is probably the major mediator of allergic inflammation, especially during the early phase. Acting at the H1 receptors, histamine can induce most of the allergic symptoms: sneezing, itching of the nose, throat, and palate, and rhinorrhea by means of stimulation of the sensory nerves, increase in vascular permeability, and mucus production. H1-antihistamines are inverse agonists, acting by stabilizing the H1-receptor on smooth muscle cells, nerve endings, and glandular cells, leading to a reduction in all the aforementioned symptoms. However, they have only a modest effect on nasal congestion [44]. Oral H1-receptor antagonists also reduce conjunctival itching, redness, and tearing but are less effective than topical agents in this class. Tolerance to the clinical effects of H1-antihistamines has not been shown to develop [45].

Oral H1-antihistamines are commonly separated into two classes: first and second generation. The first-generation antihistamines include diphenhydramine, clemastine, tripelennamine, pyrilamine, brompheniramine, chlorpheniramine, tripolidine, hydroxyzine, promethazine, and cyptoheptadine and are often referred to as *sedating*, which has been used to encompass both drowsiness and a reduction in intellectual and motor performance [46]. Sedating H1-antihistamines have been linked to pilot fatalities [47] and industrial accidents [48], as well as to significant loss of productivity at school and work [49]. Diphenhydramine given as a single 50-mg dose led to greater impairment of driving performance, as assessed in a driving simulator, than did the quantity of ethanol ingested to achieve an estimated blood alcohol level of 0.1% [50]. As in ethanol intake, there is a discrepancy between the self-perception of sedation and objective measures of drowsiness and performance [51]. Although dosing for first-generation H1-antihistamines is often undertaken several times a day, the terminal elimination of first-generation antihistamine half life varies from 9.2 to 27.9 hours [52], leading to potential daytime deficits even when the drug is administered only at bedtime. One study suggested that tolerance may develop to the sedating properties of diphenhydramine [53].

Second-generation oral H1-antihistamines include loratadine, desloratadine, fexofenadine, cetirizine, levo-cetirizine, ebastine, and mizolastine; the final three are currently not commercially available in the United States. Except for fexofenadine, all second-generation H1-antihistamines have the potential to cause increased sedation when used at more than the recommended dose. For the oral agents available in the United States, cetirizine is the only one to cause an increased incidence of sedation at its recommended dose in patients aged 12 or older (11% to 14%, versus 6% receiving placebo) [54].

In contrast to first-generation antihistamines, for which studies showing clinical efficacy are limited [55], the effectiveness of second-generation antihistamines has been established in a variety of well-designed, double-blind, placebo-controlled studies. These clinical studies provide important information regarding onset of action, peak effect, and duration of action of the antihistamine. Such information is lacking for first-generation antihistamines. Current dosing suggestions for older H1-antihistamines are based, at best, on the individual antihistamine's ability to suppress the cutaneous wheal and flare response after allergen or histamine introduction into the skin.

Currently, azelastine is the only intranasal antihistamine available in the United States, although olopatadine may become available in the near future. Azelastine appears to have mechanisms of therapeutic action in addition to its H1-receptor effect. These include interference with the vasoactive neuropeptide substance P [56], inhibited production of leukotrienes B4 and C4 [57], and a possible decrease in the nuclear factor–κB [58], a transcription factor for multiple proinflammatory substances. Azelastine has demonstrated efficacy in both seasonal rhinitis [59–61] and vasomotor rhinitis [62]. Although some studies have shown a decrease in nasal congestion, others have not been able to confirm this result. Dose-ranging trials have shown an onset of action within 3 hours after initial dosing and a persistence of efficacy over a 12-hour interval. The most common side effects at the recommended dose of two sprays per nostril twice a day are bitter taste (19.7%, versus 0.6% placebo) and sedation (11.5%, versus 5.4% placebo).

Overall efficacy of oral H1-antihistamines is of a similar magnitude to that of the mast cell stabilizers nedocromil and sodium cromoglycate; it may also, based on limited available data, resemble that of the leukotriene inhibitor montelukast.

A list of currently available oral H1-antihistamines is presented in Table 2.

## Decongestants

Vasoconstrictors exist in both topical and oral form. Topical applied vasoconstrictor sympathomimetic agents belong to the catecholamine family (eg, phenylephrine) or imidazoline family (eg, ozymetazoline), whereas

Table 2
Formulations and dosages of representative H₁-antihistamines

| Generic name (trade name) | Formulation | Recommended dose |
|---|---|---|
| *First generation* | | |
| Chlorpheniramine (Chlortrimeton) | • Tablets: 4 mg, 8 mg, 12 mg <br> • Syrup: 2.5 mg/5 mL <br> • Parenteral solution: 10 mg/mL | Adult: 8–12 mg twice daily |
| Diphenhydramine (Benadryl) | • Capsules: 25 mg or 50 mg <br><br> • Elixir: 12.5 mg/5 mL <br> • Syrup: 6.25 mg/5 mL <br> • Parenteral solution: 50 mg/mL | Adult: 25–50 mg three times daily |
| Doxepin (Zonalon) | • Capsules: 10–75 mg | Adult: 25–50 mg three times daily or every day at bedtime |
| Hydroxyine (Atarax) | • Capsules: 10 mg, 25 mg, 50 mg <br><br> • Syrup: 10 mg/5 mL | Adult: 25–50 mg three times daily or every day at bedtime |
| *Second generation* | | |
| Cetirizine (Zyrtec) | • Tablets: 10 mg <br> • Chewable tablets: 5 mg, 10 mg <br> • Syrup: 5 mg/5 mL | Adult: 5–10 mg every day |
| Desloratadine (Clarinex) | • Tablets: 5 mg <br> • Syrup: 2.5 mg/5 mL | ≥ 12 y: 5 mg every day |
| Fexofenadine (Allegra) | • Tablets: 30 mg, 60 mg, 120 mg, 180 mg | ≥ 12 y: 60 mg twice daily or 120 mg or 180 mg every day |
| Loratadine (Claritin) | • Tablets: 10 mg <br> • Rapidly disintegrating tablets (Reditabs): 10 mg <br> • Syrup: 5 mg/5 mL | Adult: 10 mg every day |

oral vasocontricting agents are primarily catecholamines (phenylephrine and pseudoephedrine). These agents exert their effect via the α1 and α2 adrenoreceptors present on nasal capacitance vessels responsible for mucosal swelling and associated nasal congestion. The reduction in blood flow to the nasal vasculature after administration leads to increased nasal patency in 5 to 10 minutes when the agent is used topically, or 30 minutes when used orally. Nasal decongestion may last as long as 8 hours with topical and 24 hours with extended-release oral decongestants. Symptoms of rhinitis other than nasal congestion are not affected [63]; hence monotherapy with vasoconstrictors has a limited role in the treatment of AR. However, when oral decongestants are combined with an antihistamine, all cardinal symptoms of AR are targeted.

The adverse effects of topical nasal decongestants include nasal burning, stinging, dryness, and, less commonly, mucosal ulceration. Tolerance and rebound congestion may occur when these agents are used for longer than 1 week and can culminate in rhinitis medicamentosa [64]. Adverse effects of oral decongestants include central nervous stimulation, such as insomnia—which may occur in as many as a third of patients—nervousness, anxiety, and tremors, as well as tachycardia, palpitations, and increases in blood pressure.

*Cromolyn and nedocromil sodium*

Cromolyn inhibits the degranulation of sensitized mast cells, thereby blocking the release of inflammatory mediators [65]. It does not interfere with either the binding of IgE to the high-affinity IgE receptor or the binding of the allergen to its specific IgE. In allergen challenge studies of individuals with AR, cromolyn sodium has proved effective in reducing both the early- and late-phase allergic reaction [66]. Cromolyn is indicated for both seasonal [67] and perennial AR [68]. The onset of relief appears during the first week of treatment, and symptoms often continue to improve as the medication is continued over subsequent weeks. The 4% intranasal solution is recommended for adults and children aged 2 and older. The frequency of dosing may lead to adherence problems, given the initial need to instill the solution four times daily. However, once symptoms are under control, a less frequent dosing regimen may suffice for adequate symptom control. Topical adverse effects, such as sneezing, nasal irritation, and unpleasant taste, are uncommon. Cromolyn is poorly absorbed systemically and therefore has an excellent safety record. Tolerance to the effects of cromolyn has not been described.

*Antileukotrienes*

Cysteinyl-leukotrienes (cys-LT) are potent lipid mediators derived from the enzymatic action on nuclear membrane phospholipids. These inflammatory molecules, first noted to play a significant role in the lower airway inflammation of asthma, also appear to play an important role in the upper airways, with high concentrations of LTC4 present in nasal secretions of atopic individuals after allergen challenge [69]. Furthermore, nasal challenge with LTD4 in normal human subjects led to a significant increase in nasal mucosal blood flow and nasal airway resistance [70]. Leukotrienes do not appear to stimulate the sensory nerves present in the nasal mucosa and hence probably do not contribute significantly to nasal itching or sneezing [71]. Blockage of the LT may be accomplished either by inhibition of synthesis using 5-lipoxygenase (5-LO) inhibitors or by receptor blockade of the cys-LT1 receptor using cys-LT receptor antagonists. Zileuton is the only drug approved for human use that blocks the 5-LO pathway. Concerns exist that the in vivo blockade of 5-LO may be significantly less than the 80% achieved in vitro [72,73]. Currently available receptor antagonists in the

United States include montelukast and zafirlukast. In general, antileuko-triene drugs are well tolerated. However, zileuton is associated with a 3% incidence of alanine transaminase elevation, so monitoring of liver function tests has been recommended for the first year [74].

Zileuton administered before nasal allergen challenge resulted in signif-icant attenuation of nasal congestion [75]. Zafirlukast performed no better than placebo in one study of patients with seasonal AR [76] and in an-other study using natural cat exposure after pretreatment with zafirlukast for 1 week [77]. However, a third study demonstrated a reduction in up-per respiratory responses to cat exposure [78]. Montelukast has been the most extensively studied antileukotriene in AR, and it has shown clinical efficacy in seasonal AR [79–81]. When montelukast is added to loratadine, the combination may be superior to either agent alone in reducing day-time nasal symptoms in patients with seasonal AR [82]. However, another study suggested that symptoms of seasonal AR were not better controlled with a combination of montelukast and loratadine than with once daily fexofenadine [83]. In summary, leukotriene antagonists do not appear to be more effective than nonsedating antihistamines. They have also been shown to be less effective than INS in the treatment of AR [84]. Nonethe-less, antileukotrienes may be an attractive alternative in individuals who have concomitant mild persistent asthma and intermittent AR.

*Omalizumab (anti-IgE)*

Omalizumab represents one of the more exciting recent developments in the treatment of atopic diseases and is probably only the first of several monoclonal antibodies aimed at modulating allergic inflammation. Unfortu-nately, at present, it is quite expensive for routine treatment of AR and is pri-marily indicated in the treatment of severe asthma. Nonetheless, studies using it provide proof-of-concept for the important roles of IgE, IgE recep-tors, and immune processes initiated by the interaction of these two mole-cules. Omalizumab is a humanized monoclonal antibody with nonhuman DNA sequences making up only 5% of the total molecule. This foreign pro-tein is murine in origin and makes up the portion binding to the IgE mole-cule. It binds to the constant region of the IgE molecule at its IgE receptor–binding portion, thereby effectively hindering IgE's interaction with the high-affinity IgE receptor present on mast cells, basophils, and den-dritic cells. Anti-IgE binds to circulating but not to cell-bound IgE, forming stable, long-lived anti-IgE–IgE complexes. After initial dosing, free IgE con-centrations decline in a rapid, dose-dependent fashion by 97% to 99%. Oma-lizumab has been shown to be effective in both allergen challenge studies and clinical trials. Multiple randomized, double-blind, placebo-controlled studies have shown efficacy of omalizumab in seasonal [85,86] and perennial AR [87,88]. In a recent open-label study of dust mite AR, even a low dose of oma-lizumab (0.015 mg/kg/IU/mL) led to reduction of the nasal mean total symptom score from 5.4 at baseline to 1.8 ($P = .002$) on day 84 and 2.1 ($P = .008$) on day 168 after nasal challenge with dust mites [89].

*Allergen immunotherapy*

Immunotherapy involves the repeated administration of increasing doses of individually selected allergens to induce immunologic tolerance and lead to symptom improvement. Multiple immunologic changes have been observed in individuals receiving allergy vaccines [90]. Over the last few years, the quantity of allergen necessary to lead to substantial clinical improvement and immunologic changes has been elucidated for many of the major standardized allergens [91]. Several placebo-controlled, double-blinded studies have shown clinical efficacy of vaccination with allergy extracts [92–94]. Furthermore, in patients receiving grass allergen vaccinations for a period of 3 to 4 years, approximately 50% continued to derive clinical benefits 3 years after immunotherapy had been discontinued. Prolonged clinical benefits in this study correlated with persistent changes in immunity and allergic inflammation. Although the theory is intellectually sound, it remains unproved whether this phenomenon applies to individuals receiving vaccinations with multiple allergens, a pattern that is more reflective of immunotherapy in the United States. Recently, it has been noted that specific immunotherapy to birch or grass in children aged 6 to 14 who were not otherwise sensitized to other allergens led to a markedly reduced risk (OR = 2.52; $P < .05$) of being newly diagnosed with asthma during the 3 years of receiving allergy vaccines [95].

Immunotherapy is most commonly reserved for patients not responding to pharmacotherapy or for those unwilling to take or unable to tolerate medications. Patients need to understand the risks and side effects of immunotherapy before commencing. First, improvement requires several months of vaccinations. It is generally accepted that a 1-year trial determines who will and will not respond to immunotherapy. Second, adverse reactions occur in both local and systemic form. Local reactions are characterized by swelling after injections and may last for days. Although they are usually scarcely more than a nuisance, local reactions may prevent certain individuals from reaching proposed maintenance doses. Systemic reactions range from mild to fatal. The risk of a fatal reaction after receiving an allergy vaccine is estimated to be 1 in 2 to 2.5 million [96,97]. It is unclear how many fatal reactions are due to human error.

**Summary**

AR is a common condition affecting individuals of all ages. Those afflicted with AR often suffer from associated inflammatory conditions of the mucosa, such as AC, rhinosinusitis, asthma, otitis media with effusion, and other atopic conditions, such as eczema and food allergies. Lack of treatment or treatment with suboptimal therapy may result in reduced quality of life and compromise productivity at work or school. Although environmental controls may prove difficult to implement, and not all controls appear adequately to mitigate symptoms of AR, they continue to represent a foundation for treatment. Many different classes of medications are now available, and they have been shown to be effective and safe in a large number of well-designed, double-blind, placebo-controlled clinical trials. Some of the over-the-counter medications have been associated with increased sedation, potentially leading to accidents and fatalities at work or while operating complex machinery, such as automobiles. Only immunotherapy with increasing doses of individually targeted allergens results in sustained changes in the immune system. Although anti-IgE is probably only the first successful immunomodulator commercially available to treat AR, monoclonal antibodies will remain too costly, at least in the near future, to find their way into routine AR treatment.

## References

[1] Bousquet J, van Cauwenberge PB, Khaltaev N, et al. Allergic rhinitis and its impact on asthma. ARIA workshop report. J Allergy Clin Immunol 2001;108:S147.

[2] Hamilton RG, Franklin Adkinson N Jr. In vitro assays for the diagnosis of IgE-mediated disorders. J Allergy Clin Immunol 2004;114(2):213–25.

[3] Ingall M, Glaser J, Meltzer RS, et al. Allergic rhinitis in early infancy. Review of the literature and report of a case in a newborn. Pediatrics 1965;35:108–12.

[4] Nathan RA, Meltzer EO, Selner JC, et al. Prevalence of allergic rhinitis in the United States. J Allergy Clin Immunol 1997;99:S808–14.

[5] Wright AL, Holberg CJ, Martinez FD, et al. Epidemiology of physician-diagnosed allergic rhinitis in childhood. Pediatrics 1994;94(6 Pt 1):895–901.

[6] Skoner DP. Allergic rhinitis: definition, epidemiology, pathophysiology, detection, and diagnosis. J Allergy Clin Immunol 2001;108(Suppl 1):S2–8.

[7] Dykewicz MS, Fineman S, Nicklas R, et al. Joint task force algorithm and annotations for diagnosis and management of rhinitis. Ann Allergy Asthma Immunol 1998;81(5 Pt 2):469–73.

[8] Ober C. Susceptibility genes in asthma and allergy. Curr Allergy Asthma Rep 2001;1(2):174–9.

[9] Evans R. Epidemiology and natural history of asthma, allergic rhinitis, and atopic dermatitis (eczema). In: Middleton E, Reed C, Ellis E, editors. Allergy: principles and practice. 4th edition. St. Louis (MO): Mosby; 1993. p. 1109–36.

[10] Tulic MK, Wale JL, Holt PG, et al. Modification of the inflammatory response to allergen challenge after exposure to bacterial lipopolysaccharide. Am J Respir Cell Mol Biol 2000; 22(5):604–12.

[11] Von Mutius E, Martinez FD. Natural history, development, and prevention of allergic disease in childhood. In: Adkinson NF Jr, Yunginger JW, Busse WW, et al, editors. Middleton's allergy: principles and practice. 4th edition. St. Louis (MO): Mosby; 2003. p. 1169–74.

[12] Leynaert B, Bousquet J, Neukirch C, et al. Perennial rhinitis: an independent risk factor for asthma in nonatopic subjects: results from the European Community Respiratory Health Survey. J Allergy Clin Immunol 1999;104(2 Pt 1):301–4.

[13] Leynaert B, Liard R, Bousquet J, et al. Lessons from the French part of the European community respiratory health survey (ECRHS). Allergy Clin Immunol Int: S World Allergy Org 1999;11:218–25.

[14] Centers for Disease Control and Prevention. Current asthma prevalence 2002. Available at: http://www.cdc.gov. Accessed February 12, 2005.

[15] Braunstahl GJ, Kleinjan A, Overbeek SE, et al. Segmental bronchial provocation induces nasal inflammation in allergic rhinitis patients. Am J Respir Crit Care Med 2000;161:2051–7.

[16] Braunstahl GJ, Overbeek SE, Kleinjan A, et al. Nasal allergen provocation induces adhesion molecule expression and tissue eosinophilia in upper and lower airways. J Allergy Clin Immunol 2001;107:469–76.

[17] Shin SH, Ponikau JU, Sherris DA, et al. Chronic rhinosinusitis: an enhanced immune response to ubiquitous airborne fungi. J Allergy Clin Immunol 2004;114(6):1369–75.

[18] Bielory LB. Allergic and immunologic disorders of the eye. Part II: Ocular allergy. J Allergy Clin Immunol 2001;106:1019–32.

[19] Chen H, Katz PP, Eisner MD, et al. Health-related quality of life in adult rhinitis: the role of perceived control of disease. J Allergy Clin Immunol 2004;114(4):845–50.

[20] Bousquet J, Bullinger M, Fayol C, et al. Assessment of quality of life in patients with perennial allergic rhinitis with the French version of the SF-36 Health Status Questionnaire. J Allergy Clin Immunol 1994;94(2 Pt 1):182–8.

[21] Bousquet J, Knani J, Dhivert H, et al. Quality of life in asthma. I. Internal consistency and validity of the SF-36 questionnaire. Am J Respir Crit Care Med 1994;149:371–5.

[22] Leynaert B, Neukirch C, Liard R, et al. Quality of life in allergic rhinitis and asthma. A population-based study of young adults. Am J Respir Crit Care Med 2000;162(4 Pt 1): 1391–6.

[23] Blanc PD, Trupin L, Eisner M, et al. The work impact of asthma and rhinitis: findings from a population-based survey. J Clin Epidemiol 2001;54(6):610–8.

[24] Terreehorst I, Hak E, Oosting AJ, et al. Evaluation of impermeable covers for bedding in patients with allergic rhinitis. N Engl J Med 2003;349:237–46.

[25] Reisman RE, Mauriello PM, Davis GB, et al. A double-blind study of the effectiveness of a high-efficiency particulate air (HEPA) filter in the treatment of patients with perennial allergic rhinitis and asthma. J Allergy Clin Immunol 1990;85(6):1050–7.

[26] Codina R, Lockey RF, Diwadkar R, et al. Disodium octaborate tetrahydrate (DOT) application and vacuum cleaning, a combined strategy to control house dust mites. Allergy 2003; 58(4):318–24.

[27] Hyndman SJ, Vickers LM, Htut T, et al. A randomized trial of dehumidification in the control of house dust mite. Clin Exp Allergy 2000;30(8):1172–80.

[28] Klucka CV, Ownby DR, Green J, et al. Cat shedding of Fel d I is not reduced by washings, Allerpet-C spray, or acepromazine. J Allergy Clin Immunol 1995;95(6):1164–71.

[29] Wood RA, Johnson EF, Van Natta ML, et al. A placebo-controlled trial of a HEPA air cleaner in the treatment of cat allergy. Am J Respir Crit Care Med 1998;158(1): 115–20.

[30] Wood RA, Eggleston PA, Rand C, et al. Cockroach allergen abatement with extermination and sodium hypochlorite cleaning in inner-city homes. Ann Allergy Asthma Immunol 2001; 87(1):60–4.

[31] Watson WT, Becker AB, Simons FE. Treatment of allergic rhinitis with intranasal corticosteroids in patients with mild asthma: effect on lower airway responsiveness. J Allergy Clin Immunol 1993;91:97–101.

[32] Fosi A, Pelucchi A, Gherson G, et al. Once daily intranasal fluticasone propionate (200 μg) reduces nasal symptoms and inflammation but also attenuates the increase in bronchial responsiveness during the pollen season in allergic rhinitis. J Allergy Clin Immunol 1996;98: 274–82.

[33] Orhan F, Sekerel BE, Adalioglu G, et al. Effect of nasal triamcinolone acetonide on seasonal variations of bronchial hyperresponsiveness and bronchial inflammation in nonasthmatic children with seasonal allergic rhinitis. Ann Allergy Asthma Immunol 2004;92(4):438–45.

[34] Pedersen B, Dahl R, Lindqvist N, et al. Nasal inhalation of the glucocorticoid budesonide from a spacer for the treatment of patients with pollen rhinitis and asthma. Allergy 1990; 45:451–6.

[35] Adams RJ, Fuhlbrigge AL, Finkelstein JA, et al. Intranasal steroids and the risk of emergency department visits for asthma. J Allergy Clin Immunol 2002;109(4):636–42.

[36] Luisi BF, Xu WX, Otwinoeski Z, et al. Crystallographic analysis of the interaction of the glucocorticoid receptor with DNA. Nature 1991;352:497–505.

[37] Diamond MI, Miner JN, Yoshinaga SK, et al. Transcription factors interactions: selectors of positive or negative regulation form a single DNA element. Science 1990;249:1266–72.

[38] Corren J. Intranasal corticosteroids for allergic rhinitis: how do different agents compare? J Allergy Clin Immunol 1999;104:S144–9.

[39] Minshall E, Ghaffar O, Cameron L, et al. Assessment by nasal biopsy of long-term use of monetasone furoate nasal spray (Nasonex) in the treatment of perennial rhinitis. Otolaryngol Head Neck Surg 1998;118:648–54.

[40] Holm AF, Fokkens WJ, Godthelp T, et al. A 1-yr placebo-controlled study of intranasal fluticasone propionate aqueous nasal spray in patients with perennial allergic rhinitis: a safety and biopsy study. Clin Otolaryngol 1998;23:69–73.

[41] Wilson AM, McFarlane LC, Lipworth BJ. Effect of repeated once daily dosing of three intranasal corticosteroids on basal and dynamic measurements of hypothalamic-pituitary-adrenal axis activity. J Allergy Clin Immunol 1998;101:470–4.

[42] Wilson AM, Sims EJ, McFarlane LC, et al. Effects of intranasal corticosteroids on adrenal, bone, and blood markers of systemic activity in allergic rhinitis. J Allergy Clin Immunol 1998;102:598–604.

[43] Suissa S, Baltzan M, Kremer R, et al. Inhaled and nasal corticosteroid use and the risk of fracture. Am J Respir Crit Care Med 2004;169(1):83–8.

[44] Van Cauwenberge P, Juniper EF. Comparison of the efficacy, safety and quality of life provided by fexofenadine hydrochloride 120 mg, loratadine 10 mg and placebo administered once daily for the treatment of seasonal allergic rhinitis. Clin Exp Allergy 2000;30:891–9.

[45] Simons FER, Simons KJ. Clinical pharmacology of H1-antihistamines. In: Simons FER, editor. Histamine and H1-antihistamines in allergic disease. 2nd edition. New York: Marcel Dekker; 2002. p. 141–78.

[46] Passalacqua G, Scordamaglia A, Ruffoni S, et al. Sedation from H1 antagonists: evaluation methods and experimental results. Allergol Immunopathol (Madr) 1993;21:79–83.

[47] Soper JW, Chaturvedi AK, Canfield DV. Prevalence of chlorpheniramine in aviation accident pilot fatalities, 1991–1996. Aviat Space Environ Med 2000;71:1206–9.

[48] Gilmore TM, Alexander BH, Mueller BA, et al. Occupational injuries and medication use. Am J Ind Med 1996;30(2):234–9.

[49] Cockburn IM, Bailit HL, Berndt ER, et al. Loss of work productivity due to illness and medical treatment. J Occup Environ Med 1999;41:948–53.

[50] Weiler JM, Bloomfield JR, Woodworth GG, et al. Effects of fexofenadine, diphenhydramine, and alcohol on driving performance: a randomized, placebo-controlled trial in the Iowa Driving Simulator. Ann Intern Med 2000;132:354–63.

[51] Goetz DW, Jacobson JM, Murnane JE, et al. Prolongation of simple and choice reaction times in a double-blinded comparison of twice-daily hydroxyzine versus terfenadine. J Allergy Clin Immunol 1989;84:316–22.

[52] Simons FER. $H_1$-antihistamines. In: Adkinson NF Jr, Yunginger JW, Busse WW, et al, editors. Middleton's allergy: principles and practice. 6th edition. Philadelphia: Mosby; 2003. p. 834–69.

[53] Richardson GS, Roehrs TA, Rosenthal L, et al. Tolerance to daytime sedative effects of H1 antihistamines. J Clin Psychopharmacol 2002;22(5):511–5.

[54] Zyrtec [prescribing information]. New York: Pfizer Laboratories; updated 2004. Available at: http://www.zyrtec.com. Accessed February 23, 2005.

[55] Druce HM, Thoden WR, Mure P, et al. Brompheniramine, Loratadine and placebo in allergic rhinitis: a placebo-controlled comparative clinical trial. J Clin Pharmacol 1998;38: 382–9.

[56] Shinoda M, Watanabe N, Suko T, et al. Effects of anti-allergic drugs on substance P (SP) and vasoactive intestinal peptide (VIP) in nasal secretions. Am J Rhinol 1997;11(3):237–41.

[57] Hamasaki Y, Shafigeh M, Yamamoto S, et al. Inhibition of leukotriene synthesis by azelastine. Ann Allergy Asthma Immunol 1996;76(5):469–75.

[58] Yoneda K, Yamamoto T, Ueta E, et al. Suppression by azelastine hydrochloride of NF-kappa B activation involved in generation of cytokines and nitric oxide. Jpn J Pharmacol 1997;73(2):145–53.

[59] Storms WW, Pearlman DS, Chervinsky P, et al. Effectiveness of azelastine nasal solution in seasonal allergic rhinitis. Ear Nose Throat J 1994;73(6):382–94.

[60] Ratner PH, Findlay SR, Hampel F Jr, et al. A double-blind, controlled trial to assess the safety and efficacy of azelastine nasal spray in seasonal allergic rhinitis. J Allergy Clin Immunol 1994;94(5):818–25.

[61] Meltzer EO, Weiler JM, Dockhorn RJ, et al. Azelastine nasal spray in the management of seasonal allergic rhinitis. Ann Allergy 1994;72(4):354–9.

[62] Banov CH, Lieberman P. Vasomotor Rhinitis Study Groups. Efficacy of azelastine nasal spray in the treatment of vasomotor (perennial nonallergic) rhinitis. Ann Allergy Asthma Immunol 2001;86(1):28–35.

[63] Malm L, McCaffrey TV, Kern EB. Alpha-adrenoceptor–mediated secretion from the anterior nasal glands of the dog. Acta Otolaryngol 1983;96:149–55.

[64] Malm L, Anggard A. Vasoconstrictors. In: Mygind N, Naclerio RM, editors. Allergic and non-allergic rhinitis: clinical aspects. Copenhagen (Denmark): Munsgaard; 1993. p. 95–100.

[65] Cos JSG. Disodium cromoglycate (FPL 670 "Intal"): a specific inhibitor of reaginic antigen–antibody mechanisms. Nature 1967;216:1328–9.

[66] Orie NGM, Booij-Nord H, Pelikan Z, et al. Protective effect of disodium cromoglycate on nasal and bronchial reactions after allergen challenge. In: Pepys J, Frankland AW, editors. Disodium cromoglycate in allergic airway disease. London: Butterworth; 1970. p. 33–41.

[67] Meltzer EO. NasalCrom Study Group. Efficacy and patient satisfaction with cromolyn sodium nasal solution in the treatment of seasonal allergic rhinitis: a placebo-controlled study. Clin Ther 2002;24(6):942–52.

[68] Cohan RH, Bloom FL, Rhoades RB, et al. Treatment of perennial allergic rhinitis with cromolyn sodium. Double-blind study on 34 adult patients. J Allergy Clin Immunol 1976; 58(1 Pt 2):121–8.

[69] Wang D, Clement P, Smitz J, et al. Concentrations of chemical mediators in nasal secretions after nasal allergen challenges in atopic patients. Eur Arch Otorhinolaryngol 1995; 252(Suppl):S40–3.

[70] Bisgaard H, Olsson P, Bende M. Effect of leukotriene D4 on nasal mucosal blood flow, nasal airway resistance and nasal secretions in humans. Clin Allergy 1986;16:289–97.

[71] Fujita M, Yonetomi Y, Shimouchi K, et al. Involvement of cysteinyl leukotrienes in biphasic increase of nasal airway resistance of antigen-induced rhinitis in guinea pigs. Eur J Pharmacol 1999;369(3):349–56.

[72] McGill KA, Busse WW. Zileuton. Lancet 1996;348:519–2419.

[73] Wenzel SE, Trudeau JB, Kaminsky DA. Effect of 5-lipoxygenase inhibition on bronchoconstriction and airway inflammation in nocturnal asthma. Am J Respir Crit Care Med 1995; 152:897–905.

[74] Liu MC, Dube LM, Lancaster J. Acute and chronic effects of a %-lipoxygenase inhibitor in asthma: a 6-month randomized multicenter trial. J Allergy Clin Immunol 1996;98: 859–71.

[75] Knapp HR. Reduced allergen-induced nasal congestion and leukotriene synthesis with an orally active 5-lipoxygenase inhibitor. N Engl J Med 1990;323(25):1745–8.

[76] Pullerits T, Praks L, Skoogh BE, et al. Randomized placebo-controlled study comparing a leukotriene receptor antagonist and a nasal glucocorticoid in seasonal allergic rhinitis. Am J Respir Crit Care Med 1999;159(6):1814–8.

[77] Corren J, Spector S, Fuller L, et al. Effects of zafirlukast upon clinical, physiologic, and inflammatory responses to natural cat allergen exposure. Ann Allergy Asthma Immunol 2001; 87(3):211–7.

[78] Phipatanakul W, Eggleston PA, Conover-Walker MK, et al. A randomized, double-blind, placebo-controlled trial of the effect of zafirlukast on upper and lower respiratory responses to cat challenge. J Allergy Clin Immunol 2000;105(4):704–10.

[79] Philip G, Malmstrom K, Hampel FC, et al. Montelukast Spring Rhinitis Study Group. Montelukast for treating seasonal allergic rhinitis: a randomized, double-blind, placebo-controlled trial performed in the spring. Clin Exp Allergy 2002;32(7):1020–8.

[80] van Adelsberg J, Philip G, Pedinoff AJ, et al. Montelukast Fall Rhinitis Study Group. Montelukast improves symptoms of seasonal allergic rhinitis over a 4-week treatment period. Allergy 2003;58(12):1268–76.

[81] Chervinsky P, Philip G, Malice MP, et al. Montelukast for treating fall allergic rhinitis: effect of pollen exposure in 3 studies. Ann Allergy Asthma Immunol 2004;92(3):367–73.

[82] Meltzer EO, Malmstrom K, Lu S, et al. Concomitant montelukast and loratadine as treatment for seasonal allergic rhinitis: a randomized, placebo-controlled clinical trial. J Allergy Clin Immunol 2000;105(5):917–22.

[83] Wilson AM, Orr LC, Coutie WJ, et al. A comparison of once daily fexofenadine versus the combination of montelukast plus loratadine on domiciliary nasal peak flow and symptoms in seasonal allergic rhinitis. Clin Exp Allergy 2002;32(1):126–32.

[84] Ratner PH, Howland WC 3rd, Arastu R, et al. Fluticasone propionate aqueous nasal spray provided significantly greater improvement in daytime and nighttime nasal symptoms of seasonal allergic rhinitis compared with montelukast. Ann Allergy Asthma Immunol 2003;90(5):536–42.

[85] Casale TB. Anti-IgE (Omalizumab) therapy in seasonal allergic rhinitis. Am J Respir Crit Care Med 2001;164:S18–21.

[86] Adelroth E, Rak S, Huahtela T, et al. Recombinant humanized mAb-E25, an anti IgE mAb, in birch pollen–induced seasonal allergic rhinitis. J Allergy Clin Immunol 2000;106:253–9.

[87] Chervinsky P, Casale T, Townley R, et al. Omalizumab, an anti-IgE antibody, in the treatment of adults and adolescents with perennial allergic rhinitis. Ann Allergy Asthma Immunol 2003;91(2):160–7.

[88] Vignola AM, Humbert M, Bousquet J, et al. Efficacy and tolerability of anti-immunoglobulin E therapy with omalizumab in patients with concomitant allergic asthma and persistent allergic rhinitis: SOLAR. Allergy 2004;59(7):709–17.

[89] Corren J, Diaz-Sanchez D, Saxon A, et al. Effects of omalizumab, a humanized monoclonal anti IgE antibody, on nasal reactivity to allergen and local IgE synthesis. Ann Allergy Asthma Immunol 2004;93(3):243–8.

[90] Till SJ, Francis JN, Nouri-Aria K, et al. Mechanisms of immunotherapy. J Allergy Clin Immunol 2004;113(6):1025–34.

[91] Joint Task Force on Practice Parameters. Allergen immunotherapy: a practice parameter. American Academy of Allergy, Asthma and Immunology. American College of Allergy, Asthma and Immunology. Ann Allergy Asthma Immunol 2003;90(1 Suppl 1):1–40.

[92] Durham SR, Walker SM, Varga EM, et al. Long-term clinical efficacy of grass-pollen immunotherapy. N Engl J Med 1999;341(7):468–75.

[93] Walker SM, Pajno GB, Lima MT, et al. Grass pollen immunotherapy for seasonal rhinitis and asthma: a randomized, controlled trial. J Allergy Clin Immunol 2001;107(1):87–93.

[94] Varney VA, Tabbah K, Mavroleon G, et al. Usefulness of specific immunotherapy in patients with severe perennial allergic rhinitis induced by house dust mite: a double-blind, randomized, placebo-controlled trial. Clin Exp Allergy 2003;33(8):1076–82.

[95] Möller C, Dreborg S, Ferdousi HA, et al. Pollen immunotherapy reduces the development of asthma in children with seasonal rhinoconjunctivitis. J Allergy Clin Immunol 2002;109:251–6.

[96] Bernstein DI, Wanner M, Borish L. Immunotherapy Committee, American Academy of Allergy, Asthma and Immunology. Twelve-year survey of fatal reactions to allergen injections and skin testing: 1990–2001. J Allergy Clin Immunol 2004;113(6):1129–36.

[97] Li JT. Immunotherapy for allergic rhinitis. Immunol Allergy Clin North Am 2000;20:381–400.

ELSEVIER
SAUNDERS

THE MEDICAL
CLINICS
OF NORTH AMERICA

Med Clin N Am 90 (2006) 39–60

# Asthma: Diagnosis and Management

Sameer K. Mathur, MD, PhD, William W. Busse, MD*

*Section of Allergy, Pulmonary, and Critical Care, Department of Medicine,
University of Wisconsin Medical School, Madison, WI, USA*

Asthma is characterized by a chronic airway inflammation that may lead to airway obstruction, hyperresponsiveness, and clinical symptoms of cough, wheeze, and shortness of breath [1]. Because the prevalence, morbidity, and perhaps mortality of asthma have been increasing worldwide [2], there is concern that asthma patients are not always readily identified and may not receive optimum treatment of their disease. To provide more effective care for patients who have asthma, physicians need to recognize asthma, diagnose it, and monitor its control. Furthermore, comorbidities associated with asthma should be considered, because they often complicate the effectiveness of asthma management. The goal of this article is to provide the physician with an overview of the approaches and tools available to diagnose and manage asthma for optimum control.

### Diagnosis of asthma

The onset of asthma often occurs in childhood and has strong associations with other allergic diseases, such as atopic dermatitis and allergic rhinitis. Asthma may also occur in adulthood in association with a history of allergic disease. Whether this represents a new onset or reactivation is often difficult to determine. The association of asthma with allergic sensitization is categorized as *allergic asthma*. However, adult-onset asthma may often be found in the absence of allergic sensitization. Rather, these individuals may have other features, such as aspirin or nonsteroidal anti-inflammatory drug (NSAID) sensitivity, nasal polyposis, or sinusitis. In the past, this class of asthma was called *intrinsic asthma*. Such classifications are artificial and are not particularly helpful to the clinician, because the end result is the

---

* Corresponding author. Section of Allergy, Pulmonary, and Critical Care, Department of Medicine, University of Wisconsin Medical School, K4/910 CSC, 600 Highland Avenue, Madison, WI 53792.

*E-mail address:* wwb@medicine.wisc.edu (W.W. Busse).

0025-7125/06/$ - see front matter © 2005 Elsevier Inc. All rights reserved.
doi:10.1016/j.mcna.2005.08.014
*medical.theclinics.com*

same in all forms of asthma: airflow obstruction that is largely reversible in most patients.

A definitive diagnostic test for asthma does not yet exist. Rather, the diagnosis of asthma is based on a clinical constellation of symptoms, the patient's personal and family history, physical examination findings (which are often absent when acute symptoms are not present), and supportive laboratory tests (Box 1). Typical asthma symptoms include any combination of wheezing, dyspnea, and cough. Although these features are nonspecific and found in many pulmonary diseases, the patient's history often relates recurrent episodes of such symptoms, frequently occurring at night or in the early morning, resulting in awakenings from sleep. There may also be specific allergic triggers, such as exposures to pollens, molds, dust mites, cockroaches, or pets, that give seasonal or environmental clues to the diagnosis. Nonallergic triggers, such as tobacco smoke, weather changes, cold air, aspirin/NSAID use, aerosolized irritants, or exercise, may also be reported. A frequent trigger for many asthma patients is a viral upper respiratory infection (URI); this can lead to an asthma exacerbation and an increase in asthma symptoms that may persist for weeks following resolution of the URI symptoms. Finally, there is often a significant family history of atopic diseases (ie, atopic dermatitis, allergic rhinitis, or asthma).

Physical examination of the chest during an asthma exacerbation usually reveals wheezing and prolongation of the expiratory phase on auscultation.

---

**Box 1. Clinical characteristics of asthma**

*Symptoms*
- Dyspnea
- Wheezing
- Cough

*Patient history*
- Allergic or cold air triggers
- Viral upper respiratory infection trigger
- Nocturnal symptoms
- History of atopic disease
- Family history of allergy or asthma

*Physical examination findings (acute)*
- Expiratory wheezing
- Prolonged expiratory phase
- Tachypnea
- Tachycardia
- Pulsus paradoxus
- Accessory muscle use
- Evidence for other atopic disease (eg, eczema)

Tachypnea and tachycardia may also be present. A pulsus paradoxus can occur and represents the changes in intrathoracic pressure associated with the obstruction from asthma. With more severe symptoms, the patient may exhibit accessory muscle use with respiration. In the absence of acute symptoms, there may be no abnormal findings on physical examination.

Because the presentation of asthma is variable, any given patient may exhibit a variety of the clinical characteristics listed in Box 1 that are dependent on the severity of asthma when evaluated. The presence of these findings is suggestive of the diagnosis of asthma. However, there are additional disorders to consider in the differential diagnosis of asthma, as noted in Box 2. Chronic obstructive pulmonary disease typically has symptoms similar to asthma but is accompanied by a long-standing history of tobacco smoking or, in rare circumstances, α1-antitrypsin deficiency. Asthma may coexist with cystic fibrosis, which has numerous additional complications—including recurrent lower respiratory bacterial infections and bronchiectasis—that can be noted on a CT scan of the chest. Vocal cord dysfunction (VCD) is an inappropriate closure of the vocal cords during inspiration or expiration. VCD may occur alone or as a coexisting condition with asthma, as will be discussed later. The pulmonary congestion from congestive heart failure (CHF) may present with symptoms similar to asthma: worse at night and more intense with physical activity. However, CHF often has additional findings, such as pleural effusions, lower extremity edema, and an abnormal cardiac examination. An echocardiogram can assist in the diagnosis of CHF in this setting. A mechanical obstruction of the airway from a tumor mass or foreign body can mimic the obstruction of asthma; however, other systemic manifestations or radiographic findings will suggest these possibilities as the cause of wheezing.

Asthma may also represent a component of a systemic disorder. For example, airflow obstruction and asthma are part of both Churg-Strauss vasculitis and allergic bronchopulmonary aspergillosis. Further discussion of these disorders is beyond the scope of this article.

### Evaluation of asthma severity

Several tests and procedures can assist in the diagnosis of asthma, assess its severity, and monitor its control. The most common assessment is pulmonary function testing, which can assist in the diagnosis, assess the severity

---

**Box 2. Differential diagnosis in asthma**

Chronic obstructive pulmonary disease
Cystic fibrosis
Vocal cord dysfunction
Congestive heart failure
Mechanical obstruction of airways (eg, tumors)

of airflow obstruction, and monitor response to treatment. A methacholine bronchoprovocation is a variation of the pulmonary function testing that is typically used to determine the airway hyperresponsiveness that is a component of asthma. Allergy testing by skin prick or radioabsorbent serologic testing is typically performed to identify allergic sensitization and allergens that might contribute to asthma symptoms. Asthma questionnaires are now recommended and are becoming commonly used as an assessment of subjective control of asthma. Two additional tests are currently being investigated for routine use in monitoring asthma control: exhaled nitric oxide and exhaled breath condensates. Of the tests described here, the current National Heart, Lung, and Blood Institute (NHLBI) Guidelines for the Diagnosis and Management of Asthma recommend the evaluation of pulmonary function testing and symptoms to define asthma severity (Table 1) [3].

*Pulmonary function testing*

Two characteristic features of asthma are airflow obstruction, which is reversible or partially reversible, and airway hyperresponsiveness. The airway obstruction may be quantitated by pulmonary function testing. Pulmonary function testing has two components: spirometry and plethysmography. For the initial evaluation of asthma, spirometry is necessary and typically sufficient to provide information on the forced expiratory volume in 1 second

Table 1
Classification of asthma severity

| Severity | Symptoms | Nocturnal symptoms | Lung function |
| --- | --- | --- | --- |
| Mild intermittent | Symptoms occur<br>  < 2 times per week<br>Asymptomatic between<br>  exacerbations | < 2 times per month | FEV1 or PEF<br>  > 80% predicted<br>PEF variability<br>  < 20% |
| Mild persistent | Symptoms occur<br>  > 2 times per week | > 2 times per month | FEV1 or PEF<br>  > 80% predicted<br>PEF variability<br>  20%–30% |
| Moderate persistent | Daily symptoms<br>Daily use of short<br>  acting $\beta_2$-agonist | > once per week | FEV1 or PEF<br>  > 60% and<br>  < 80% predicted<br>PEF variability<br>  > 30% |
| Severe persistent | Continuous<br>  symptoms | Frequent | FEV1 or PEF<br>  < 60% predicted<br>PEF variability<br>  > 30% |

*Adapted from* National Institutes of Health: National Heart, Lung, and Blood Institute. Guidelines for the diagnosis and management of asthma. Bethesda (MD): National Institutes of Health; 1997.

(FEV1), forced vital capacity (FVC), midexpiratory flow rate (FEF25-75), peak expiratory flow rate (PEF), and the flow-volume loop plotting flow rate (y-axis) versus lung volume (x-axis). The presence of airway obstruction results in a characteristic appearance of the flow-volume loop, often described as a scooped appearance of the expiratory phase of the loop (Fig. 1A). In symptomatic asthma, the FEV1 is typically reduced (less than 80% of predicted for age and sex), whereas the FVC remains relatively normal. This spirometric pattern results in a diminished FEV1 to FVC ratio, with less than 0.8 being suggestive of obstruction. Measures that may reflect the smaller airways (eg, FEF25-75) are also decreased and often remain abnormal, even with a normal FEV1 and absence of symptoms.

A second component of the evaluation of asthma by pulmonary function testing is the determination of bronchodilator response to a $\beta_2$-agonist such as albuterol. Following bronchodilator administration, there is often a significant improvement in the FEV1, FVC, or FEF25-75. The flow-volume loop exhibits significant reversibility following the bronchodilator administration, which may approximate normal lung function (Fig. 1B) or reduced obstruction (Fig. 1C). Based on criteria established by the American Thoracic Society, a 12% increase in the FEV1 or FVC representing at least 200 mL of volume constitutes a significant bronchodilator response [4]. For the FEF25-75, a significant response is considered a 25% increase in volume. Such responses to bronchodilator are suggestive of a diagnosis of asthma. However, some patients with severe airway inflammation do not exhibit a significant bronchodilator response because the underlying obstruction is largely caused by airway inflammation. In these patients, a short trial of corticosteroids to reduce airway inflammation may demonstrate their reversibility.

In addition to pulmonary function testing or spirometry, it is possible to measure the PEF with a portable, handheld device. Patients can be given

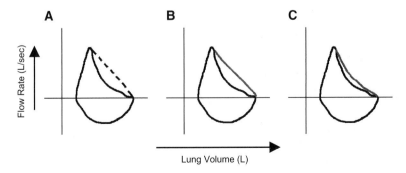

Fig. 1. Flow-volume loops in asthma. (*A*) The typical scooped appearance of the flow-volume loop in asthma is shown as the solid black line. The predicted normal flow-volume loop is shown by the dashed black line. (*B*) The scooped appearance of the initial flow-volume loop (*black line*) may exhibit complete reversal following use of a bronchodilator (*red line*). (*C*) In some cases, the reversal of the scooped appearance following use of a bronchodilator is partial (*red line*).

such a device for home use and are able to monitor the relative status of their lung function compared with baseline or personal best PEF. As will be discussed later, this measure of pulmonary function can be part of an action plan to guide self-management of asthma.

## Methacholine challenge

The presence of airway hyperresponsiveness may be determined by a methacholine bronchoprovocation challenge [5]. With this procedure, patients inhale increasing concentrations of methacholine, which is a cholinergic agonist capable of stimulating muscarinic receptors on smooth muscle cells in the airway to cause their constriction. In patients who have asthma, the airway smooth muscle is more sensitive to methacholine than in normal patients and hence contracts at lower concentrations of this medication. The results from this test are typically expressed as a provocative concentration of methacholine that causes a 20% decline in FEV1 (denoted as $PC_{20}$). A methacholine $PC_{20}$ of less than 8 mg/dL has a sensitivity for asthma of 100%, specificity of 93%, and negative predictive value of 100%, but a positive predictive value of only 29% [6]. The high sensitivity associated with the methacholine challenge indicates that virtually all patients who have asthma will have a positive response to this stimulus. However, the low specificity and low positive predictive values indicate that a positive test does not necessarily indicate a diagnosis of asthma. Based on the high negative predictive value of the methacholine challenge test, it is more clinically useful as a tool to exclude the diagnosis of asthma. With a negative test, it is possible to be confident that asthma is not present. A $PC_{20}$ between 2 and 8 mg/dL is considered mild asthma, although other conditions representing false positives may result in this intermediate hyperreactivity (Box 3). This test may also be performed using alternative modes of bronchoprovocation, including histamine, cold air, and exercise challenge [7].

## Allergy testing

Asthma is often associated with allergic disease, and many patients exhibit a progression of allergic diseases from atopic dermatitis to allergic rhinitis

---

**Box 3. Conditions with false-positive methacholine challenges**

Allergic rhinitis (without coexisting asthma)
Cystic fibrosis
Chronic obstructive pulmonary disease
Congestive heart failure
Tobacco use
Postviral upper respiratory infection

to asthma, known as the allergic march. Allergy skin-prick testing is usually performed and confirms the presence of IgE antibody to aeroallergens and their potential role in asthma. The presence of allergic sensitivities does not make the diagnosis of asthma, but the identification of a patient's allergic status to specific aeroallergens may guide recommendations regarding seasons with potential for difficulties and home avoidance efforts. For example, allergic sensitization to pets often corresponds with the development of symptoms on exposure to the animal, implying the potential benefit of pet avoidance. A recent study demonstrated that measures to reduce dust mite and cockroach allergen exposure in allergic children resulted in significant improvement of asthma symptoms [8], providing evidence for the benefit of home avoidance measures in asthma control.

The use of a complete blood cell count with a differential assessment may also be helpful. In asthma, there may be mild eosinophilia, but no data suggest that monitoring the serum eosinophil count has a role in following asthma. Nonetheless, the existence of peripheral blood eosinophilia with airway obstruction is almost diagnostic of asthma.

*Asthma questionnaires*

Recent studies have evaluated whether asthma patients are well controlled by monitoring specific symptoms. The use of such questionnaires has been validated in asthma as showing a correlation between symptom scores and level of asthma control [9,10]. An example of an asthma questionnaire is shown in Box 4. Studies indicate that, when patients are given specific questions regarding the severity of symptoms, a significant disparity between the perceived and actual control of asthma often appears [11–13]. The regular use of these questionnaires, in conjunction with the objective measures already described, should provide a more complete and quantitative assessment of asthma control.

---

**Box 4. Sample asthma questionnaire: asthma control test**

1. Asthma keeps you from getting as much done at work or home (1 = none of the time, 5 = all of the time).
2. Rate your asthma control (1 = completely controlled, 5 = not controlled at all).
3. How often have you had shortness of breath? (1 = not at all, 5 = more than once a day).
4. Do asthma symptoms wake you up at night or earlier than usual? (1 = not at all, 5 = four or more nights per week).
5. How often have you used your rescue inhaler or nebulizer solution? (1 = not at all, 5 = three or more times per day).

---

*Exhaled nitric oxide*

Because asthma has a prominent inflammatory component in airways, which reflects disease activity and the therapeutic target, efforts have been made to measure the extent of bronchial inflammation. One method is the measurement of exhaled nitric oxide, a byproduct of the inflammatory process. Exhaled nitric oxide ($FE_{NO}$) has been proposed as a diagnostic tool for asthma based on significant correlations between airway hyperresponsiveness and $FE_{NO}$ in corticosteroid-naïve patients [14]. However, after the initiation of inhaled corticosteroid therapy, the correlation does not always persist, because $FE_{NO}$ is rapidly reduced by inhaled corticosteroids. In addition, the baseline levels of exhaled nitric oxide can vary significantly due to age [15], sex [16], viral infections, smoking, allergic rhinitis, and genetic polymorphisms in the nitric oxide synthetase genes [17].

Although $FE_{NO}$ has not been fully validated for the diagnosis of asthma, it functions well as an indicator of disease activity. In several studies, $FE_{NO}$ decreases with use of anti-inflammatory therapy and increases on exacerbation when compared with an individual patient's baseline value [18–21]. In addition, elevated baseline $FE_{NO}$ predicts a favorable response to corticosteroids [22]. A recent study also demonstrates the use of $FE_{NO}$ to monitor asthma control and direct changes in inhaled corticosteroid dose [23]. The patients with $FE_{NO}$–guided inhaled corticosteroid therapy had an equivalent level of asthma control; however, this was achieved at lower corticosteroid doses. Thus, the utility of $FE_{NO}$ may reside in monitoring asthma control, guiding therapy, and providing an indication of corticosteroid sensitivity [24].

*Exhaled breath condensates*

Recently, there has also been interest in analyzing exhaled breath condensates (EBC). Because EBC is collected by having a patient breathe through a condensing apparatus, this test is noninvasive and has the potential to provide detailed information on airway inflammation. Analyses of the EBC have revealed the capacity to detect many inflammatory mediators, including cytokines, leukotrienes, and prostaglandins [25,26]. In addition, the condensate pH, levels of hydrogen peroxide, and other reduction-oxidation intermediates have been found to differ in the EBC of asthma patients, either at baseline or with exacerbations [27–30]. The EBC is currently a research tool, with investigative efforts directed at its clinical use, perhaps in conjunction with spirometry, both to diagnose and provide predictive information for asthma.

## Comorbidities in asthma

Several disorders can complicate asthma management, including gastroesophageal reflux disease, allergic rhinitis, chronic rhinosinusitis, and VCD.

It is often difficult to gain optimum control of asthma symptoms unless these coexisting disorders have also been treated.

*Gastroesophageal reflux*

Gastroesophageal reflux disease (GERD) is a common disorder characterized by the reflux of gastric contents into the esophagus and possibly into the oropharynx. Typical symptoms include heartburn, cough, and an acid taste in the mouth. Several studies have found an increased prevalence of GERD in patients who have asthma; for example, one study found symptoms of heartburn in 77% of asthmatic patients compared with 50% of the control group [31]. Whether symptoms of GERD can induce changes in the airway was also addressed in several studies. A strong correlation was observed in asthma patients between the number of reflux episodes measured by esophageal pH monitoring and the airway hyperresponsiveness measured by methacholine challenge, suggesting that GERD was enhancing existing airway inflammation [32]. In addition, a correlation was found between nighttime esophageal acidity and lower airway resistance [33].

The precise mechanism of pulmonary manifestations of GERD in asthma is not known, although there are suggestions that a neuro-reflex or microaspirations may be involved. Of particular interest are demonstrations that GERD treatment can improve asthma control. For example, one cross-over, placebo-controlled study showed that 8 weeks of proton-pump inhibitor therapy improved nighttime asthma symptoms and FEV1 [34]. Also, a study that examined corticosteroid-dependent asthma found that improved control of asthma followed initiation of therapy for GERD, regardless of whether symptoms of reflux were experienced [35]. Collectively, the studies on the benefits of gastric acid–suppression suggest that there is a subset of asthma patients with coexisting GERD. Therefore, in patients with incomplete control of asthma, with or without symptoms of GERD, a trial of an $H_2$-blocker or proton-pump inhibitor therapy may be of benefit.

*Allergic rhinitis*

Allergic rhinitis is a common condition coexisting with asthma and may worsen asthma control. It has been hypothesized that there is a common inflammatory pathway with communication between the nose and lung [36]. This relationship is typically referred to as the one airway or unified hypothesis. Support for this relationship was provided by a study in which patients with seasonal allergic rhinitis and asthma were given antigen in the nose and subsequently developed increased lower airway hyperresponsiveness, as measured by a change in methacholine $PC_{20}$ [37]. In a follow-up study, patients who had allergic rhinitis and asthma were treated with intranasal corticosteroids or placebo during ragweed season. Although FEV1, peak flows, and symptoms were not significantly different in the two groups, airway hyperresponsiveness decreased in the treatment group [38]. Thus, treatment of allergic rhinitis may have a beneficial effect on asthma control.

*Chronic rhinosinusitis*

Rhinosinusitis and asthma often coexist, leading to consideration of a common pathophysiology akin to the one airway model in allergic rhinitis. Patients with chronic rhinosinusitis may exhibit a chronic inflammatory process in the sinuses with features in common with the lower airway inflammation in asthma [39,40]. In children, studies demonstrate improved control of asthma following antibiotic treatment for chronic rhinosinusitis [41,42]. In adults, surgical treatment of chronic rhinosinusitis also was accompanied by improved asthma control, although a concern of the study was the lack of a control group who had not received surgery [43]. Thus, treatment of rhinosinusitis contributes to the level of asthma control.

*Vocal cord dysfunction*

VCD is a condition characterized by an inappropriate adduction of the vocal cords during respiration that results in upper airway obstruction and symptoms similar to asthma: wheezing, cough, dyspnea, and chest tightness. The diagnosis of VCD is suggested by the following features: sudden onset and sudden resolution of symptoms, an attenuated or absent response to standard asthma therapy, and symptoms localized to the vocal cords (eg, hoarseness). A definitive diagnosis of VCD may be established by visualization of the vocal cords and observation of the paradoxical vocal cord movement; however, in the absence of active symptoms, this may not be observed. Another characteristic of VCD is the demonstration of a cut-off on the inspiratory portion of the flow-volume loop (Fig. 2), which represents an extrathoracic obstruction from a complete or partial paradoxical closure

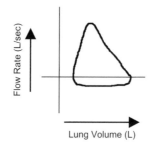

Fig. 2. Flow-volume loop in VCD. Patients who have VCD may exhibit a cut-off or flattening of the inspiratory portion of the flow-volume loop (below the x-axis), in contrast to the typical rounded appearance during inspiration.

of the vocal cords during inspiration. This inspiratory cutoff may not be observed in the absence of symptoms.

It is common for asthma and VCD to coexist. As many as 50% of patients with a diagnosis of VCD also have airway hyperresponsiveness [44]. Moreover, for unclear reasons, VCD occurs more commonly in women [44]. Interestingly, other comorbidities for asthma are also associated with VCD, including rhinitis and GERD. Thus, the rhinitis and GERD should be treated to minimize their contribution to irritation of the vocal cords. Referral to speech therapy for instruction on breathing exercises during direct visualization of the vocal cords can also be effective in managing symptoms [45].

## Management of asthma

Once the diagnosis of asthma has been made, medical treatment may be initiated based on an initial assessment of disease severity (see Table 1) [3]. The NHLBI asthma guidelines were updated in 2002, with revised recommendations for initiation of asthma therapy based on the classification of disease severity (Table 2) [46]. The goal of asthma therapy is to reduce the frequency and severity of both symptoms and exacerbations, maintain normal levels of activity, and achieve optimum lung function. Two aspects of asthma therapy must be addressed: baseline controller therapy and a plan for modification of the therapeutic regimen based on changes in asthma control, often referred to as an *asthma action plan*.

As indicated in Table 2, for mild intermittent asthma, daily controller therapy is usually not required, because symptoms occur infrequently. Thus, use of a rescue inhaler such as albuterol, as needed, may be sufficient

Table 2
Guidelines for initiation of asthma therapy

| Severity | Therapy | |
| --- | --- | --- |
| | Controller | Rescue |
| Mild intermittent | None | Short-acting $\beta_2$-agonist |
| Mild persistent | Low dose inhaled corticosteroid *or* Alternate controller therapy | Short-acting $\beta_2$-agonist |
| Moderate persistent | Low-to-medium dose inhaled corticosteroid plus long-acting $\beta_2$-agonist *or* Medium dose inhaled corticosteroid plus alternate controller therapy | Short-acting $\beta_2$-agonist |
| Severe persistent | High dose inhaled corticosteroid plus long acting $\beta_2$-agonist | Short-acting $\beta_2$-agonist |

*Adapted from* National Institutes of Health. National Heart, Lung, and Blood Institute. Update on selected topics 2002. Bethesda (MD): National Institutes of Health; 2003.

for asthma control. However, it is important to recognize that patients with mild intermittent asthma can have severe exacerbations of asthma. For persistent asthma, in contrast, whether mild, moderate, or severe, daily use of an inhaled corticosteroid is recommended as initial or baseline therapy. The initial dose of the corticosteroid is dependent on severity of the underlying persistent asthma: mild—low dose, moderate—medium dose, and severe—high dose. The addition of a long-acting $\beta_2$-agonist is recommended for both moderate and severe persistent asthma. Inhaled corticosteroids are the preferred initial treatment; however, the NHLBI guidelines do acknowledge the use of alternative controller medications, such as monteleukast, nedocromil, or theophylline. These alternative therapies may replace inhaled corticosteroids in mild persistent asthma or may be used in conjunction with low-dose inhaled corticosteroids to enhance control of symptoms in moderate persistent asthma. No recommendation has been made regarding use of alternative controller therapy in severe persistent asthma; rather, the addition of oral corticosteroids is the usual approach mentioned as a consideration.

Once therapy has been initiated, there is often a need to adjust medications for continued symptoms or change in status of asthma: either a "step-up" or a "step-down" approach. When there is complete control of asthma symptoms, consideration is given to a step-down in therapy, involving either a decrease in dosage of medications or the discontinuation of adjunctive medications. By contrast, when asthma symptoms persist or escalate despite initiation of therapy, there should be consideration of a step-up in therapy, involving either an increase in dosage of medications or the initiation of adjunctive medications. Previously, only anecdotal evidence suggested that increasing the corticosteroid dose would improve asthma control. However, a recent study demonstrates that titration of the dose of corticosteroid or combination corticosteroid with long-acting $\beta_2$-agonist can be effective in improving symptoms and lung function [47].

*Asthma action plans*

It is possible and appropriate in most cases to instruct patients and empower them with the ability to manage their own asthma symptoms. Asthma action plans are considered an effective tool to provide guidance for appropriate interventions for given levels of symptoms. However, well-designed studies to document the efficacy of asthma action plans are lacking. Nevertheless, a Cochrane review of the existing studies does favor the use of written asthma action plans in the care of asthma patients [48]. Typically, there are three zones—green, yellow, and red, as shown in Table 3—that are defined by the severity of symptoms and peak flow or spirometry measures. The green zone indicates well-controlled or stable asthma and continued use of current therapy. The yellow zone describes measures to be introduced for an increase in symptoms. The red zone describes immediate measures to

Table 3
Asthma action plan

| Zone | Criteria | Recommendation |
|------|----------|----------------|
| Green | Peak flow rate >80% of baseline<br>Mild-to-no symptoms | Continue controller therapy with<br>as needed rescue inhaler use |
| Yellow | Peak flow rate 50%–80% of baseline<br>Moderate symptoms, some interference<br>with normal activity, possible<br>nocturnal awakenings | Initiate increased dose of<br>inhaled corticosteroid<br>*or*<br>Add an adjunctive medication<br>(eg, long-acting $\beta_2$-agonist) |
| Red | Peak flow rate <50% of baseline<br>Moderate-to-severe symptoms, definite<br>impact on normal activities | Initiate short-term course of<br>corticosteroids |

address either failure of yellow zone therapy to achieve control or an increase in severity of symptoms. One of the most common reasons for a worsening of asthma control is a viral URI. Studies indicate that, with the onset of URI symptoms, a prophylactic progression into a yellow zone plan, consisting of at least a fourfold increase in inhaled corticosteroid dose, is usually required for a measurable benefit in the susceptible patient [49]. As will be discussed, data also suggest that as-needed use of the budesonide/formoterol combination medication will be effective, once it is available in the United States [50]. Progressive worsening of symptoms into the red zone typically necessitates the use of an oral corticosteroid burst.

**Classes of medications**

A number of medications are available for the management of asthma, and each targets specific pathways or mediators involved in asthma pathophysiology (Box 5). The drugs used in the treatment of asthma are categorized as either *controller* or *rescue* medications, which reflects their use as baseline therapy (ie, anti-inflammatory) or add-on therapy (ie,

---

**Box 5. Classes of asthma medications**

$\beta_2$-Agonists
Corticosteroids
Combined corticosteroid and $\beta_2$-agonists
Anticholinergics
Mast cell stabilizers
Methylxanthines
Leukotriene modifiers
Monoclonal antibody immunomodulators

bronchodilator) for acute worsening of asthma control, respectively. The evidence for the benefit in asthma of each class of medication and its proposed role in the management of asthma will be discussed.

### $\beta_2$-Agonists

The $\beta_2$-adrenergic receptor is found on airway smooth muscle in addition to several other cell types. Bronchoconstriction in asthma may be relieved with the use of $\beta_2$-selective agonists that act primarily on $\beta_2$-adrenergic receptors to relax bronchial smooth muscle contraction. The $\beta_2$-agonists are delivered by a meter dose inhaler, dry powder inhaler, or nebulizer.

The most commonly used $\beta_2$-agonist meter dose inhalers in the United States are albuterol and pirbuterol. Their action begins within 5 minutes of use and lasts as long as 4 hours. These medications are typically used as rescue inhalers for acute symptoms of asthma. Some studies have compared the scheduled use of short-acting $\beta_2$-agonists with use on an as-needed basis and found no significant beneficial or adverse effects, although there was some suggestion of improved evening peak flows and decreased rescue inhaler use with scheduled use [51,52].

Long-acting preparations of $\beta_2$-agonists are also available with salmeterol and formoterol and have significantly longer half lives than albuterol, requiring dosing only every 12 hours. Notably, formoterol has a quicker onset of action than salmeterol and is comparable to albuterol, suggesting that formoterol may be effective as both a rescue inhaler and a controller medication. However, one caution about the use of long-acting $\beta_2$-agonists arose initially from a trial in which salmeterol was compared with salbutamol. A higher mortality, though not a statistically significant one, was observed in patients using salmeterol [53]. Another study compared salmeterol alone with salmeterol plus fluticasone. Increased mortality was observed in the salmeterol-alone group, although, again, the study was not adequately powered to address a significant increase in mortality [54]. These results have led to the current recommendation of long-acting $\beta_2$-agonist use only in conjunction with an inhaled corticosteroid, not as monotherapy.

### Corticosteroids

Corticosteroids are the most potent anti-inflammatory agents available and are considered an essential component of the management of an acute asthma exacerbation, in conjunction with quicker-onset $\beta_2$-agonists. The use of intravenous corticosteroids following an acute exacerbation has been shown to provide a significant improvement in FEV1 compared with a saline control [55]. However, the long-term use of systemic corticosteroids has potential adverse effects, including cataracts, osteoporosis, avascular necrosis, and diabetes mellitus. Thus, it is essential to closely monitor severe asthma patients who require daily systemic corticosteroid therapy for these adverse events with routine surveillance, including bone density scans and ophthalmology evaluations.

The delivery of topical corticosteroids to the lung as an aerosol was initially described in 1972 with beclomethasone [56]. Since that time, numerous studies have described the use of inhaled corticosteroids as an effective means to control asthma symptoms with far reduced adverse reactions compared with systemic corticosteroids. The effectiveness of inhaled corticosteroids has resulted in NHLBI guidelines recommending their use as baseline controller therapy in persistent asthma (see Table 2).

*Combination of inhaled corticosteroid and long-acting β₂-agonist*

Improved asthma outcome measures are derived from combined use of corticosteroids and $\beta_2$-agonists. As a result, formulations have been developed to combine inhaled corticosteroids (ICS) and long-acting $\beta_2$-agonists. The addition of a long-acting $\beta_2$-agonist to ICS therapy improves symptom control, reduces risk for severe exacerbations, and improves lung function measures such as FEV1 and peak flows [57–61]. These benefits are equivalent to or greater than that observed with an increase in the ICS dose. Further evidence to support the beneficial effect of combining ICS and a long-acting $\beta_2$-agonist was provided by a study that demonstrated a successful reduction in ICS dose in patients using combination therapy, whereas those patients using ICS alone had increased treatment failures on reduction of corticosteroid dose [62].

The two combination medications currently in use are salmeterol/fluticasone and formoterol/budesonide, with the latter not currently available in the United States. As mentioned previously, formoterol has a more rapid onset of action than salmeterol; consequently, the combination of budesonide and formoterol is being examined as possible asthma monotherapy (ie, use of the same medication as a controller and rescue treatment). To evaluate this possibility, a recent study compared three treatment protocols: (1) use of budesonide/formoterol as monotherapy, (2) use of budesonide/formoterol as a controller with terbutaline as a rescue inhaler, and (3) use of high-dose budesonide with terbutaline as a rescue inhaler [50]. The use of budesonide/formoterol as both a controller and a rescue inhaler resulted in a prolonged time until first exacerbation, a reduced rate of severe exacerbations, improved symptoms, and improved lung function compared with both other treatment arms.

*Anticholinergics*

Anticholinergics, such as ipratropium bromide, promote smooth muscle relaxation. The use of inhaled ipratropium for acute asthma exacerbations has been evaluated in several studies with mixed outcomes, although one significant measure of improvement is a reduction in hospitalizations admitted from the emergency room following the exacerbation [63]. Although use of anticholinergics has not been shown to have long-term benefit for treatment of asthma, it can provide a subjective relief of symptoms in an acute setting. Thus, ipratropium is usually combined with albuterol in nebulizer treatments for acute exacerbations.

*Mast cell stabilizers*

Cromolyn and nedocromil are believed to function, in part, by stabilizing mast cells. In vitro studies have shown that they prevent release of potent inflammatory mediators, including histamine, leukotrienes, and prostaglandins. Several clinical studies have demonstrated modest benefit with the use of cromolyn or nedocromil for asthma [64]. However, the efficacy of nedocromil was markedly inferior to that observed for ICS in a head-to-head trial conducted in children [65]. Thus, preference is given to use of ICS, with the possibility of including mast cell stabilizers as adjunctive medications.

*Leukotriene antagonists*

An important mediator in the pathogenesis of asthma is a family of lipid-derived substances, the leukotrienes (LT), which include $LTB_4$, $LTC_4$, $LTD_4$, and $LTE_4$. Leukotrienes are produced by several cell types, including eosinophils and mast cells. The leukotrienes produce bronchoconstriction and the recruitment of inflammatory cells, including neutrophils and eosinophils. The leukotriene pathways may be blocked by inhibiting the synthesis of leukotrienes with 5-lipoxygenase inhibitors or by using leukotriene receptor antagonists. Use of the leukotriene modifiers has been shown to result in clinical improvements in asthma, including increases in FEV1, decrease in symptoms, decrease in use of rescue medications, and decrease in asthma exacerbations [66–68]. Although the leukotriene modifiers do improve asthma control, the efficacy is usually less than is observed with ICS [69]. Thus, preference is given to use of ICS with the inclusion of leukotriene modifiers as adjunctive medications. The priority of these agents is still undergoing evaluation.

*Methylxanthines*

Theophylline functions as a phosphodiesterase inhibitor and may have multiple effects on components of asthma, including a reduction in airflow obstruction. Inconsistent evidence suggests that the addition of theophylline can have a corticosteroid-sparing effect. One study compared budesonide with theophylline versus high-dose budesonide alone and found that the addition of theophylline to budesonide was accompanied by significant improvement in FEV1 and FVC compared with high-dose budesonide alone [70]. However, another study compared the same two treatments and found no differences in outcome measures, including FEV1, peak flows, asthma symptoms, and rescue medication use [71]. Thus, controversy remains as to the efficacy of adding theophylline to ICS. In addition, one of the difficulties with the use of methylxanthines is their low therapeutic index. Commonly, there are gastrointestinal side effects of nausea and vomiting and potential for cardiac arrythmias; thus, the safety of theophylline use remains a concern.

Currently there is renewed interest in the phosphodiesterase inhibitors, particularly in inhibiting specific isoforms of phosphodiesterase activity to achieve the benefits of theophylline without the side effects. Recently, inhibitors of phosphodiesterase-4 have been studied, with some encouraging preliminary results [72].

*Anti-IgE*

A characteristic feature of allergic asthma is an elevated serum IgE level, which, in conjunction with mast cell IgE receptors, is believed to play a significant role in asthma pathogenesis. This concept led to the development of a humanized anti-IgE monoclonal antibody. Studies of the use of anti-IgE therapy have demonstrated clinical improvement in asthma control, including improved symptoms, reduced rescue inhaler use, and fewer exacerbations [73–77]. Although anti-IgE does not confer significant improvement in objective measures of lung function, such as FEV1, it makes possible a reduction in doses of other medications, particularly oral and inhaled corticosteroids. Thus, its current primary role is that of a corticosteroid-sparing therapy for use in severe asthma.

*Pharmacogenetics*

An area of recent interest in many fields of medicine, and most recently in the treatment of asthma, is pharmacogenetics. This term refers to differential responses to pharmacotherapy due to genetic encoded isoforms of molecular targets. For example, a polymorphism in the $\beta_2$-adrenergic receptor, homozygous Arg/Arg at amino acid 16, has been found in retrospective analyses to be associated with a decline in lung function or asthma control with regular use of albuterol [78,79]. This effect has been examined prospectively, comparing subjects with Arg/Arg versus Gly/Gly at amino acid 16 of the $\beta_2$-adrenergic receptor [80]. Arg/Arg subjects were found to have lower peak flow values, lower FEV1, and more symptoms; they required more reliever medication use while using albuterol regularly during the treatment period. Thus, an interpretation of these studies is that regular use of $\beta_2$-agonists should be avoided in patients with an Arg/Arg genotype at amino acid 16 of the $\beta_2$-adrenergic receptor. This concept, however, is still under investigation.

Recently, it was also demonstrated that children with asthma symptoms responsive to ICS exhibited phenotypic differences from those with symptoms responsive to leukotriene modifiers [81]. This finding suggests that there may also be genotypic markers that reflect responsiveness to these medications. As more phenotype-genotype relationships are identified with respect to response to asthma medications, it is possible that therapy will be customized for each patient.

## Summary

The diagnosis and management of asthma continue to be of critical importance, as recent trends have demonstrated its increasing prevalence, morbidity, and perhaps mortality. Because current treatments for asthma are effective and safe, it is important to diagnose asthma early and to use treatments effectively, particularly those directed toward airway inflammation. The diagnostic measures and array of medications, both those currently available and on the horizon, provide an armamentarium for effective diagnosis, management, and monitoring of asthma. In the coming years, it is expected that additional testing modalities will be available for more precise monitoring of asthma control, and an increased understanding of pharmacogenetics will enable the tailoring of asthma medications to specific patients, providing customized therapy to maximize asthma control.

## References

[1] Busse WW, Lemanske RF. Advances in immunology—asthma. N Engl J Med 2001;344: 350–62.

[2] Masoli M, Fabian D, Holt S, et al. The global burden of asthma: executive summary of the GINA Dissemination Committee Report. Allergy 2004;59:469–78.

[3] National Institutes of Health: National Heart, Lung, and Blood Institute. Guidelines for the diagnosis and management of asthma. Bethesda (MD): National Institutes of Health; 1997.

[4] Anonymous. Standardization of spirometry—1994 update. Am J Respir Crit Care Med 1995;152:1107–36.

[5] Parker CD, Bilbo RE, Reed CE. Methacholine aerosol as test for bronchial asthma. Arch Intern Med 1965;115:452–8.

[6] Cockcroft DW, Murdock KY, Berscheid BA, et al. Sensitivity and specificity of histamine PC20 determination in a random selection of young college-students. J Allergy Clin Immunol 1992;89:23–30.

[7] O'Connor GT, Sparrow D, Weiss ST. The role of allergy and nonspecific airway hyperresponsiveness in the pathogenesis of chronic obstructive pulmonary-disease. Am Rev Respir Dis 1989;140:225–52.

[8] Morgan WJ, Crain EF, Gruchalla RS, et al. Results of a home-based environmental intervention among urban children with asthma. N Engl J Med 2004;351:1068–80.

[9] Juniper EF, Guyatt GH, Ferrie PJ, et al. Measuring quality-of-life in asthma. Am Rev Respir Dis 1993;147:832–8.

[10] Nathan RA, Sorkness CA, Kosinski M, et al. Development of the asthma control test: a survey for assessing asthma control. J Allergy Clin Immunol 2004;113:59–65.

[11] Osborne ML, Vollmer WM, Pedula KL, et al. Lack of correlation of symptoms with specialist-assessed long-term asthma severity. Chest 1999;115:85–91.

[12] Adams RJ, Fuhlbrigge A, Guilbert T, et al. Inadequate use of asthma medication in the United States: results of the Asthma in America national population survey. J Allergy Clin Immunol 2002;110:58–64.

[13] Fuhlbrigge AL, Adams RJ, Guilbert TW, et al. The burden of asthma in the United States—level and distribution are dependent on interpretation of the National Asthma Education and Prevention Program guidelines. Am J Respir Crit Care Med 2002;166:1044–9.

[14] Dupont LJ, Rochette F, Demedts MG, et al. Exhaled nitric oxide correlates with airway hyperresponsiveness in steroid-naïve patients with mild asthma. Am J Respir Crit Care Med 1998;157:894–8.

[15] Franklin PJ, Taplin R, Stick SM. A community study of exhaled nitric oxide in healthy children. Am J Respir Crit Care Med 1999;159:69–73.

[16] Tsang KW, Ip SK, Leung R, et al. Exhaled nitric oxide: the effects of age, gender and body size. Lung 2001;179:83–91.

[17] Henriksen AH, Sue-Chu M, Holmen TL, et al. Exhaled and nasal NO levels in allergic rhinitis: relation to sensitization, pollen season and bronchial hyperresponsiveness. Eur Respir J 1999;13:301–6.

[18] Bratton DL, Lanz MJ, Miyazawa N, et al. Exhaled nitric oxide before and after montelukast sodium therapy in school-age children with chronic asthma: a preliminary study. Pediatr Pulmonol 1999;28:402–7.

[19] Silkoff PE, McClean PA, Slutsky AS, et al. Exhaled nitric oxide and bronchial reactivity during and after inhaled beclomethasone in mild asthma. J Asthma 1998;35:473–9.

[20] Silkoff PE, McClean P, Spino M, et al. Dose-response relationship and reproducibility of the fall in exhaled nitric oxide after inhaled beclomethasone dipropionate therapy in asthma patients. Chest 2001;119:1322–8.

[21] Jones SL, Kittelson J, Cowan JO, et al. The predictive value of exhaled nitric oxide measurements in assessing changes in asthma control. Am J Respir Crit Care Med 2001;164:738–43.

[22] Little SA, Chalmers GW, MacLeod KJ, et al. Non-invasive markers of airway inflammation as predictors of oral steroid responsiveness in asthma. Thorax 2000;55:232–4.

[23] Smith AD, Cowan JO, Brassett KP, et al. Use of exhaled nitric oxide measurements to guide treatment in chronic asthma. N Engl J Med 2005;352:2163–73.

[24] Bates CA, Silkoff PE. Exhaled nitric oxide in asthma: from bench to bedside. J Allergy Clin Immunol 2003;111:256–62.

[25] Scheideler L, Manke HG, Schwulera U, et al. Detection of nonvolatile macromolecules in breath—a possible diagnostic-tool. Am Rev Respir Dis 1993;148:778–84.

[26] Montuschi P, Barnes PJ. Exhaled leukotrienes and prostaglandins in asthma. J Allergy Clin Immunol 2002;109:615–20.

[27] Hunt JF, Fang KZ, Malik R, et al. Endogenous airway acidification—implications for asthma pathophysiology. Am J Respir Crit Care Med 2000;161:694–9.

[28] Emelyanov A, Fedoseev G, Abulimity A, et al. Elevated concentrations of exhaled hydrogen peroxide in asthmatic patients. Chest 2001;120:1136–9.

[29] Loukides S, Bouros D, Papatheodorou G, et al. The relationships among hydrogen peroxide in expired breath condensate, airway inflammation, and asthma severity. Chest 2002;121:338–46.

[30] Ganas K, Loukides S, Papatheodorou G, et al. Total nitrite/nitrate in expired breath condensate of patients with asthma. Respir Med 2001;95:649–54.

[31] Field SK, Underwood M, Brant R, et al. Prevalence of gastroesophageal reflux symptoms in asthma. Chest 1996;109:316–22.

[32] Vincent D, Cohen-Jonathan AM, Leport J, et al. Gastro-oesophageal reflux prevalence and relationship with bronchial reactivity in asthma. Eur Respir J 1997;10:2255–9.

[33] Cuttitta G, Cibella F, Visconti A, et al. Spontaneous gastroesophageal reflux and airway patency during the night in adult asthmatics. Am J Respir Crit Care Med 2000;161:177–81.

[34] Kiljander TO, Salomaa ERM, Hietanen EK, et al. Gastroesophageal reflux in asthmatics—a double-blind, placebo-controlled crossover study with omeprazole. Chest 1999;116:1257–64.

[35] Irwin RS, Curley FJ, French CL. Difficult-to-control asthma—contributing factors and outcome of a systematic management protocol. Chest 1993;103:1662–9.

[36] Bousquet J, van Cauwenberge P, Khaltaev N. Allergic rhinitis and its impact on asthma (ARIA); executive summary of the workshop report 7–10 December 1999, Geneva, Switzerland. Allergy 2002;57:841–55.

[37] Corren J, Adinoff AD, Irvin CG. Changes in bronchial responsiveness following nasal provocation with allergen. J Allergy Clin Immunol 1992;89:611–8.

[38] Corren J, Adinoff AD, Buchmeier AD, et al. Nasal beclomethasone prevents the seasonal increase in bronchial responsiveness in patients with allergic rhinitis and asthma. J Allergy Clin Immunol 1992;90:250–6.

[39] Harlin SL, Ansel DG, Lane SR, et al. A clinical and pathologic study of chronic sinusitis—the role of the eosinophil. J Allergy Clin Immunol 1988;81:867–75.

[40] Newman LJ, Plattsmills TAE, Phillips CD, et al. Chronic sinusitis—relationship of computed tomographic findings to allergy, asthma, and eosinophilia. JAMA 1994;271: 363–7.

[41] Rachelefsky GS, Katz RM, Siegel SC. Chronic sinus disease with associated reactive airway disease in children. Pediatrics 1984;73:526–9.

[42] Friedman R, Ackerman M, Wald E, et al. Asthma and bacterial sinusitis in children. J Allergy Clin Immunol 1984;74:185–9.

[43] Nishioka GJ, Cook PR, Davis WE, et al. Functional endoscopic sinus surgery in patients with chronic sinusitis and asthma. Otolaryngol Head Neck Surg 1994;110:494–500.

[44] Newman KB, Mason UG, Schmaling KB. Clinical features of vocal cord dysfunction. Am J Respir Crit Care Med 1995;152:1382–6.

[45] Martin RJ, Blager FB, Gay ML, et al. Paradoxic vocal cord motion in presumed asthmatics. Semin Respir Crit Care Med 1987;8:332–7.

[46] National Institutes of Health. National Heart, Lung, and Blood Institute. Update on selected topics 2002. Bethesda (MD): National Institutes of Health; 2003.

[47] Bateman ED, Boushey HA, Bousquet J, et al. Can guideline-defined asthma control be achieved? The Gaining Optimal Asthma Control study. Am J Respir Crit Care Med 2004; 170:836–44.

[48] Gibson PG, Coughlan J, Wilson AJ, et al. Self-management education and regular practitioner review for adults with asthma. Cochrane Database Syst Rev 2000;2:CD001117 [update in Cochrane Database Syst Rev 2003;1:CD001117].

[49] Foresi A, Morelli MC, Catena E. Low-dose budesonide with the addition of an increased dose during exacerbations is effective in long-term asthma control. Chest 2000; 117:440–6.

[50] O'Byrne PM, Bisgaard H, Godard PP, et al. Budesonide/formoterol combination therapy as both maintenance and reliever medication in asthma. Am J Respir Crit Care Med 2005;171: 129–36.

[51] Drazen JM, Israel E, Boushey HA, et al. Comparison of regularly scheduled with as-needed use of albuterol in mild asthma. N Engl J Med 1996;335:841–7.

[52] Dennis SM, Sharp SJ, Vickers MR, et al. Regular inhaled salbutamol and asthma control: the TRUST randomised trial. Lancet 2000;355:1675–9.

[53] Castle W, Fuller R, Hall J, et al. Serevent Nationwide Surveillance Study—comparison of salmeterol with salbutamol in asthmatic patients who require regular bronchodilator treatment. BMJ 1993;306:1034–7.

[54] Wooltorton E. Salmeterol (Serevent) asthma trial halted early. CMAJ 2003;168:738.

[55] Fanta CH, Rossing TH, McFadden ER Jr. Glucocorticoids in acute asthma. A critical controlled trial. Am J Med 1983;74:845–51.

[56] Brown HM, Storey G, George WH. Beclomethasone dipropionate: a new steroid aerosol for the treatment of allergic asthma. BMJ 1972;1:585–90.

[57] Wilding P, Clark M, Coon JT, et al. Effect of long term treatment with salmeterol on asthma control: a double blind, randomised crossover study. BMJ 1997;314:1441–6.

[58] Pauwels RA, Lofdahl CG, Postma DS, et al. Effect of inhaled formoterol and budesonide on exacerbations of asthma. N Engl J Med 1997;337:1405–11.

[59] O'Byrne PM, Barnes PJ, Rodriguez-Roisin R, et al. Low dose inhaled budesonide and formoterol in mild persistent asthma—the OPTIMA randomized trial. Am J Respir Crit Care Med 2001;164:1392-7.

[60] Strand AM, Luckow A. Initiation of maintenance treatment of persistent asthma: salmeterol/fluticasone propionate combination treatment is more effective than inhaled steroid alone. Respir Med 2004;98:1008-15.

[61] Greening AP, Ind PW, Northfield M, et al. Added salmeterol versus higher-dose corticosteroid in asthma patients with symptoms on existing inhaled corticosteroid. Lancet 1994;344: 219-24.

[62] Lemanske RF, Sorkness CA, Mauger EA, et al. Inhaled corticosteroid reduction and elimination in patients with persistent asthma receiving salmeterol—a randomized controlled trial. JAMA 2001;285:2594-603.

[63] Rodrigo GJ, Rodrigo C. The role of anticholinergics in acute asthma treatment—an evidence-based evaluation. Chest 2002;121:1977-87.

[64] Schwartz HJ, Blumenthal M, Brady R, et al. A comparative study of the clinical efficacy of nedocromil sodium and placebo—how does cromolyn sodium compare as an active control treatment? Chest 1996;109:945-52.

[65] Szefler S, Weiss S, Tonascia A, et al. Long-term effects of budesonide or nedocromil in children with asthma. N Engl J Med 2000;343:1054-63.

[66] Gaddy JN, Margolskee DJ, Bush RK, et al. Bronchodilation with a potent and selective leukotriene-D4 (LTD4) receptor antagonist (MK-571) in patients with asthma. Am Rev Respir Dis 1992;146:358-63.

[67] Spector SL, Smith LJ, Glass M, et al. Effects of 6 weeks of therapy with oral doses of ICI-204,219, a leukotriene D-4 receptor antagonist, in subjects with bronchial asthma. Am J Respir Crit Care Med 1994;150:618-23.

[68] Israel E, Cohn J, Dube L, et al. Effect of treatment with zileuton, a 5-lipoxygenase inhibitor, in patients with asthma—a randomized controlled trial. JAMA 1996;275: 931-6.

[69] Busse W, Wolfe J, Storms W, et al. Fluticasone propionate compared with zafirlukast in controlling persistent asthma—a randomized double-blind, placebo-controlled trial. J Fam Pract 2001;50:595-602.

[70] Evans DJ, Taylor DA, Zetterstrom O, et al. A comparison of low-dose inhaled budesonide plus theophylline and high-dose inhaled budesonide for moderate asthma. N Engl J Med 1997;337:1412-8.

[71] Ukena D, Harnest U, Sakalauskas R, et al. Comparison of addition of theophylline to inhaled steroid with doubling of the dose of inhaled steroid in asthma. Eur Respir J 1997; 10:2754-60.

[72] Lipworth BJ. Phosphodiesterase-4 inhibitors for asthma and chronic obstructive pulmonary disease. Lancet 2005;365:167-75.

[73] Milgrom H, Fick RB, Su JQ, et al. Treatment of allergic asthma with monoclonal anti-IgE antibody. N Engl J Med 1999;341:1966-73.

[74] Busse W, Corren J, Lanier BQ, et al. Omalizumab, anti-IgE recombinant humanized monoclonal antibody, for the treatment of severe allergic asthma. J Allergy Clin Immunol 2001; 108:184-90.

[75] Soler M, Matz J, Townley R, et al. The anti-IgE antibody omalizumab reduces exacerbations and steroid requirement in allergic asthmatics. Eur Respir J 2001;18:254-61.

[76] Buhl R, Hanf G, Soler M, et al. The anti-IgE antibody omalizumab improves asthma-related quality of life in patients with allergic asthma. Eur Respir J 2002;20:1088-94.

[77] Finn A, Gross G, van Bavel J, et al. Omalizumab improves asthma-related quality of life in patients with severe allergic asthma. J Allergy Clin Immunol 2003;111:278-84.

[78] Green SA, Turki J, Innis M, et al. Amino-terminal polymorphisms of the human beta(2)-adrenergic receptor impart distinct agonist-promoted regulatory properties. Biochemistry 1994;33:14368.

[79] Israel E, Drazen JM, Liggett SB, et al. The effect of polymorphisms of the beta(2)–adrenergic receptor on the response to regular use of albuterol in asthma. Am J Respir Crit Care Med 2000;162:75–80.

[80] Israel E, Chinchilli VM, Ford JG, et al. Use of regularly scheduled albuterol treatment in asthma: genotype-stratified, randomised, placebo-controlled cross-over trial. Lancet 2004; 364:1505–12.

[81] Szefler SJ, Phillips BR, Martinez FD, et al. Characterization of within-subject responses to fluticasone and montelukast in childhood asthma. J Allergy Clin Immunol 2005;115:233–42.

ELSEVIER
SAUNDERS

THE MEDICAL
CLINICS
OF NORTH AMERICA

Med Clin N Am 90 (2006) 61–76

# Differential Diagnosis of Adult Asthma

## Stephen A. Tilles, MD*

*Department of Medicine, University of Washington School of Medicine, Seattle, WA, USA*

Asthma is a common syndrome that affects approximately 5% of the adult population in the United States. In recent years asthma management guidelines have consistently emphasized therapeutic goals that include minimizing symptoms and normalizing both pulmonary function and physical activity levels [1]. There is also increasing evidence that asthma severity and asthma control are independent concepts [2]. For example, it is appropriate to increase treatment in a patient with mild asthma who has normal lung function but reports having frequent symptoms that disrupt his or her life. It is of critical importance to establish that asthma is the correct diagnosis. This article focuses on the differential diagnosis of adult asthma, including a discussion of reasonable clinical approaches to determining the correct diagnosis. Chronic obstructive pulmonary disease (COPD) and vocal cord dysfunction (VCD) are discussed in the most detail because these are more likely to be mistaken for asthma in clinical practice (Table 1). Less common asthma masqueraders are then discussed (Table 2), including those that also may confound or aggravate asthma. Uncommon asthma masqueraders are listed in Box 1.

### Hallmarks of asthma

Although asthma is a heterogeneous disease with a variety of clinical presentations, there are several general asthma clinical hallmarks that apply to all asthma phenotypes [3,4]. First, asthma symptoms typically include some combination of wheezing, dyspnea, chest tightness, and cough. Chronic symptoms may also include sputum production. Second, asthma symptoms are episodic. When asthma is not well-controlled, symptoms are typically worse in the early morning hours between the hours of 2 and 5 AM. Asthma symptoms are also typically provoked in response to one or more of the

---

* Department of Medicine, University of Washington School of Medicine, 4540 Sand Point Way NE, Suite 200, Seattle, WA 98105.

*E-mail address:* stilles@nwasthma.com

0025-7125/06/$ - see front matter © 2005 Elsevier Inc. All rights reserved.
doi:10.1016/j.mcna.2005.08.004

Table 1
Comparison of asthma, chronic obstructive pulmonary disease, and vocal cord dysfunction

| Criteria | Asthma | COPD | VCD |
|---|---|---|---|
| Age of onset | Any age | Elderly smokers | Adolescents and young adults |
| Classic symptoms | Wheezing, dyspnea, cough, which worsen at night | Dyspnea on exertion | Dyspnea, chest tightness, and stridor |
| Relation of symptoms to the respiratory cycle | Exhalation > inhalation | Exhalation > inhalation | Inhalation > exhalation |
| Localization of symptoms | Deep in chest | Deep in chest | Upper chest, throat |
| Physical examination findings during symptoms | Expiratory wheezing (posterior chest) | Expiratory wheezing (posterior chest) | Inspiratory wheezing or stridor, upper chest |
| Chest radiograph | Hyperinflation | Hyperinflation and hyperlucency | Normal |
| Pulmonary function testing | Increased lung volumes, reversible airflow obstruction, and normal or increased DLCO | Increased lung volumes, irreversible airflow obstruction, and decreased DLCO | Normal lung volumes, extrathoracic airflow obstruction, and normal DLCO |
| Response to corticosteroids | Good | Poor | Poor |
| Response to bronchodilators | Good | Modest | Poor |

Significant overlap in clinical presentation is possible. This is a guide to represent the most common presentations of isolated disease.

*Reproduced from* Tilles SA, Nelson HS. Asthma diagnosis and differential diagnosis. In: Kaliner MA, editor. Current review of asthma. Philadelphia: Current Medicine; 2003. p. 44; with permission.

following triggers: exercise; cold air; viral upper respiratory infections; irritants (eg, perfumes, passive smoke, air pollution); inhalant allergens (eg, dust mites, animal dander, pollens); weather changes; and emotional stress. Third, asthma symptoms are accompanied by intrathoracic airflow obstruction (Fig. 1), and this obstruction should be at least partially reversible. Airflow obstruction may be documented using office spirometry, a peak expiratory flow monitor, or formal pulmonary function testing. During symptomatic asthma, there is a decrease in the forced expiratory volume in 1 second ($FEV_1$) and the peak expiratory flow rate, a normal or somewhat reduced forced vital capacity, and an increase in lung volumes. Asthma patients usually have a normal or increased diffusing capacity for carbon monoxide (DLCO) [5].

Table 2
Less common asthma masqueraders

| Diagnosis | Presentation | Key to differentiating from asthma |
|---|---|---|
| Congestive heart failure | • Dyspnea on exertion, paroxysmal nocturnal dyspnea, occasionally wheezing, bronchial hyperreactivity<br>• Cardiac risk factors | • Examination findings: rales, edema, gallop rhythm<br>• Chest radiograph<br>• ECG<br>• Echocardiogram |
| Pulmonary embolism | • Dyspnea, occasionally wheezing<br>• Pulmonary embolus risk factors: oral contraceptive use, history of deep venous thrombosis, pregnancy, hypercoagulable state, immobility | • Unilateral rales, leg edema, cord<br>• V/Q scan<br>• Spiral CT scan |
| Cystic fibrosis | • Dyspnea, cough, gastrointenstinal complaints<br>• Airflow obstruction<br>• Infertility<br>• Poor growth | • Sweat chloride test<br>• DNA analysis |
| Bronchiolitis obliterans | • Cough, dyspnea<br>• Irreversible airflow obstruction | • Bronchoscopy with bronchioalveolar lavage<br>• Transbronchial biopsy |
| Bronchiecstasis | • Cough, dyspnea unresponsive to bronchodilator or corticosteroid<br>• Recurrent pneumonia | • High resolution CT of the chest |
| Hypersensitivity pneumonitis | • Dyspnea after chronic exposure to organic antigen (eg, moldy hay, birds)<br>• Restriction on spirometry | • Resolution of symptoms upon removal from exposure<br>• Precipitating antibodies |
| Aspiration gastroesophageal reflux disease | • Recurrent pneumonia<br>• Pulmonary fibrosis | • Overnight esophageal pH probe<br>• Barium yellow<br>• High resolution CT of the chest |
| Central airway obstruction | • Dyspnea, expiratory wheezing<br>• Symptoms not episodic<br>• No diurnal variation | • Symptoms improve with heliox inhalation<br>• Bronchoscopy |
| Extrahtoracic obstruction | • Dyspnea, stridor, inspiratory wheezing<br>• Truncation of the inspiratory portion of the flow volume loop | • Laryngoscopy |

*Reproduced from* Tilles SA, Nelson HS. Asthma diagnosis and differential diagnosis. In: Kaliner MA, editor. Current review of asthma. Philadelphia: Current Medicine; 2003. p. 47; with permission.

> **Box 1. Uncommon asthma masqueraders**
>
> Pulmonary infiltration with eosinophilia
> Tropical eosinophilia
> Löffler's syndrome
> Chronic eosinophilic pneumonia
> Idiopathic hypereosinophilic syndrome
> Allergic bronchopulmonary aspergillosis
> Churg-Strauss syndrome
> Metastatic carcinoid
> Systemic mastocytosis
> Lymphangioleiomyomatosis
>
> ---
>
> *From* Tilles SA, Nelson HS. Asthma diagnosis and differential diagnosis. In:
> Kaliner MA, editor. Current review of asthma. Philadelphia: Current Medicine;
> 2003. p. 48; with permission.

Asthma symptoms and airflow obstruction usually respond to appropriate therapy, such as inhaled β-adrenergic agonists and corticosteroids, and an assessment of the response to treatment aids in confirming the diagnosis. Inhaled β-adrenergic agonists typically provide relief within minutes, whereas a maximal response to systemic corticosteroids usually takes several days to a week. A trial of either prednisone, 20 mg twice daily for 2 weeks, or high-dose inhaled corticosteroid for 1 month (eg, fluticasone propionate, 220 µg/puff, two puffs twice daily) usually reverses airflow obstruction caused by asthma.

When the diagnosis of asthma is in doubt, bronchoprovocation studies, such as methacholine challenge or exercise challenge, may be performed. A standardized methacholine challenge protocol is quite sensitive (but not specific) for the diagnosis of asthma. Fig. 2 outlines an algorithm for establishing the diagnosis of asthma.

## Common asthma masqueraders

### Chronic obstructive pulmonary disease

COPD is a common disease in adult smokers. Emphysema and chronic bronchitis are the two classic COPD phenotypes, and either may be misdiagnosed as asthma. Because COPD and asthma are both common, some patients have both diseases. COPD is a disease of the elderly, although emphysema in $\alpha_1$-antitrypsin deficiency may become symptomatic in young adulthood.

Both COPD and asthma often present with dyspnea, wheezing, or cough. The expected pattern of these symptoms, however, and their triggering

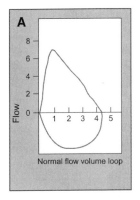

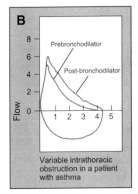

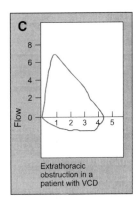

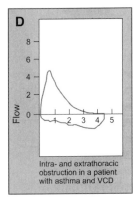

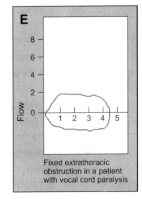

Fig. 1. Flow volume loops and airflow obstruction. (*A*) Normal flow volume loop. (*B*) Variable intrathoracic obstruction in a patient with severe asthma. (*C*) Variable extrathoracic obstruction in a patient with vocal cord dysfunction (VCD). (*D*) Variable intrathoracic and extrathoracic obstruction in a patient with both asthma and VCD. (*E*) Fixed extrathoracic obstruction in a patient with vocal cord paresis. (*From* Tilles SA, Nelson HS. Asthma diagnosis and differential diagnosis. In: Kaliner MA, editor. Current review of asthma. Philadelphia: Current Medicine; 2003. p. 43; with permission.)

factors differs. For example, COPD tends to develop gradually over a period of years in a subset of individuals with an extensive smoking history, and patients with COPD typically have little day-to-day variability in their baseline symptoms. Asthma patients commonly feel well at baseline but may become acutely symptomatic within minutes of exposure to a relevant trigger, such as an allergen (eg, cat) or an irritant (eg, perfume).

Both COPD and asthma patients typically report symptoms with exercise, although these patterns also differ. The classic exercise-induced bronchospasm response requires a minimum of 5 minutes of vigorous exercise followed by a peak in bronchospasm within 20 minutes regardless of whether the exercise continues or stops [6]. Exercise-induced bronchospasm symptoms subsequently gradually resolve and are followed by a relative

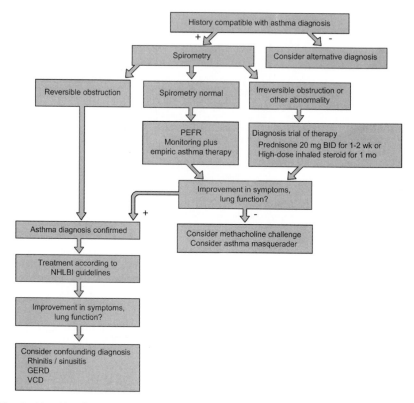

Fig. 2. Algorithm for establishing the diagnosis of asthma. BID, twice a day; GERD, gastro-esophageal reflux disease; NHLBI, National Heart, Lung, and Blood Institute; PEFR, peak expiratory flow rate. (*From* Tilles SA, Nelson HS. Asthma diagnosis and differential diagnosis. In: Kaliner MA, editor. Current review of asthma. Philadelphia: Current Medicine; 2003. p. 45; with permission.)

refractory period of several hours during which additional exercise provokes little or no bronchospasm. Exercise-induced bronchospasm is usually prevented using a prophylactic regimen, such as two puffs of inhaled albuterol 15 minutes before exercise. In contrast, the symptoms induced by exercise in COPD patients tend more closely to parallel oxygen demand and often reflect hypoxemia. For example, a patient with COPD might report he or she is able to walk no more than three blocks on level ground without rest. Exercise challenge testing with monitoring of spirometry and either oximetry or arterial blood gas measurements may be helpful when the diagnosis is in question.

Pulmonary function testing may also help differentiate asthma from COPD. Both diseases result in intrathoracic airflow obstruction and lung hyperinflation with increased lung volumes. In general, airflow obstruction caused by COPD is poorly reversible, and the most common way to measure this is to document the $FEV_1$ before and after administration of an inhaled bronchodilator. An increase in $FEV_1$ of greater than 15% (as a percent of baseline) is a commonly used criterion for identifying asthma, although many asthma patients do not reverse to this degree, especially if their pre-bronchodilator $FEV_1$ is near its predicted value at the time of the test [7]. In addition, defining reversibility as an increase in $FEV_1$ as a percent of baseline has poor specificity for asthma versus COPD. In contrast, defining reversibility as the increase in percent predicted $FEV_1$ is a better way to discriminate asthma from COPD [2,3]. One study [8] reported that an improvement in the percent predicted $FEV_1$ of 10% had a specificity of 0.95 for asthma versus chronic bronchitis. An increase of 15% of the predicted value had a specificity of 1 for asthma.

DLCO measurement may also help discriminate asthma from COPD. Because the measured DLCO increases as lung volumes increase, it is important to focus on the DLCO corrected for alveolar volume rather than the measured DLCO. In COPD the DLCO corrected for alveolar volume is usually decreased, reflecting impaired gas exchange. In asthma the DLCO corrected for alveolar volume is either normal or increased.

Methacholine challenge testing has an excellent negative predictive value for asthma and, in selected cases, may help discriminate asthma from COPD. Expressed as the provocative concentration of inhaled methacholine that results in a 20% fall in $FEV_1$ (PC20), methacholine challenge excludes asthma as the diagnosis when the 20% fall in $FEV_1$ is greater than 8 mg/mL. Patients with COPD may also have bronchial hyperresponsiveness, however, particularly when their baseline $FEV_1$ is below 70% of predicted [9]. In addition, for safety reasons methacholine challenges are contraindicated in patients with severe airflow obstruction. Methacholine challenge testing is most useful for differentiating mild to moderate asthma from relatively mild COPD.

Radiographic imaging studies may reveal abnormalities that discriminate COPD from asthma. Although lung hyperinflation is present with both diseases, bullous changes on a chest radiograph or CT scan are characteristic of emphysema.

## Vocal cord dysfunction

VCD is a common and frequently unrecognized masquerader and confounder of asthma. More properly termed "paradoxical laryngeal dysfunction," VCD is a heterogeneous disorder that involves intermittent unintentional adduction of the vocal cords or arytenoids during the respiratory cycle. VCD is classically present during inspiration only [10], although symptoms may also (or alternatively) occur during the expiratory phase. Patients often localize VCD symptoms to their throat during inspiration (with or without stridor), although some report symptoms in their chest (see Table 1). Spirometry during VCD symptoms often reveals classic signs of extrathoracic airflow obstruction (see Fig. 1), including truncation of the inspiratory portion of the flow volume loop and an increase in the ratio of midexpiratory airflow to midinspiratory airflow ($MEF_{50}/MIF_{50} > 1$). In the absence of symptoms, the flow volume loop is usually normal.

There is a spectrum of severity with VCD. Some patients report relatively mild symptoms, whereas others have histories of multiple ambulance transfers to emergency departments, intubation, or even tracheostomy. Polypharmacy with asthma medications (including in some cases long-term systemic corticosteroids) is common and VCD should be suspected as a possible diagnosis in any asthma patient who has failed to respond to aggressive asthma therapy, especially in the absence of a documented pulmonary function test abnormality.

VCD is not believed to have a primary organic basis. Although the pathophysiology of VCD is not known, anxiety and depression are common features reported in the literature, and in some patients VCD seems to be a conversion disorder [11]. Postnasal drip and laryngopharyngeal acid reflux have also been reported as either causing or confounding VCD. There is a paucity of controlled data in the literature, however, to establish any firm mechanistic conclusions. For example, a large case series description from the National Jewish Immunology and Respiratory Research Center [12] described 95 cases of laryngoscopically confirmed VCD, 53 of which also had asthma. There was a very strong association between VCD and psychiatric illness, although this association did not differ from control subjects with asthma.

VCD primarily affects women and adolescent girls, and there are two main phenotypes of VCD that are commonly confused with asthma. The first tends to occur in adolescent athletes and is exclusively provoked by exercise [13,14]. These patients typically experience symptoms only with intense exercise, often during competitions, and they also tend to be high achievers academically. The other general phenotype tends to occur in middle adulthood in patients with a history of psychiatric illness or a history of major psychologic trauma. A disproportionate number of adult VCD patients are employed in a health-related field.

The primary therapy for VCD is speech therapy [11] focusing on laryngeal relaxation techniques. Appropriate treatment of associated conditions, such as anxiety, depression, or acid reflux, may also improve VCD symptoms. An important goal of therapy in VCD is to reduce or discontinue unnecessary asthma medications. In patients with both VCD and asthma, asthma medications should be reduced or withdrawn gradually.

## Less common asthma masqueraders

### Cardiac asthma

Pulmonary edema caused by congestive heart failure (CHF) is often accompanied by wheezing, cough, and dyspnea. Dyspnea on exertion and paroxysmal nocturnal dyspnea are also characteristic features of chronic, suboptimally controlled CHF. Pulmonary function test abnormalities may include intrathoracic obstruction during acute flares, and a gradually progressive restrictive pattern with chronic disease. Bronchial hyperresponsiveness with inhaled methacholine is also common with nonasthmatic patients with CHF [15]. This is likely caused by vagally mediated reflex bronchospasm that occurs with distal airway edema [16].

There are several clinical clues that help distinguish CHF from asthma. First, bronchospasm caused by CHF only partially responds to inhaled bronchodilators, such as albuterol [17]. In one study, treatment of methacholine-induced bronchoconstriction with inhaled albuterol resulted in only a 43% improvement in $FEV_1$ [15]. Second, although both CHF and asthma may result in nocturnal awakening caused by dyspnea, both paroxysmal nocturnal dyspnea and orthopnea from CHF improve acutely with positional changes, such as sitting up or standing. Nocturnal asthma symptoms typically persist despite positional changes unless a bronchodilator is administered. Finally, as with COPD, the pattern of exercise-induced symptoms in CHF patients tends to parallel oxygen demand rather than resemble the classic exercise-induced bronchospasm response.

Physical examination findings that help distinguish CHF from asthma include the presence of inspiratory rales, a third heart sound, pitting edema, distended neck veins, and hepatomegaly. These findings, however, and chest radiographic findings of CHF, may be absent with mild left ventricular dysfunction. When the diagnosis remains in question, it is appropriate to proceed with echocardiography or a gated blood pool study.

*Pulmonary embolism*

Pulmonary embolism (PE) is a common and potentially fatal condition that in some circumstances can masquerade as asthma. The list of possible symptoms caused by PE is quite long, although its classic presentation includes some combination of tachypnea, dyspnea, new-onset wheezing, pleuritic chest pain, fever, or hemoptysis [18]. PE may also cause cardiac arrhythmias, such as atrial fibrillation, syncope, or seizures. Many patients with PE are minimally symptomatic, however, and chronic PE manifesting primarily with dyspnea may be difficult to distinguish from asthma. Clinical suspicion for PE versus asthma should be high when the classic hallmarks of asthma are not present or when respiratory symptoms occur in the setting of PE risk factors, such as having a prior history of PE or deep venous thrombosis, pregnancy, oral contraceptive use, hypercoagulable state, immobility, prior trauma, or obesity.

Physical examination findings suggestive of PE include a loud pulmonic component of the second heart sound, unilateral rales, unilateral lower leg edema, or a palpable cord. Chest radiographic abnormalities are not always seen, although findings characteristic of PE include unilateral volume loss, an enlarged proximal pulmonary artery, an enlarged cardiac silhouette, and a localized decrease in vascular markings. Ventilation-perfusion scanning is a highly sensitive way of detecting PE, although indeterminant results are often seen [19]. On occasion, a classic ventilation-perfusion mismatch may also be seen in chronic stable asthma [20]. Pulmonary angiography or high-resolution helical CT angiography (spiral CT scan) should be considered when clinical suspicion for PE remains high after inconclusive screening tests [21].

*Intrathoracic central airway obstruction*

The list of causes of central airway obstruction is long and includes several potentially life-threatening diagnoses, such as endobronchial *Mycobacterium tuberculosis,* malignancy, and sarcoidosis [3]:

Broncholithiasis
Endobronchial granulomatous disease
*M tuberculosis*
Sarcoidosis
Bronchomalacia
Foreign body
Web or stricture
Vascular ring
Tumor
Relapsing polychondritis
Extrinsic compression
Tumor
Vascular structure

Central airway obstruction usually presents with expiratory wheezing, dyspnea, and an obstructive pattern on spirometry, and may easily be misdiagnosed as asthma. Symptoms are typically much less episodic, however, and fail to respond to bronchodilators or corticosteroids. Because airflow in large airways is subject to turbulence, breathing a low-density mixture of oxygen and helium (heliox) may improve both symptoms and spirometry. Confirming the cause of central airway obstruction requires direct visualization by bronchoscopy. Biopsy is often also required.

*Extrathoracic airway obstruction*

Extrathoracic obstruction typically presents with dyspnea, inspiratory wheezing, or stridor. Some patients also experience symptoms and airflow obstruction during expiration (see Fig. 1E). Although VCD is the most common form of upper airway obstruction that masquerades as asthma, a variety of other causes should be kept in mind, particularly when symptoms are less episodic than asthma or VCD [3]:

Angioedema
Laryngeal spasm

Vocal cord dysfunction
Vocal cord paresis
Cricoarytenoid joint arthritis
Lymph node enlargement
Tumor
Tracheomalacia
Epiglottitis
Tracheal stricture
Extrinsic compression
Edema
Hemorrhage
Thyroid enlargement
Tumor

The diagnostic evaluation of upper airway obstruction other than VCD typically requires consultation with an otolaryngologist. Flexible or rigid laryngoscopy usually confirms the location of the obstruction, although additional diagnostic studies (eg, biopsy, CT, or MRI) may be required to confirm the diagnosis.

## Cystic fibrosis

Cystic fibrosis is the most common fatal hereditary disorder affecting whites in the United States [22]. In cystic fibrosis, defects in a membrane protein called the cystic fibrosis transmembrane conductance regulator impair several physiologic processes, including chloride ion transport and fatty acid metabolism. The clinical manifestations of cystic fibrosis include recurrent lower respiratory tract infections, bronchiectasis, sinusitis and nasal polyposis, pancreatic insufficiency, steatorrhea, arthritis, and male infertility. Although 70% of cystic fibrosis patients are diagnosed by age 12 months, less severe forms of cystic fibrosis may present in midadulthood, often in a context of long-standing asthma. Cystic fibrosis should be suspected in young to middle aged adults with a history of one or more of the following: recurrent respiratory infections, recurrent pancreatitis, a relative failure to respond to asthma treatment, and a family history of either cystic fibrosis or male infertility. The sweat chloride test is an effective screening tool, although establishing the diagnosis requires documenting two cystic fibrosis mutations.

## Bronchiolitis obliterans

Bronchiolitis obliterans is a nonspecific clinicopathologic pulmonary syndrome involving chronic scarring and eventual obliteration of the small airways resulting in dry cough, dyspnea, wheezing, and progressive airflow obstruction [23]. A variety of disease processes may result in the development of bronchiolitis obliterans, including connective tissue diseases, toxic inhalational exposures, respiratory infections, and chronic graft versus host disease in transplant recipients. There is also an idiopathic form of bronchiolitis obliterans [24]. Occasionally, bronchiolitis obliterans also involves intraluminal granulation tissue of the alveolar ducts and alveoli. This syndrome is referred to as "cryptogenic organizing pneumonia" or "bronchiolitis obliterans with organizing pneumonia" and commonly presents with dry cough, dyspnea, and fever.

Bronchiolitis obliterans masquerading as asthma is most likely to present with cough, dyspnea, and airflow obstruction that does not respond to empiric asthma treatment, especially if there is a history of an associated condition (eg, connective tissue disease, organ transplant, and so forth) in a lifelong nonsmoker. Pulmonary function studies typically reveal irreversible intrathoracic airflow obstruction and, in advanced cases, a decreased DLCO. The diagnosis often requires video-assisted thoracoscopic lung biopsy.

*Bronchiectasis*

Bronchiectasis is a syndrome of medium-sized bronchi that results from abnormal airway dilation and resultant bacterial superinfection [25]. As with bronchiolitis obliterans, there are a variety of distinct causes of bronchiectasis. These include allergic bronchopulmonary aspergillosis (ABPA), cystic fibrosis, recurrent pneumonias, and focal mechanical obstructive processes (eg, tumor or aspirated foreign body) that result in postobstructive bronchiectasis. Cough and dyspnea that do not respond well to bronchodilators or corticosteroids help distinguish bronchiectasis from asthma, although bronchiectasis sometimes complicates asthma. High-resolution CT of the chest is a sensitive way to confirm the presence of bronchiectasis. Chest percussion and postural drainage combined with judicious use of antibiotics are the treatments of choice.

*Aspiration and gastroesophageal reflux*

Gastroesophageal acid reflux (GER) is a common cause of respiratory symptoms in adults. A patient presenting with a primary complaint of chronic cough is the most common scenario in which GER may be mistaken for asthma [26]. An extensive literature investigating the causes of chronic cough suggests that GER is a contributing factor in roughly half of the cases, and is the sole cause in approximately 20% [27,28]. When GER masquerades as asthma, the patient history may reveal additional symptoms of heartburn or regurgitation. GER is frequently otherwise silent, however, and differentiating cough variant asthma from cough caused by GER may be difficult, because both tend to occur intermittently during the day and night [29]. Spirometry, methacholine challenge, or overnight esophageal pH monitoring are all appropriate diagnostic tests to consider. An empiric treatment trial with a proton pump inhibitor (eg, omeprazole, 20 mg twice a day for 3 months) is also reasonable, especially if initial testing does not reveal objective evidence of asthma.

Although GER may be mistaken for asthma, it is a much more common confounder of asthma. The effect of GER on asthma is believed to be caused by a vagally mediated reflex bronchoconstriction [30]. Approximately three fourths of asthma patients have GER, GER has been shown experimentally to trigger asthma symptoms, and multiple GER treatment trials have reported improvements in asthma symptoms. It is not surprising that the National Heart Lung and Blood Institute's Guidelines for asthma management recommend considering an evaluation for GER in any patient with poorly controlled asthma [1]. As with GER masquerading as asthma, patients with refractory asthma caused in part by GER may also deny GER symptoms, and objective documentation of GER or an empiric trial of GER treatment should be considered [30]. It also should be kept in mind that the presence of GER in an asthma patient does not necessarily mean that the patient's asthma improves with GER treatment. In fact, a recent Cochrane Database Review of trials studying the effects of GER treatment in patients with both asthma and GER concluded that such treatment did not consistently result in improvements in asthma outcomes [31]. The authors note that subgroups may respond but that predicting responders is difficult, especially in patients who do not report a clear history of reflux-associated respiratory symptoms.

*Hypersensitivity pneumonitis*

Hypersensitivity pneumonitis is a pulmonary syndrome resulting from an immunologic response to mold or other inhaled organic antigen. Hypersensitivity pneumonitis is an important cause of occupational lung disease (eg, farmer's lung, malt-workers lung) and also may occur in other settings of unusually high exposures to organic matter (eg, bird fancier's disease, humidifier lung). A recent workshop convened by the National Institutes of Health concluded that HP is likely underdiagnosed, currently diagnostic strategies are imperfect, and it is not always necessary to identify the causative agent if the diagnosis is highly suggested [32]. There are acute, subacute, and chronic forms of hypersensitivity pneumonitis, each characterized by dyspnea and cough. Acute hypersensitivity pneumonitis also commonly presents with fever, weight loss, and malaise. Lung examination findings include either bibasilar or diffuse crackles. Pulmonary function testing typically reveals a restrictive pattern and a decrease in the DLCO, although airflow obstruction is sometimes present in subacute or chronic hypersensitivity pneumonitis. Serum IgG ELISA to the suspected antigen is a sensitive but somewhat nonspecific laboratory test. High-resolution CT findings are more sensitive than chest radiography. During acute hypersensitivity pneumonitis, high-resolution CT findings include round, poorly defined centrilobular nodules. Bronchial biopsy findings include chronic, lymphocytic interstitial inflammation of the bronchioles.

*Allergic bronchopulmonary aspergillosis*

*Aspergillus fumigatus* is a ubiquitous mold that has the potential to sensitize atopic patients. Although usually resulting in no more than minor IgE-mediated triggering of rhinitis or asthma, *A fumigatus* exposure sometimes results in the development of ABPA, a distinct and potentially disabling immunologic syndrome that confounds asthma [33]. ABPA involves growth of the fungus within mucus plugs in asthma patients, and usually presents as refractory asthma with recurrent pulmonary infiltrates. Diagnostic criteria include having asthma, an elevated total IgE level, specific IgE and IgG to *A fumigatus*, and central bronchiectasis. End-stage ABPA often involves lung fibrosis. On rare occasion, an ABPA-like syndrome is caused by a different *Aspergillus* species or another fungus, such as *Fusarium*. In these cases the diagnosis depends on high index of suspicion together with recovery of the fungus in sputum.

## Summary

Although the term "all that wheezes is not asthma" is not new, and the long list of asthma masqueraders has remained essentially the same for several decades, the importance of knowing when to question the accuracy of a diagnosis of asthma has remained critical for physicians who care for patients with respiratory symptoms. The concepts of "asthma control" and "asthma severity" are currently evolving, although the fundamental hallmarks that define the syndrome of asthma endure and should be mastered by asthma specialists. Asthma masqueraders, including several that may confound a correct diagnosis of asthma, are important to consider when either the presentation of asthma is atypical or the response of the patient to treatment is suboptimal. COPD and VCD head the list of diagnoses most likely to be confused with asthma in everyday practice. Correctly identifying the diagnosis of COPD enables implementation of an up-to-date treatment plan that differs from asthma management. VCD is a vastly underrecognized syndrome whose existence is widely accepted but whose pathophysiology is poorly understood, and correctly identifying a VCD component to asthma symptoms enables both a reduction in costly and potentially harmful asthma medications and focus on specific VCD treatment, such as speech therapy. For less common and uncommon asthma masqueraders, it is important to be familiar with their typical clinical presentation and basic diagnostic approaches.

## References

[1] National Institutes of Health/National Heart, Lung, and Blood Institute. National Asthma Education and Prevention Program Expert Panel. Clinical practice guidelines. Expert Panel

report 2: guidelines for the diagnosis and management of asthma. Publication No. 97–4051. Bethesda (MD): National Institutes of Health/National Heart, Lung, and Blood Institute; 1997.

[2] Cockcroft DW, Swystun VA. Asthma control versus asthma severity. J Allergy Clin Immunol 1996;98(6 Pt 1):1016–8.

[3] Tilles SA, Nelson HS. Differential diagnosis of adult asthma. Immunol Allergy Clin North Am 1996;16:19–34.

[4] Tilles SA, Nelson HS. Asthma diagnosis and differential diagnosis. In: Kaliner MA, editor. Current review of asthma. Philadelphia: Current Medicine; 2003. p. 41–50.

[5] Irvin CG, Cherniac RM. Pathophysiology and physiologic assessment of the asthmatic patient. Semin Respir Med 1987;8:201–15.

[6] Silverman M, Anderson SD. Standardization of exercise tests in asthmatic children. Arch Dis Child 1972;47:882–9.

[7] Nicklaus TM, Burgin W, Taylor JR. Spirometric tests to diagnose suspected asthma. Am Rev Respir Dis 1969;100:153–9.

[8] Ramsdale EH, Morris MM, Roberts RS. Bronchial responsiveness to methacholine in chronic bronchitis: relationship to airflow obstruction and cold air responsiveness. Thorax 1984;39:912–8.

[9] Sterk PJ, Bel EH. The shape of the dose-response curve to inhaled bronchoconstrictor agents in asthma and chronic obstructive pulmonary disease. Am Rev Respir Dis 1991; 143:1433–7.

[10] Wood RP, Milgrom H. Vocal cord dysfunction. J Allergy Cin Immunol 1996;98:481–5.

[11] Christopher KL, Wood RP II, Eckert RC, et al. Vocal-cord dysfunction presenting as asthma. N Engl J Med 1983;308:1566–70.

[12] Newman KB, Mason UG, Schmaling KB. Clinical features of vocal cord dysfunction. Am J Respir Crit Care Med 1995;152:1382–6.

[13] Landwehr LP, Wood RP II, Blager FB, et al. Vocal cord dysfunction mimicking exercise-induced bronchospasm in adolescents. Pediatrics 1997;99:971.

[14] Tilles SA. Vocal cord dysfunction in children and adolescents. Curr Allergy Asthma Rep 2003;3:467–72.

[15] Cabanes LR, Weber SN, Matran R, et al. Bronchial hyperresponsiveness to methacholine in patients with impaired left ventricular function. N Engl J Med 1989;320:1317–22.

[16] Roberts AM, Bhattacharya J, Schultz HD, et al. Stimulation of vagal afferent C-fibers by lung edema in dogs. Circ Res 1986;58:512–22.

[17] Krieger BP. When wheezing may not mean asthma. Postgrad Med 2002;112:101–11.

[18] Raskob GE, Hull RD. Diagnosis of pulmonary embolism. Curr Opin Hematol 1999;6:280–4.

[19] Stein PD, Hull RD, Saltzman HA. Strategy for diagnosis of patients with suspected acute pulmonary embolism. Chest 1993;103:1553–9.

[20] Wagner PD, Hedenstierna G, Bylin G. Ventilation-perfusion inequality in chronic asthma. Am Rev Respir Dis 1987;136:605–12.

[21] Quiroz R, Kucher N, Zou KH, et al. Clinical validity of a negative computed tomography scan in patients with suspected pulmonary embolism: a systematic review. JAMA 2005; 293:2012–7.

[22] Yankaskas JR, Marshall BC, Sufian B, et al. Cystic fibrosis adult care: consensus report. Chest 2004;125:1S–39S.

[23] King TE. Overview of bronchiolitis. Clin Chest Med 1993;14:607–10.

[24] Afessa B, Litzow MR, Tefferi A. Bronchiolitis obliterans and other late onset non-infectious pulmonary complications in hematopoietic stem cell transplantation. Bone Marrow Transplant 2001;28:425–34.

[25] Luce JM. Bronchiectasis. In: Murray JF, Nadel JA, editors. Textbook of respiratory medicine. Philadelphia: WB Saunders; 1994. p. 1398–413.

[26] Napierkowski J, Wong RKH. Extraesophageal manifestations of GERD. Am J Med Sci 2003;326:285–99.

[27] Irwin RS, Corrao WM, Pratter MR. Chronic persistent cough in the adult: the spectrum and frequency of causes and successful outcome of specific therapy. Am Rev Respir Dis 1981;123: 413–7.

[28] Irwin RS, Curley FJ, French CL. Chronic cough: the spectrum and frequency of causes, key components of the diagnostic evaluation, and outcome of specific therapy. Am Rev Respir Dis 1990;141:640–7.

[29] Mello CJ, Irwin RS, Curley FJ. Predictive values of the character, timing, and complications of chronic cough in diagnosing its cause. Arch Intern Med 1996;156:997–1003.

[30] Harding SM. Gastroesophageal reflux and asthma: insight into the association. J Allergy Clin Immunol 1999;104(2 Pt 1):251–9.

[31] Gibson PG, Henry RL, Coughlan JL. Gastro-oesophageal reflux treatment for asthma in adults and children. Cochrane Database Syst Rev 2003;2:CD001496.

[32] Fink JN, Ortega HG, Reynolds HY, et al. Needs and opportunities for research in hypersensitivity pneumonitis. Am J Respir Crit Care Med 2005;171:792–8.

[33] Slavin RG, Hutcheson PS, Chauhan B, et al. An overview of allergic bronchopulmonary aspergillosis with some new insights. Allergy Asthma Proc 2004;25:395–9.

ELSEVIER
SAUNDERS

THE MEDICAL
CLINICS
OF NORTH AMERICA

Med Clin N Am 90 (2006) 77–95

# Anaphylaxis

## Phillip Lieberman, MD*

*Division of Allergy and Immunology, Departments of Medicine and Pediatrics,
University of Tennessee College of Medicine, Memphis, TN, USA*

The exact incidence of anaphylaxis is unknown [1]. Perhaps the best insight into incidence is obtained from assessing prescriptions for automatic epinephrine injectors. Using such prescription data, Simons [2] found an overall incidence of approximately 1% of the population of Manitoba, Canada. Regardless of the exact incidence, the incidence of anaphylactic episodes seems to be increasing based on the assessment of admissions to the emergency room in the United Kingdom [3]. Factors affecting incidence are listed in Box 1:

Atopy is a risk factor in all general series of anaphylactic events [1]. This is particularly true for agents administered by the mucosal route (eg, food). This is not surprising because atopy is a mucosally expressed and usually mucosally sensitized disease. Atopy, however, does not seem to be a risk factor for agents administered parenterally (eg, penicillin, insulin). It is interesting to note, however, that atopy is even a risk factor for episodes normally considered anaphylactoid (not IgE mediated). This includes anaphylactoid reactions to radiocontrast material and exercise. The reasons for this have not been established, but are thought to be caused by the cytokine milieu with increased production of interleukin-4, -5, and -13 in atopics as compared with nonatopic individuals. These cytokines not only enhance the releasability of mast cells and basophils, but also sensitize the target organs to mediators, such as histamine [4].

Sex clearly exerts an effect on the incidence of anaphylaxis. Males under the age of 16 experience anaphylaxis more frequently than females that age [2], whereas after the age of 30, the incidence is higher in females [5]. The female predominance after puberty may be related to hormonal differences in that progesterone enhances susceptibility to anaphylaxis in animal models

* Division of Allergy and Immunology, Departments of Medicine and Pediatrics, University of Tennessee College of Medicine, 7205 Wolf River Boulevard, Suite 200, Memphis, TN 38138.

*E-mail address:* aac@allergymemphis.com

0025-7125/06/$ - see front matter © 2005 Elsevier Inc. All rights reserved.
doi:10.1016/j.mcna.2005.08.007          *medical.theclinics.com*

---

**Box 1. Factors affecting the incidence of anaphylactic episodes**

*Risk factors*
  Atopy
  Sex
  Age
  Route of administration
  Constancy of administration
  Time since previous reaction
  Economic status
  Season of the year

*Not a risk factor*
  Race
  Geography
  Chronobiology

---

and progesterone-related (catamenial) anaphylactic events have been described in humans [6]. As a rule, anaphylactic events seem to be more common in adults than children, probably because of increased use of drugs in the older population [1]. In some series, however, children predominate [2].

In atopic individuals the route of administration is important in that the mucosal route is more sensitizing. The constancy of administration is also important. For example, insulin allergy is more likely to occur after recurrent administrations of insulin with interruptions between each administration as often occur in gestational diabetes [1]. The time since the previous reaction is important in that the longer the duration since the last administration of antigen, the less the likelihood of a recurrence.

An unusual observation, but one that has been confirmed, is that there seems to be an increased incidence of anaphylaxis in individuals of higher socioeconomic status. This cannot be related to access to medical care [7]. Anaphylactic episodes show a seasonal predisposition because of the seasonality of insect sting reactions. Anaphylactic reactions are more common in the summer and early fall.

Race, geographic location, and chronobiology seem to play no role. As opposed to other atopic conditions, which seem to worsen at night (eg, allergic asthma), there seems to be no increased incidence of anaphylactic episodes at this time [5].

**Pathophysiology**

Anaphylactic events can be defined as acute, generalized reactions caused by the release of mediators from mast cells and basophils secondary to the union of IgE antibody and antigen. Anaphylactoid episodes are clinically similar but do not involve IgE. Most of these episodes seem to be caused by direct histamine release, not requiring IgE antibody (eg, reactions to opiates or radiocontrast media). There are a number of other mechanisms, however, responsible for anaphylactoid events as listed in Box 2:

The mediators of anaphylactic episodes are the well-known contents of mast cells and basophils. These contents and their activities are seen in Table 1.

Histamine is probably the most important mediator of the most rapidly occurring symptoms. Histamine acts through both $H_1$ and $H_2$ receptors. The overall effect in the vascular bed is vasodilatation with increased vascular permeability. This causes flushing with a lowering of peripheral resistance along with a shift in fluid to the extravascular space. Vasodilatation is mediated by both $H_1$ and $H_2$ receptors. The $H_2$ receptors exert their effect by direct action on vascular smooth muscle. $H_1$ receptors act indirectly by stimulating the production of nitric oxide by endothelial cells [1].

The cardiac effects of histamine are primarily mediated through the $H_2$ receptor but the $H_1$ receptor also plays a role. $H_2$ receptor stimulation increases both the rate and force of atrial and ventricular contraction, probably by enhancing calcium influx. This also increases cardiac oxygen demand. $H_1$ receptor activity increases the heart rate by hastening diastolic depolarization at the sinoatrial node. $H_1$ receptor stimulation also can produce coronary artery vasospasm, which can result in myocardial infarction in spite of normal coronary arteries (the Kounis syndrome) [8].

Histamine produces varying effects on extravascular smooth muscle. It can cause contraction in the bronchial tree, mediated entirely by the $H_1$ receptor. The $H_1$ receptor also produces modest contraction of the human

---

**Box 2. Mechanisms responsible for anaphylactoid events**

*Anaphylaxis: IgE-mediated events*
  Drugs
  Food
  Insect bites and stings

*Anaphylactoid events*
  Direct release of mediators from mast cells and basophils
    Drugs (eg, opiates and radiocontrast media)
    Idiopathic
    Physical causes (cold, heat, sunlight, exercise)
  Arachidonic acid metabolic abnormalities (nonsteroidal
    anti-inflammatory drug-induced events)
  Activation of contact and complement systems
    Reactions caused by first use of membranes during dialysis
    Some reactions caused by radiocontrast material

Table 1

Mast cell and basophil mediators and their roles in producing anaphylactic and anaphylactoid
events

| Mediators | Pathophysiologic activity | Clinical correlates |
|---|---|---|
| Histamine and products of arachidonic acid metabolism (leukotrienes, thromboxane, prostaglandins, and platelet-activating factor) | Smooth muscle spasm, mucus secretion, vasodilatation, increased vascular permeability, activation of nociceptive neurons, platelet adherence, eosinophil activation, eosinophil chemotaxis | Wheeze, urticaria, angioedema, flush, itch, diarrhea and abdominal pain, hypotension, rhinorrhea, and bronchorrhea |
| Neutral proteases: tryptase, chymase, carboxypeptidase, cathepsin G | Exert activity via PAR receptors (protease activated cell surface receptors). Cleavage of complement components, chemoattractants for eosinophils and neutrophils, further activation and degranulation of mast cells, cleavage of neuropeptides, conversion of angiotensin I to angiotensin II. | May recruit complement by cleaving C3, may ameliorate symptoms by invoking a hypertensive response through the conversion of angiotensin I to angiotensin II and by inactivating neuropeptides. Also, can magnify response because of further mast cell activation. |
| Proteoglycans: heparin, chondroitin sulphate | Anticoagulation, inhibition of complement, binding phospholipase A2, chemoattractant for eosinophils, inhibition of cytokine function, activation of kinin pathway. | Can prevent intravascular coagulation and the recruitment of complement. Also can recruit kinins increasing the severity of the reaction. |
| Chemoattractants: chemokines, eosinophil chemotactic factors | Calls forth cells to the site | May be partly responsible for recrudescence of symptoms in late phase reaction or extension and protraction of reaction. |

uterus, whereas $H_2$ receptor stimulation can produce uterine relaxation. The predominant effect of histamine on gastrointestinal smooth muscle is contraction by the $H_1$ receptor.

Glandular secretion is mediated by both the $H_1$ and $H_2$ receptor. Glycoprotein secretion from goblet cells in bronchial glands is produced by stimulation of the $H_2$ receptor, whereas stimulation of the $H_1$ receptor increases mucous viscosity.

Infusion of histamine into humans causes symptoms similar to those observed during anaphylaxis. It is important to note that for maximal inhibition of flushing, headaches, hypotension, and tachycardia, a combination of $H_1$ and $H_2$ receptor blockade is required [1]. Other mast cell and basophil contents are important in that they recruit the activation of other inflammatory pathways. In protracted cases of anaphylaxis, one can see activation of the contact system with the formation of kinins; the coagulation pathway (both clotting and clot lysis); and the complement cascade. During severe and protracted episodes, evidence for activation of all of these occurs as summarized in Table 2. Severe disseminated intravascular coagulation can occur and has been reported as the cause of death in several instances [9]. Successful treatment of this manifestation has been reported with the administration of tranexamic acid [10].

It has recently been recognized that nitric oxide is also produced in large quantities during anaphylactic events. This molecule has both potentially beneficial and detrimental effects. It can cause bronchodilatation, vasodilatation of the coronary arteries, and reduced mast cell degranulation. These are salutary in nature. Based on studies using nitric oxide synthesis inhibitors in both animal models and humans [1], however, the sum total of the effects of nitric oxide is detrimental. This molecule produces vasodilatation in the vascular bed and also enhances vascular permeability, worsening shock [1].

The mechanism of production of shock during anaphylaxis is complex. Most cardiovascular parameters progress as one expects. Systemic vascular resistance, however, does not always behave according to expectations. While blood pressure declines, pulse increases, cardiac output declines, and intravascular volume diminishes as shock progresses from the onset of the reaction to a more severe state. Peripheral vascular resistance, however, can vary. One might expect that peripheral vascular resistance, based on the reduction in intravascular volume and vasodilatation, falls as shock progresses; however, in many instances it increases. This increase is presumably caused by the elicitation of endogenous compensatory responses, which include the release of epinephrine, the conversion of angiotensin I to angiotensin II,

Table 2
Findings during anaphylactic events that indicate the activation of multiple inflammatory cascades

| Coagulation pathway | Complement cascade | Contact system (kinin formation) |
|---|---|---|
| Decreased factor V | Decreased C4 | — |
| Decreased factor VIII | Decreased C3 | Decreased high-molecular-weight kininogen |
| Decreased fibrinogen | Decreased C3a | Formation of kallikrein–C1–inhibitor complexes, factor XIIa-C1–inhibitor complexes |

and the production of endothelin (all of which are vasoconstrictive) or the administration of exogenous vasoconstrictors (eg, epinephrine, dopamine). One can be maximally vasoconstricted in the face of shock. The clinical importance of this observation is that patients in this state do not respond to the administration of further vasoconstrictor agents and require large volumes of fluid for resuscitation.

## Signs and symptoms

The signs and symptoms of anaphylaxis are listed according to frequency in Table 3. As can be seen, cutaneous symptoms are by far the most common manifestations. In fact, the absence of cutaneous symptoms (unless shock is present) casts doubt on the diagnosis. In the presence of shock, presumably because blood flow is diverted away from the skin, cutaneous symptoms are often absent. In addition, severe respiratory obstruction with death can occur in the absence of reported cutaneous symptoms.

It is of note that episodes can present in a biphasic manner. That is, there can be an acute episode, followed by abatement of symptoms, and then a recurrence of manifestations after the asymptomatic period. This is important in that biphasic events impact the duration of observation after successful treatment of the initial phase [11]. Characteristics of biphasic events are listed in Box 3.

## Differential diagnosis

The diagnosis of the acute event rarely presents a problem when seen in a medical setting (eg, after the administration of a drug in office). The causes

Table 3
Signs and symptoms of anaphylaxis

| Signs and symptoms | Approximate percent of cases |
|---|---|
| *Cutaneous* | > 90 |
| Urticaria and angioedema | 88 |
| Flush | 26 |
| Pruritus without rash | 5 |
| *Respiratory* | |
| Dyspnea and wheeze | 55–60 |
| Upper airway angioedema | > 25 |
| *Dizziness, syncope, hypotension, blurred vision* | 30–35 |
| *Abdominal: nausea, vomiting, diarrhea, cramping pain* | 25–30 |
| *Miscellaneous* | |
| Headache | 5–8 |
| Substernal pain | 5 |
| Seizure | 1–2 |

*Data from* Webb L, Green E, Lieberman P. Anaphylaxis: a review of 593 cases. J Allergy Clin Immunol 2004;113(2):S240.

---

**Box 3. Characteristics of biphasic reactions**

- Incidence up to 20%; more common when antigen is food
- May be results of too small a dose of epinephrine or a delay in the administration of epinephrine administered to treat the first phase
- Manifestations can be identical, worse, or less severe than initial phase
- Fatalities have occurred
- Most episodes occur within the first 8 hours after resolution of the first event, but recurrences have been recorded as late as 72 hours after
- There is no consistent clinical presentation that predicts the recurrence of symptoms (biphasic reactions)
- The cause of biphasic reactions is unknown
- Clinical importance relates to the length of time patients are observed after successful treatment of the initial reaction; recommendations have ranged from 2- to 24-hour observation

---

of shock must be considered. The usual cutaneous manifestations and the frequent occurrence of bronchospasm, however, make most episodes easily diagnosable when the patient is seen during the acute event. The most common condition to be confused with anaphylaxis if the patient is seen during the acute event is a vasodepressor (vasovagal) reaction. The mechanisms underlying the vasodepressor response have not been definitively clarified, but such reactions seem to be caused by the activation of the Bezold-Jarisch reflex. This reflex is thought to be initiated by excessive venous pooling, with resulting decrease in venous ventricular return and the subsequent activation of sensory receptors that respond to wall tension in the inferoposterior portions of the left ventricle. Stimulation of these receptors results in activation of the vagus nerve consequently producing bradycardia with further vasodilatation, hypotension, and quite often syncope. Characteristic features of the vasodepressor reaction are hypotension, pallor, weakness, nausea, vomiting, and diaphoresis. Vasodepressor reactions can be distinguished from anaphylaxis in many instances in that the latter has, as noted, frequent cutaneous manifestations that are absent during the vasodepressor response. The characteristic bradycardia that occurs during vasodepressor reactions has been classically cited as a feature differentiating these from anaphylactic events. More recently, however, it has been found that bradycardia occurs more often than previously expected during anaphylactic events. In a study of anaphylaxis caused by insect stings, the presence of hypotension was always accompanied by a relative bradycardia [12]. Bradycardia may not be as helpful in differentiating vasodepressor versus anaphylactic events as previously thought.

The differential diagnosis is more complex in patients seen after the event, in office, to solidify the diagnosis and identify the culprit. The differential diagnosis for such episodes is seen in Box 4. Episodes of flushing can occur in association with anaphylaxis, but such episodes more often occur with other conditions. Flush can occur in a wet and dry form. In the wet form, there is sweating. In the dry form, the skin remains dry. The wet form is mediated by sympathetic cholinergic nerves that supply the sweat glands and is the type that characteristically occurs in postmenopausal flushes.

Certain tumors secrete substances that also are present in anaphylactic events. These tumors include the gastrointestinal vasointestinal peptide–secreting tumors (eg, from the pancreas) and carcinoid tumors and medullary carcinomas of the thyroid.

Alcohol-induced flush occurs quite often in the Asian population (incidence 47%–85%) and can also occur in non-Asians (incidence ranging from 3%–29%) [1]. This can be related to the simultaneous administration of drugs along with alcohol, but can occur independent of the ingestion of such drugs. In the drug-independent form, it is quite often caused by null alleles for the mitochondrial enzyme aldehyde dehydrogenase-2. This enzyme catabolizes acetaldehyde (a metabolic product of alcohol metabolism). In its absence, acetaldehyde accumulates and produces degranulation of mast cells, resulting in what is, in essence, an anaphylactoid reaction.

Histamine poisoning (scombroidosis) has become the most common cause of restaurant-induced events. Histamine poisoning is caused by the ingestion of spoiled fish. Most episodes are mild, but severe episodes can occur and can mimic anaphylactic events. Histamine and *cis*-urocanic acid are produced by bacteria that proliferate within fish stored at elevated temperature. A number of different bacteria are capable of producing these substances. When they are present in large amounts, symptoms of histamine poisoning, which are similar to those of anaphylaxis, can occur. Cutaneous manifestations, as in anaphylaxis, are the most common. A clue leading to this diagnosis is that more than one person eating at the same table may have symptoms. Secondly, the cutaneous symptoms are often somewhat different than those produced during anaphylaxis. They can consist of a prolonged flush without urticaria. Thirdly, these episodes can be distinguished from anaphylactic events because they are accompanied by elevations of plasma histamine and urinary histamine metabolites, but not by elevated levels of tryptase. In anaphylaxis both tryptase and histamine are elevated (see below).

The laboratory may assist in establishing the differential diagnosis. Tests that may be considered are seen in Table 4. Serum tryptase is probably the most useful test to confirm a diagnosis of anaphylaxis. Serum tryptase exists in two forms. α-Protryptase is secreted constitutively and β (mature) tryptase is released during mast cell degranulation. Serum tryptase levels remain elevated for 6 hours, and occasionally longer. They are usually more useful than plasma histamine determinations, which remain elevated for only up to

**Box 4. Differential diagnosis of anaphylaxis and anaphylactoid reactions**

*Anaphylaxis and anaphylactoid reactions*
  To exogenously administered agents
  Caused by physical factors
  Idiopathic
*Vasodepressor (vasovagal) reactions*
*Flush syndromes*
  Carcinoid
  Postmenopausal
  Chlorpropamide: alcohol
  Medullary carcinoma thyroid
  Epilepsy
  Vasointestinal polypeptide–secreting tumors
*"Restaurant syndromes"*
  Monosodium glutamate
  Sulfites
  Scombroidosis
*Other forms of shock*
  Hemorrhagic
  Cardiogenic
  Endotoxic
*Excess endogenous production of histamine syndromes*
  Systemic mastocytosis
  Urticaria pigmentosa
  Basophilic leukemia
  Acute promyelocytic leukemia (tretinoin treatment)
  Hydatid cyst
*Nonorganic disease*
  Panic attacks
  Munchausen stridor
  Vocal cord dysfunction syndrome
  Globus hystericus
  Undifferentiated somatoform anaphylaxis
*Miscellaneous*
  Hereditary angioedema
  Progesterone anaphylaxis
  Urticarial vasculitis
  Pheochromocytoma
  Hyperimmunoglobulin E, urticaria syndrome
  Neurologic (seizure, stroke)
  Pseudoanaphylaxis
  Red-man syndrome (vancomycin)
  Capillary leak syndrome

60 minutes. Elevation of baseline tryptase (the α-protryptase or immature
form) indicates the presence of mastocytosis as a cause of an anaphylactic
episode because the increased mast cell burden results in secretion of constitutively elevated amounts. The other tests, such as metanephrine and serotonin, seen in Table 4 are useful in ruling out conditions that mimic
anaphylaxis.

## Prevention of the acute event

In patients predisposed to anaphylactic episodes, preventive measures as
noted in Box 5 are indicated. A thorough history for drug allergy is necessary. Proper interpretation of this history requires knowledge of the immunologic and biochemical cross-reactivity among drugs. Whenever possible, if
the history suggests a reaction to a specific agent, a substitute, non–cross-
reactive drug should be administered. Parenteral administration usually

Table 4
Laboratory tests to be considered in establishing the differential diagnosis of anaphylaxis and
anaphylactoid events

| Test | Comment |
| --- | --- |
| Serum tryptase | Levels peak 60–90 min after the onset of anaphylaxis and can persist several hours ($\geq$ 6). Levels usually peak between 1–2 h after the intiation of symptoms, this is the ideal time to obtain a serum sample. |
| Plasma histamine | Levels rise more rapidly than serum tryptase, 5–10 min after symptom onset. They remain elevated for a very limited period of time, however, usually only 30–60 min, and are usually less useful than serum tryptase because more patients are seen after histamine levels decline. They are of little help if the patient is seen as long as an hour after the onset of the event. |
| 24-h Urinary histamine metabolites (methylhistamine) | May be found in the urine for up to 24 h after symptom onset. |
| Plasma-free metanephrine | Rules out paradoxical pheochromocytoma. |
| Urinary vanillylmandelic acid | Also useful in ruling out paradoxical response to pheochromocytoma. |
| Serum serotonin | Carcinoid syndrome |
| Urinary 5-hydroxindoleacetic acid | Rules out carcinoid syndrome |
| Serum vasointestinal polypeptide hormone panel: pacreastatin, vasintestinal polpeptide hormone, substance P, neurokinin | Rules out gastrointestinal tumor or medullary carcinoma of the thyroid, both of which can secrete vasoactive peptides. |

---

**Box 5. Measures to reduce the incidence of anaphylaxis and anaphylactic deaths**

*General measures*
Obtain thorough history for drug allergy.
Avoid drugs with immunologic or biochemical cross-reactivity with any agents to which the patient is sensitive.
Administer drugs orally rather than parenterally when possible.
Check all drugs for proper labeling.
Keep patients in office 20 to 30 minutes after injections.
Consider a waiting period of 2 hours if the patient has been given the drug in office, which they have never before received, by mouth.

*Measures for patients at risk*
Have patient wear and carry warning identification.
Teach self-injection of epinephrine and caution patients to keep epinephrine kit with them.
Discontinue β-adrenergic blocking agents, angiotensin-converting enzyme inhibitors, angiotensin-converting enzyme blockers, monoamine oxidase inhibitors, and certain tricyclic antidepressants when possible.
Use preventive techniques when patients are required to undergo a procedure or take an agent that places them at risk. Such techniques include pretreatment, provocative challenge, and desensitization.

---

produces a more severe reaction than oral administration, and the latter is the route of choice in reference to preventing anaphylactic episodes. When receiving a drug in office, the patient should remain a minimum of 20 to 30 minutes after the drug is given if it is administered by injection, and 2 hours if the drug is administered orally.

Patients subject to anaphylaxis (eg, those with recurrent idiopathic episodes, caused by foods or insect stings) should wear MedicAlert jewelry (available at: http//www.medicalert.org) and should keep an identification card in their wallet or purse. Such patients should also be supplied with automatic epinephrine injectors and should be told clearly to keep the injector with them at all times and renew the prescription when the expiration date is reached.

Certain drugs diminish the effect of endogenous compensatory responses (the endogenous production of epinephrine or the formation of angiotensin) and worsen episodes. In addition β-blockers tend to block the effect of exogenously administered epinephrine. Monoamine oxidase inhibitors, which prevent the metabolism of epinephrine, and tricyclic antidepressants, which prevent the reuptake of catecholamines at peripheral nerve endings, can complicate therapy by exaggerating the effect of epinephrine given for treatment. Although this, at first blush, may not seem to be important, it is of note that epinephrine overdoses have been the cause of death in some instances [9].

In patients who are required to take medications or receive diagnostic agents to which they have experienced previous reactions, specific preventive measures should be considered. They include pretreatment protocols, provocative challenges, or desensitization. In most instances, with the possible exception of the institution of a pretreatment regimen, such procedures should be performed by an allergist or immunologist. An example of a pretreatment regimen that has proved effective in diminishing the severity or preventing reactions to the readministration of radiocontrast and the prevention of cold-induced anaphylactic events during bypass surgery is seen in Box 6.

## Management of the acute event

An algorithm for management of the acute episode of anaphylaxis is seen in Fig. 1. Box 7 summarizes the actions to be taken on diagnosis of the acute event.

---

**Box 6. Treatment protocol to prevent a recurrence of anaphylaxis or diminish symptoms during an occurrence when a patient must receive a diagnostic agent to which they have previously reacted**

Prednisone, 50 mg by mouth given 13, 7, and 1 hour before the procedure.
Diphenhydramine, 50 mg intramuscularly (IM) given 1 hour before the procedure.
Consider ephedrine, 25 mg by mouth given 1 hour before the procedure.
Consider an $H_2$ antagonist, such as ranitidine, 300 mg given 3 hours before the procedure.[a]

---

Has been shown to be effective for the readministration of radiocontrast material and to prevent cold-induced anaphylactic episodes during bypass surgery. It is not always effective, and has been shown to be ineffective in other venues (eg, prevention of latex-induced reactions during surgery).

[a] It should be noted that the use of an $H_2$ antagonist is controversial in that in some instances it has proved beneficial and in others has increased the frequency of events [1].

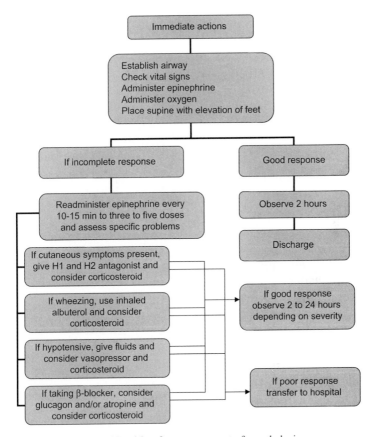

Fig. 1. Algorithm for management of anaphylaxis.

The initial step in the management of anaphylaxis is rapid assessment of the patient's status with emphasis on evaluation of the airway and the state of consciousness. If the airway is compromised, it should be secured immediately. Blood pressure and pulse measurements should be obtained. The patient should be placed in the supine position with feet elevated. This is extremely important because recently it has been noted that assuming the sitting position can be associated with fatality [9]. It is presumed that this occurs because there is no venous return to the heart when the sitting position is assumed. This in turn produces pulseless mechanical contraction of the heart and predisposes to arrhythmias. In several instances death occurred immediately after assuming the sitting position [13].

It has been suggested that if the antigen was injected a tourniquet should be placed proximal to the injection site and that site infiltrated with 0.3 mL epinephrine to slow absorption. There are no data, however, to confirm the efficacy of either of these two procedures. If a tourniquet is used, care should

---

**Box 7. Therapy of the anaphylactic event**

*Immediate action*
  Assessment
  Check airway and secure if needed
  Rapid assessment of level of consciousness
  Vital signs

*Treatment*
  Epinephrine
  Supine position, legs elevated
  Oxygen
  Tourniquet proximal to injection site

*Dependent on evaluation*
  Start peripheral intravenous (IV) fluids
  $H_1$ and $H_2$ antagonist
  Vasopressors
  Corticosteroids
  Aminophylline
  Glucagon
  Atropine
  Electrocardiographic monitoring
  Transfer to hospital

*Hospital management*
  Medical antishock trousers
  Continued therapy with previously noted agents and
    management of complications

---

be taken to release it every 5 minutes (for a minimum of 3 minutes) during therapy.

Epinephrine is the drug of choice and the mainstay of therapy. It has been shown that IM injection in the lateral thigh (vastus lateralis muscle) results in a more rapid rise in serum levels than subcutaneous or IM (deltoid) injection in the arm. It has been recommended that lateral thigh injection (as one does with automatic epinephrine injectors) is the route of choice [2]. It should be noted, however, that there are no outcome studies to date that compare various routes of administration.

Regardless of the route, epinephrine should be administered simultaneously while the patient is being assessed. It is clear that delays in administration have been associated with worse outcomes. The IM dose of epinephrine in adults is 0.3 mL to 0.5 mL (0.3–0.5 mg) of a 1:1000 solution. In children the dose is 0.1 mg/kg. This initial dose can be repeated two to three times at 10- to 15-minute intervals.

Table 5
Drugs and other agents used to treat anaphylaxis

| Drug/agent | Dose and route of administration | Comment |
|---|---|---|
| Epinephrine | 1:1000 0.3–0.5 mL IM (adult); 1:1000 0.01 mg/kg or 0.1–0.3 mL IM (child) | Initial drug of choice for all episodes; should be given immediately; may repeat every 10–15 min |
| | 0.1–1.0 mL of 1:1000 aqueous epinephrine diluted in 10 mL normal saline IV (see text for details) | If no response to IM administration and patient in shock with cardiovascular collapse |
| *Antihistamines* | | |
| Diphenhydramine | 25–50 mg IM or IV (adult); 12.5–25 mg PO, IM, or IV (child) | Route of administration depends on severity of episode |
| Ranitidine, cimetidine | 1 mg/kg IV ranitidine; 4 mg/kg IV cimetidine | Cimetidine should be administered slowly because rapid administration has been associated with hypotension; doses shown are for adults; dose in children less well-established |
| *Corticosteroids* | | |
| Hydrocortisone | 100 mg–1 g IV or IM (adult); 10–100 mg IV (child) | Exact dose not established; other preparations such as methyl-prednisolone can be used as well; for milder episodes, prednisone 30–60 mg may be given (see text) |
| *Drugs for resistant bronchospasm* | | |
| Aerosolized β-agonist (albuterol, metaproterenol) | Dose as for asthma (0.25–0.5 mL in 1.5–2 mL saline every 4 h, when needed) | Useful for bronchospasm not responding to epinephrine |
| Aminophylline | Dose as for asthma | Rarely indicated for recalcitrant bronchospasm; β-agonist is drug of choice |
| *Volume expanders* | | |
| Crystalloids (normal saline or Ringer's lactate) | 1000–2000 mL rapidly (adults); 30 mL/kg in first hour (child) | Rate of administration titrated against blood pressure response for IV volume expander; after initial infusion, further administration requires tertiary care monitoring; in patients who are β-blocked, larger amounts may be needed. |

(*continued on next page*)

Table 5 (*continued*)

| Drug/agent | Dose and route of administration | Comment |
|---|---|---|
| Colloids (hydroxyethyl starch) | 500 mL rapidly followed by slow infusion (adult) | |
| *Vasopressors* | | |
| Dopamine | 400 mg in 500 mL; dextrose 5% in water as IV infusion; 2–20 mcg/kg/min | Dopamine is probably the drug of choice; the rate of infusion should be titered against the blood pressure response; continued infusion requires intensive care monitoring |
| *Drugs used in patients who are β-blocked* | | |
| Atropine sulfate | 0.3–0.5 mg IV; may repeat every 10 min to a maximum of 2 mg (adult) | |
| Glucagon | Initial dose of 1–5 mg IV followed by infusion of 5–15 mcg/min titrated against blood pressure | Glucagon is probably the drug of choice with atropine useful only for treatment of bradycardia. |
| Ipratropium | | Ipratropium might be considered as an alternative or added to inhaled beta-adrenergics for wheezing. |

*Abbreviations:* IM, intramuscular; IV, intravenous; PO, by mouth.

If there is no response after several injections, IV epinephrine should be considered. There is no definitively established dose and numerous regimens have been suggested. The amount administered depends on the severity of the episode and should be titrated against the response. During the administration of IV epinephrine constant monitoring with whatever means are available is necessary. A suggested dose for IV preparation can be prepared by diluting 0.1 mL (0.1 mg) of a 1:1000 aqueous epinephrine solution in 10 mL of normal saline. This 10-mL preparation can be infused over 5 to 10 minutes and repeated depending on the response. The dose can be increased in more critical situations to 1 mL (1 mg) of a 1:1000 solution of epinephrine diluted in 10 mL of normal saline (for a concentration of 0.1 mg/ mL) and a dose of 1 to 2 mL (0.1–0.2 mg) administered every 5 to 20 minutes by bolus. An alternative is to prepare an epinephrine infusion by adding 1 mL (1 mg) of a 1:1000 dilution of epinephrine to 250 mL of dextrose 5% in water to yield a concentration of 4 µg/mL. This 1:250,000 solution is infused at a rate of 1 to 4 µg per minute (15–60 drops/min with a microdrop apparatus [60 drops per minute = 1 mL = 60 mL/h]). The dose can be increased to a maximum of 10 µg per minute.

Antihistamine therapy can be useful as adjunctive treatment but should not be administered as monotherapy. Based on the known effects of histamine on the $H_1$ and $H_2$ receptors as previously mentioned, a combination

---

**Box 8. Equipment and medication suggested to be kept in office for potential use in the management of an anaphylactic event**

*Primary*
Tourniquet
1-mL and 5-mL disposable syringes
Oxygen tank and mask or nasal prongs
Epinephrine solution (aqueous) 1:1000 (1-mL amps and multidose vials)
Epinephrine solution (aqueous) 1:10,000 (commercially available preloaded in a syringe)
Diphenhydramine injectable
Ranitidine or cimetidine injectable
Injectable corticosteroids
Ambu-bag, oral airway, laryngoscope, endotracheal tube, No. 12 needle
IV setup with large-bore catheter
IV fluids, 2000 mL crystalloid, 1000 mL hydroxyethyl starch
Aerosol beta-II bronchodilator and compressor nebulizer
Glucagon
Electrocardiogram
Normal saline 10-mL vial for epinephrine dilution

*Supporting*
Suction apparatus
Dopamine
Sodium bicarbonate
Aminophylline
Atropine
IV set-up with needles, tape, and tubing
Nonlatex gloves

*Optional*
Defibrillator
Calcium gluconate
Neuroleptics for seizures
Lidocaine

---

of an $H_1$ and $H_2$ antagonist is often superior to an $H_1$ antagonist alone. This is especially true for symptoms of flush, hypotension, and urticaria. Diphenhydramine can be administered at a dose of 1 to 2 mg/kg or 25 to 50 mg given parenterally (IM or IV). Ranitidine, as an $H_2$ antagonist, is given at a dose of 1 mg/kg. Ranitidine can be diluted in 5% dextrose to a total volume of 20 mL and injected IV over 5 minutes. Cimetidine at a dose of 4 mg/kg can also be used in adults.

Shock can be caused by fluid shifts from the intravascular to the extravascular space. In these instances vasoconstrictor agents may not be effective and volume resuscitation is necessary. There is no clear preference for a colloid or a crystalloid. The most important component of fluid therapy is the volume of the fluid itself. Large volumes of crystalloid are often required. A total of 1000 to 2000 mL of lactated Ringer's or normal saline should be given rapidly in an adult, depending on the blood pressure, at a rate of 5 to 10 mL/kg in the first 5 minutes. An alternative to crystalloids is hydroxyethyl starch. Adults should receive rapid infusion of 500 mL followed by a slow infusion thereafter. In patients who are taking a β-blocker, the amount of fluid may be greater (5–7 L) before stabilization occurs. Such large volumes of fluid require transfer as soon as possible to an ICU where extensive monitoring can be performed.

The role of corticosteroids in the management of anaphylaxis has not been clearly established. Based on extrapolation of their effects in other allergic diseases, however, their administration is indicated. Patients with severe anaphylactic episodes and those patients who have received systemic corticosteroids in the past several months should be given IV corticosteroids. The exact time of onset of activity of corticosteroids is unknown, and it is unclear whether they prevent a biphasic response, but there is theoretic rationale for their use.

β-Adrenergically blocked patients may also require glucagon as a substitute for epinephrine. The initial dose is 1 to 5 mg IV followed by an infusion of 5 μg/min to 15 μg/min titrated against the blood pressure response. For bradycardia, atropine sulfate can be used at a dose of 0.3 mg to 0.5 mg IV repeated every 10 minutes to a maximum of 2 mg in adults. This dose may also be helpful in treating a vasodepressor (vasovagal) reaction.

Table 5 suggests possible agents to be used to treat an anaphylactic event, giving the doses and comments regarding the use of each drug. Although there is no clear-cut consensus as to the equipment one needs in an office to prepare to treat anaphylactic reactions, Box 8 presents suggestions in this regard.

## References

[1] Lieberman P. Anaphylaxis and anaphylactoid reactions. In: Middleton E, editor. Allergy: principles and practice, Vol. 2, 6th edition. Philadelphia: Mosby; 2003. p. 1497–522.

[2] Simons E. Epinephrine in the first-aid out-of-hospital treatment of anaphylaxis. In: Anaphylaxis. London: John Wiley & Sons; 2004. p. 228–43.

[3] Gupta R, Sheikh A, Strachen D, et al. Increasing hospital admissions for systemic allergic disorders in England: analysis of National Admissions Data. BMJ 2003;327:1142–3.

[4] Strait R, Morris SC, Finkelman FD. Cytokine enhancement of anaphylaxis. In: Anaphylaxis. London: John Wiley & Sons; 2004. p. 80–97.

[5] Webb L, Green E, Lieberman P. Anaphylaxis: a review of 593 cases. J Allergy Clin Immunol 2004;113:S240.

[6] Heinly TL, Lieberman P. Anaphylaxis in pregnancy. Immunol Clin North Am 2000;20:831.

[7] Simons FER, Peterson S, Black CD. Epinephrine dispensing pattern for an out-of-hospital population: a novel approach to studying the epidemiology of anaphylaxis. J Allergy Clin Immunol 2002;110:647–51.

[8] Zavras GM, Papadaki PJ, Kokkinis CE, et al. Kounis syndrome secondary to allergic reaction following shellfish ingestion. Int J Clin Pract 2003;57:622–4.

[9] Pumphrey R. Fatal anaphylaxis in the UK 1992–2001. In: Anaphylaxis. London: John Wiley & Sons; 2004. p. 116–28.

[10] DeSousa RL, Short T, Warmin GR, et al. Anaphylaxis with associated fibrinolysis reversed with tranexamic acid and demonstrated by thromboelastography. Anaesth Intensive Care 2004;32:580–7.

[11] Lieberman P. Biphasic anaphylaxis. Journal of the World Allergy Organization 2004;16: 241–8.

[12] Brown SGA, Blackman KE, Stenleke V, et al. Insect sting anaphylaxis: prospective evaluation of treatment with intravenous adrenaline and volume resuscitation. Emerg Med J 2004; 21:149–54.

[13] Pumphrey R. Anaphylaxis: Can we tell who is at risk of a fatal reaction? Cur Opin Allergy Clin Immunol 2004;4:285–90.

ELSEVIER
SAUNDERS

THE MEDICAL
CLINICS
OF NORTH AMERICA

Med Clin N Am 90 (2006) 97–127

# Adverse Reactions to Foods

Anna Nowak-Wegrzyn, MD[a,b],
Hugh A. Sampson, MD[a,b],*

[a]Division of Allergy and Immunology, Department of Pediatrics,
Mount Sinai School of Medicine, New York, NY, USA
[b]Jaffe Food Allergy Institute, New York, NY, USA

Over the past 20 years, food allergy has emerged as an important clinical problem in Westernized countries. Not only has food allergy prevalence almost doubled but its severity and scope have increased. Consequently, research focusing on characterization, mapping, and cloning of food allergens, as well as on deciphering the nature of immune responses to food allergens and the mechanisms of oral tolerance, has blossomed. It is hoped that this research will lead to the development of therapeutic modalities for food allergy in the near future. This article discusses the pathomechanism of food allergic reactions, classification and manifestations of clinical food allergic disorders, and an approach to diagnosis and management.

## Definition

Food allergy is defined as an immune-mediated adverse reaction to foods. Food allergy must be distinguished from a variety of adverse reactions to foods that do not have an immune basis but may resemble it in clinical manifestations. Examples of such adverse food reactions are presented in Table 1.

## Prevalence

Food allergy affects about 6% to 8% of infants and young children and approximately 3.5% to 4% of adults [1,2]. Children with moderate to severe persistent atopic dermatitis have a higher prevalence of IgE-mediated food

This article was supported by National Institutes of Health Grants AI43668, AI44236, and M01-RR-00071 to Dr. Sampson.
* Corresponding author. Division of Allergy and Immunology, Department of Pediatrics, Mount Sinai Hospital, Box 1198, One G. Levy Place, New York, NY 10029.
E-mail address: hugh.sampson@mssm.edu (H.A. Sampson).

0025-7125/06/$ - see front matter © 2005 Elsevier Inc. All rights reserved.
doi:10.1016/j.mcna.2005.08.012          *medical.theclinics.com*

Table 1
Adverse reactions to foods mimicking food allergy

| Condition | Symptoms | Mechanism |
|---|---|---|
| Lactose intolerance | Bloating, abdominal pain, diarrhea (dose-dependent) | Lactase deficiency |
| Fructose intolerance | Bloating, abdominal pain, diarrhea (dose-dependent) | Fructase deficiency |
| Pancreatic insufficiency | Malabsorption | Deficiency of pancreatic enzymes |
| Gallbladder/liver disease | Malabsorption | Deficiency of liver enzymes |
| Food poisoning | Pain, fever, nausea, emesis, diarrhea | Bacterial toxins in food |
| Scombroid fish poisoning | Flushing, angioedema, hives, abdominal pain | In spoiled fish histidine is metabolized to histamine |
| Caffeine | Tremors, cramps, diarrhea | Pharmacologic effects of caffeine in susceptible individuals |
| Thyramine | Migraine | Pharmacologic effects of thyramine in susceptible individuals |
| Auriculo-temporal syndrome (Freye syndrome) | Facial flush in trigeminal nerve distribution associated with spicy foods | Neurogenic reflex, frequently associated with birth trauma to trigeminal nerve (forceps delivery) |
| Gustatory rhinitis | Profuse watery rhinorrhea associated with spicy foods | Neurogenic reflex |
| Panic disorder | Subjective reactions, fainting upon smelling or seeing the food | Psychologic |
| Anorexia nervosa | Reactions to multiple foods, weight loss | Psychologic |
| Allergy to contaminants in foods | Hives, pruritus, angioedema, coughing, vomiting | IgE-mediated reactions to dust mites and molds contaminating flour, *Anisakis* parasite in fish |

allergy, estimated at about 35% [3]. The most common food allergens in the pediatric population include cow's milk, eggs, peanuts, tree nuts, soy, wheat, fish, and shellfish, whereas peanuts, tree nuts, fish, and shellfish predominate in adults. Recent studies report doubling of peanut allergy in young children. A 5-year follow-up study of peanut and tree nut allergy using a random-digit dial telephone survey found that, in comparison with the 0.4% prevalence of peanut allergy in American children aged 5 years or younger in 1997, there was an increase to 0.8% in 2002 [4]. Similarly, results reported from the Isle of Wight in the United Kingdom indicate a doubling of clinical peanut allergy and a tripling of IgE peanut sensitization in young children over a period of 10 years [5].

Food allergy remains the leading single cause of anaphylaxis outside the hospital, and an increasing trend has been noted in recent years [6,7]. In addition, there has been a significant increase in reports of eosinophilic gastroenteropathies, such as allergic eosinophilic esophagitis and allergic eosinophilic gastroenteritis, which are due to dietary food protein hypersensitivity in a subset of patients [8,9]. Finally, it has recently been appreciated that as many as 50% of episodes of gastroesophageal reflux in infants younger than 1 year are caused by hypersensitivity to dietary food proteins, primarily cow's milk and soybean [10].

The reasons for the increase in food allergy prevalence are not known, but, considering the short period over which the change occurred, environmental factors are clearly more relevant than genetic factors [11]. The hygiene hypothesis has been proposed as an explanation for the increase in prevalence of all allergic diseases and may also apply to food allergy. The hygiene hypothesis postulates that decreased early life-exposures to immunomodulatory factors, such as certain viral infections and endotoxins, may be responsible for the increasing prevalence of allergic disorders, including asthma, allergic rhinitis (AR), and food allergy [12]. It is likely that additional factors play an important role, such as early introduction of solid foods into infants' diets, diversification of diet to include a variety of tree nuts, seeds, and fish, propagation of peanut/peanut butter as a healthy nutritional supplement for pregnant and lactating women and young children, and alternative, noningestion routes of sensitization resulting from application of skin care products that contain food allergens (eg, peanut oil, milk protein) [1,13,14].

Recent reports demonstrate development of food–IgE antibodies and clinical reactivity in mice and in adult patients receiving medications that lower gastric pH [15,16]. These findings highlight a possibility that liberal use of antacids may contribute to development of hypersensitivity reactions to foods, because reduced protein digestion in the stomach results in increased food protein allergenicity, both in pediatric and adult patients.

**Pathophysiology**

Immaturity of the immune system and gastrointestinal tract predisposes young infants to food allergy. Compared with older children and adults, infants and young children have an immature glycocalyx, decreased gastric acidity, and decreased intestinal and pancreatic enzyme activity [17]. The intestinal permeability is increased, resulting in higher concentrations of intact food proteins in the circulation and most likely leading to stimulation of the immune system and development of IgE-sensitization [17]. The mucosal immune response is immature; surface secretory IgA concentration is lower, but T-lymphocyte reactivity to food proteins is increased. Early introduction of food allergens has been shown to stimulate IgE antibody production [18] and induce allergic conditions in predisposed infants [19]. Impaired mucosal gut barrier together with the resulting increased intestinal permeability has been proposed as an important factor contributing to the development of food allergy in infants and young children. During the first 2 years of life, gradual maturation of the intestinal barrier corresponds to decreased prevalence of food allergy and may be associated with the process of outgrowing food allergy [17].

Even in the mature gut, about 2% of ingested food allergens are absorbed and transported throughout the body in an immunologically intact form [20,21]. However, in most individuals these food proteins do not cause clinical symptoms because of oral tolerance—the physiologic mucosal immune response to soluble antigens such as those in foods, resulting in a state of unresponsiveness. Oral tolerance is hypothesized to result from T-cell anergy or induction of regulatory T cells. Intestinal epithelial cells act as nonprofessional antigen-presenting cells and induce tolerance [22,23]. In addition, intestinal dendritic cells express interleukin (IL)-10 and IL-4, which favor the generation of tolerance in vivo. The regulatory T cells that are potent sources of tumor growth factor-β (TGF-β) are generated in mucosal lymphoid tissue in response to low-dose antigen. The gut flora are also believed to play a significant role in the induction of normal mucosal immunity, because animals raised in a germ-free environment fail to develop normal tolerance [24]. Childhood food allergy therefore may be viewed as a failure to develop oral tolerance in the setting of immature gastrointestinal and immune systems.

When immune tolerance fails, sensitization to ingested food allergens occurs. In genetically predisposed, atopic individuals, sensitization leads to the generation of allergic IgE antibodies that facilitate immediate reactions, such as food-induced anaphylaxis, urticaria, angioedema, bronchospasm, or gastrointestinal symptoms of emesis and diarrhea. In others, allergic sensitization affects primarily T lymphocytes without generation of IgE antibody. Such non-IgE, cell-mediated food allergic disorders are represented by allergic proctocolitis and food protein-induced enterocolitis syndrome. Atopic dermatitis and allergic eosinophilic gastroenteritis are examples of disorders with mixed mechanism, in which both IgE antibody and cell immunity may play a role [25].

## Characterization of food allergens

In spite of the tremendous diversity of the human diet, a few foods account for the majority of food allergies. In the United States, milk, egg, peanut, wheat, and soybean are the most common culprits in children, whereas peanut, tree nuts, fish, and shellfish are the most common culprits in adults [25]. Raw fruits and vegetables are responsible for the oral allergy syndrome that affects approximately 50% of adults with rhinitis caused by birch pollen [26]. Modern diets that routinely include exotic foods as well as a variety of fresh fruits and vegetables have resulted in an increase in allergic reactions to fruits, such as kiwi and papaya, and seeds, such as sesame, poppy, mustard, and rape (canola).

Traditional or class 1 food allergens induce allergic sensitization by way of the gastrointestinal tract and are responsible for systemic reactions (traditional or class 1 food allergy). Type 1 food allergens are typically heat- and low pH–stable, water-soluble glycoproteins ranging in size from 10 to 70 kD. Type 2 food allergens are heat-labile and susceptible to digestion. Type 2 food allergens are highly homologous with proteins in pollens, and sensitization occurs in the respiratory tract as a consequence of sensitization to the cross-reactive pollen allergens (oral allergy syndrome or class 2 food allergy). Cooking can reduce the allergenicity of fruits and vegetables responsible for the oral allergy syndrome, or that of raw or undercooked egg and fish, by destroying heat-labile conformational allergenic epitopes. In contrast, high temperatures (eg, roasting) may increase allergenicity of certain allergens, such as peanut, through the induction of covalent binding that leads to new antigens or improved stability.

## Clinical food allergic disorders

Food allergic disorders may be classified based on the role of IgE antibody as IgE-mediated, non-IgE, cell-mediated, or mixed, IgE- and cell-mediated (Table 2).

IgE-mediated food allergy reactions typically start within minutes to 1 hour (rarely past 2 hours) and may affect skin (urticaria, angioedema, morbilliform eruptions, flushing, pruritus), the respiratory tract (sneezing, rhinorrhea, congestion, cough, wheezing, difficulty breathing), and the gastrointestinal tract (oral allergy syndrome, nausea, vomiting, diarrhea, cramping abdominal pain). Generalized reactions involving the cardiovascular system (tachycardia, hypotension) are called anaphylactic shock. Mixed and cell-mediated mechanisms typically have delayed onset of symptoms (>2 hours) and a chronic, relapsing course.

### Food-induced anaphylaxis

Anaphylaxis represents the most severe form of IgE-mediated food allergy and is clinically defined as a food-allergic reaction involving two or more organ systems [27]. In extremely sensitive individuals, reactions may be triggered by minute amounts of food proteins [28]. Symptoms start within seconds to 2 hours following allergen ingestion and include feelings of impending doom, throat tightness, coughing or wheezing, abdominal pain, vomiting, diarrhea, and loss of consciousness. Cutaneous symptoms of flushing, urticaria, and angioedema are present in most anaphylactic reactions; however, the most rapidly progressive anaphylaxis may involve no cutaneous manifestations.

Risk factors for fatal anaphylaxis in teenagers and young adults include allergy to peanut, asthma of any severity, and delayed administration of epinephrine [6]. Anaphylaxis may have a biphasic course in as many as 20% to

Table 2
Food allergy disorders

| Disorder | IgE-mediated | Mixed mechanism:<br>IgE- and cell-mediated | Non–IgE-mediated |
|---|---|---|---|
| Generalized | Anaphylactic shock, food-dependent exercise-induced anaphylaxis | — | — |
| Cutaneous | Urticaria, angioedema, flushing, morbilliform rash, acute contact urticaria | Atopic dermatitis, contact dermatitis | Dermatitis herpetiformis |
| Gastrointestinal | Oral allergy syndrome, immediate gastrointestinal food allergy | Allergic eosinophilic esophagitis, allergic eosinophilic gastroenteritis | Allergic proctocolitis, food protein-induced enterocolitis syndrome, celiac disease, infantile colic |
| Respiratory | Acute rhinoconjunctivitis, bronchospasm | Asthma | Pulmonary hemosiderosis (Heiner's syndrome) |

25% of cases, with initial improvement with or without treatment followed by recurrence of severe symptoms within 1 to 2 hours. Severity of late symptoms cannot be predicted based on the early symptoms—for instance, mild early symptoms may be followed by anaphylactic shock. Given this potential for late-phase reactions, an observation period of at least 4 hours following a reaction is recommended. Rarely, anaphylaxis may have a protracted course, with symptoms lasting for days [28]. Peanut, tree nuts (eg, almond, cashew, hazelnut, pecan, and walnut), fish, and shellfish are most often responsible for food-induced anaphylaxis (Box 1).

Food-dependent, exercise-induced anaphylaxis (FDEIA) has been reported in young, athletic individuals (especially women in late teens to mid-30s) and occurs in two forms: anaphylaxis may occur when exercise follows the ingestion of a particular food to which IgE-sensitivity can be identified (eg, wheat, shellfish, fish, celery) or, less commonly, 2 to 4 hours after the ingestion of any food (postprandial anaphylaxis). Affected patients frequently identify hot and humid weather as an additional factor. Ingestion of the incriminated food or exercise alone does not provoke symptoms, although occasionally patients have a history of reacting to the food when they were younger. Patients generally (60%) have asthma and other atopic disorders. The pathogenesis of FDEIA is not known. In the case of wheat FDEIA, the putative mechanism may involve reduced splanchnic blood flow, resulting in transient intestinal ischemia and increased intestinal permeability, with subsequent activation of tissue transglutaminase and formation of high-molecular-weight complexes of ω-5 gliadin (an alcohol-soluble fraction of gluten) that have increased allergenicity. An alternative (or additional) pathway of tissue transglutaminase activation might involve exercise-

> **Box 1. Key points about food-induced anaphylaxis**
>
> - IgE-mediated massive release of mediators affecting two or more target organ systems
> - Flushing, pruritus, generalized urticaria and angioedema, rhinitis, throat tightness/swelling, dyspnea, cough, wheezing, vomiting, cramping abdominal pain, uterine contractions, hypotension, shock, collapse, metallic taste in mouth, feeling of impending doom
> - In approximately 20% to 30% of food-anaphylactic episodes, symptoms recur within 2 to 4 hours (biphasic anaphylaxis); rarely, prolonged reactions may last for a few days.
> - An estimated 200 people die in the United States each year from food anaphylaxis; food anaphylaxis is responsible for an estimated 30,000 emergency room visits every year.
> - Risk factors: asthma, age (late teen to young adult), peanut and tree nut allergy, no treatment or delayed treatment with epinephrine

induced generation of cytokines (IL-6, IL-1β, tumor necrosis factor–α [TNF-α]), hormones (cortisol, growth hormone), reactive oxygen species, and catecholamines [29]. Management involves avoiding exercise or any intense physical activity for 4 to 6 hours following a meal of the incriminated food, carrying emergency medication (EpiPen, cetirizine, or diphenhydramine), exercising with a partner, wearing a Medic Alert bracelet, and avoiding exercise in hot and humid weather.

## Cutaneous food allergic disorders

### IgE-mediated cutaneous food allergy disorders

Acute urticaria and angioedema are the most common manifestations of acute allergic reactions to ingested foods in children and adults. Onset of symptoms may be rapid, within minutes of ingesting the responsible food. Skin involvement may be isolated or associated with other organ systems in food anaphylaxis. Acute IgE-mediated urticaria can be induced by skin contact with cow's milk, raw egg white, raw meats, fish, vegetables, and fruits. Skin contact reactions are typically local in nature, but contact with oral mucous membranes (eg, kissing) or conjunctiva (eg, eye rubbing) may lead to generalized reactions [30,31]. Chronic urticaria (symptoms lasting longer than 6 weeks) is rarely caused by food allergy (Table 3).

### Mixed IgE-mediated and cell-mediated cutaneous food allergy disorders

Food allergy is frequently seen in children with atopic dermatitis (AD) but infrequently in adults. AD is a chronic inflammatory disease of the

Table 3
Cutaneous food allergic disorders

| Disorder | Age group | Characteristics | Diagnosis | Prognosis/course |
|---|---|---|---|---|
| *IgE-mediated* | | | | |
| Acute urticaria and angioedema | Any | Pruritic, evanescent skin rash (hives) and swelling within minutes to 2 h after food ingestion; food identified as a culprit in 20% | History, positive PST, and/or serum food-IgE; confirmed by OFC if necessary | Variable, food-dependent; milk, soy, egg, and wheat typically outgrown; peanut, tree nuts, seeds, and shellfish typically persistent |
| Chronic urticaria and angioedema | Any | Hives and swelling on and for > 6 wk; only 2% caused by food | History, positive PST, and/or serum food-IgE; confirmed by OFC if necessary | Variable |
| *IgE and cell-mediated* | | | | |
| Atopic dermatitis | Infant and child; 90% start < 5 y | Relapsing pruritic vesiculo-papular rash; generalized in infants, localized to flexor areas in older children; food allergy in 35% of children with moderate–severe AD | History, PST, and/or serum food-IgE, elimination diet and OFC | 60%–80% improve significantly or resolve by adolescence |
| *Cell-mediated* | | | | |
| Contact dermatitis | Any; more common in adults | Relapsing pruritic eczematous rash, frequently on hands or face; often in occupational contact with food stuff | History, patch testing | Variable |
| Dermatitis herpetiformis | Any | Intensely pruritic vasicular rash on extensor surfaces and buttocks | Biopsy diagnostic: IgA granule deposits at the dermo-epidermal junction; resolves with dietary gluten avoidance | Life-long |

skin characterized by marked pruritus and a remitting and relapsing course. The vesiculopapular rash of AD has a typical distribution, with generalized involvement in infants and young children and localization to flexural areas in older children. AD starts before age 5 years in more than 95% of patients. In a study of 63 children with moderate to severe AD referred to a pediatric dermatologist in a tertiary medical center who underwent 1613 double-blind, placebo-controlled food challenges, 37% of patients were allergic to at least one food [3]. In the presence of extensive chronic eczematous skin lesions, acute skin symptoms are not easily appreciated, and identification of the responsible food allergen is notoriously difficult, if not impossible. However, following a 2-week strict dietary elimination period, reintroduction of the causative food results in clear-cut, immediate cutaneous reactions. In some adults with birch pollen sensitivity, ingestion of birch pollen–related foods (eg, apple, carrot, celery) causes immediate or late eczematous reactions or both [32,33]. Strict elimination of the causative food allergen results in significant improvement in dermatitis (Box 2) [3,34].

*Gastrointestinal food allergic disorders*

*IgE-mediated gastrointestinal food allergy*
  Gastrointestinal anaphylaxis (immediate gastrointestinal hypersensitivity) is an IgE-mediated gastrointestinal reaction that frequently accompanies

---

**Box 2. Key points about food allergy in atopic dermatitis**

- Approximately 35% to 40% of children with moderate–severe persistent AD refractory to medical treatment have food allergy; food allergy is uncommon in adult-onset AD.
- Egg is the single most common allergen in children with AD; egg, milk, and peanut account for about 80% of food allergy in children with AD; more than 30% of children are allergic to more than one food.
- Extremely pruritic papulo-vesicular rash that waxes and wanes
- Difficult to identify offending foods in chronic AD based on history
- Avoidance of the food for 2 weeks and reintroduction under supervision results in acute skin reactions that may be accompanied by respiratory and/or gastrointestinal symptoms.
- Removal of the offending foods from diet results in significant improvement of skin rash in most children with AD.
- Most children improve by teenage years; many grow into respiratory allergy: ~50% risk in children with AD and egg allergy

allergic manifestations in other target organs (eg, skin and lungs) and presents with a variety of symptoms, including oral pruritus, nausea, abdominal pain, colic, vomiting, and diarrhea (Table 4) [25].

*Oral allergy syndrome*

Oral allergy syndrome (OAS) is a form of contact allergy to raw fruits and vegetables that is confined to the oropharyngeal mucous membranes and affects subjects allergic to pollens such as birch (apple, cherry, peach, carrot), grass (tomato, kiwi), ragweed (melon, banana, tomato), and mugwort (carrot, celery) (Box 3) [35]. OAS affects approximately 50% of pollen-allergic adults and represents the most common adult food allergy. It results from the cross-reactivity between the allergenic proteins in the pollens and plant foods [26]. Local IgE-mediated mast cell activation provokes the rapid onset of pruritus, tingling, and angioedema of the lips, tongue, palate, and throat, occasionally accompanied by a sensation of pruritus in the ears, tightness in the throat, or both. These symptoms resolve promptly when the food is swallowed or removed. Patients typically tolerate cooked or baked forms of fruits and vegetables in which unstable allergens are destroyed by high temperature. Symptoms of OAS are typically mild, but in a small subset of patients, allergy to fruits and vegetables may progress to systemic reactions [36]. Risk factors for systemic reaction are not well delineated but may involve sensitization to heat-stable and protease-resistant lipid transfer proteins and storage proteins, such as globulins (7S and 11S) and albumins (2S). Other possible risk factors include lack of pollen allergy, peach hypersensitivity, positive allergy tests with commercial extracts (64% rate of systemic reaction versus 6%; $P < .001$), history of systemic reaction to one of the related foods, and reactions to cooked foods.

*Mixed IgE- and cell-mediated gastrointestinal food allergy disorders*

Allergic eosinophilic esophagitis (AEE) and gastroenteritis (AEG) are characterized by infiltration of the gastrointestinal tract with eosinophils, basal zone hyperplasia, papillary elongation, and absence of vasculitis. The eosinophilic infiltrates may involve the mucosal, vascular, or serosal layers of the esophagus, stomach, or small intestine. The underlying pathophysiology of these disorders is poorly understood, but both T-lymphocyte and food-specific IgE antibody are implicated. Clinical symptoms correlate with the extent of eosinophilic infiltration of the bowel wall [9]. AEE is seen most frequently in infants, children, and adolescents and presents with symptoms of gastroesophageal reflux, such as nausea, dysphagia, emesis, and epigastric pain, that fail to resolve with standard antireflux therapy. Patients typically have a negative pH probe; on esophageal biopsy, more than 10 to 20 eosinophils per $40\times$ high-power field are seen [8]. AEG may occur at any age, including early infancy, and failure to thrive is common. In young infants, AEG may cause gastric outlet obstruction with pyloric stenosis. Patients also present with abdominal pain, emesis, diarrhea, blood loss in the stool, anemia, and protein-losing gastroenteropathy [37].

As many as 50% of patients with these eosinophilic disorders are atopic and have detectable IgE sensitization to food allergens (by prick skin test [PST] or radioallergosorbent test [RAST]). However, food-induced IgE-mediated immediate reactions are uncommon. Furthermore, results of PST and RAST correlate poorly with clinical response to elimination of the food and thus must be interpreted with caution. Resolution of symptoms typically occurs within 3 to 8 weeks following the elimination of the responsible food allergen (frequently multiple foods, most commonly cow's milk, soy, wheat, and egg). Because patients who have AEE and AEG may be sensitive to trace amounts of the offending foods in the diet, and testing may fail to identify all relevant food allergens, an elemental diet based on an amino acid formula may be needed to achieve improvement (Box 4) [38–40].

*Non–IgE-mediated gastrointestinal food allergy disorders*

Allergic proctocolitis typically starts in the first few months of life, with blood-streaked stools in otherwise healthy-looking infants, and is considered a major cause of colitis before age 1 year; more than 50% of infants in published reports are exclusively breastfed [41]. Food protein-induced proctocolitis typically presents in the first 4 months of life, usually at 1 to 4 weeks of age, with intermittent blood-streaked normal to moderately loose stools. Pathologic findings are limited to the colon and include focal acute inflammation with epithelial erosions and eosinophilic infiltration of the lamina propria, the epithelium, and lamina muscularis. After 9 to 12 months of age, the infants typically tolerate an unrestricted diet.

Food protein-induced enterocolitis syndrome (FPIES) is most frequently seen in young infants who present with irritability, protracted vomiting, and diarrhea [42,43]. Twenty percent of cases may result in shock, presumably due to intense intestinal inflammation leading to third-spacing and intravascular volume depletion. Vomiting generally occurs 1 to 3 hours after feeding, but continued exposure may result in bloody diarrhea, anemia, abdominal distention, and failure to thrive. FPIES is most frequently due to cow's milk and soy, but other foods, such as grains (rice, oat), meats (turkey, chicken), and vegetables (pea), have also been reported [44,45]. Breast-feeding appears to have a protective effect [45]. The pathophysiology of FPIES may involve depressed TGF-β expression in intestinal mucosa and increased secretion of TNF- α by circulating milk-specific T cells, resulting in increased intestinal permeability [46–48].

Celiac disease (CD) is a dietary protein enteropathy characterized by an extensive loss of absorptive villi and hyperplasia of the crypts; it leads to malabsorption, chronic diarrhea, steatorrhea, abdominal distention, flatulence, and weight loss or failure to thrive [49]. Oral ulcers and a linear papular, intensely pruritic rash of dermatitis herpetiformis may occur, occasionally in the absence of gastrointestinal symptoms. Patients who

Table 4
Gastrointestinal food allergic disorders

| Disorder | Age group | Characteristics | Diagnosis | Prognosis/course |
|---|---|---|---|---|
| *IgE-mediated* | | | | |
| Gastrointestinal anaphylaxis | Any | Onset: minutes to 2 h; nausea, abdominal pain, emesis, diarrhea; typically in concert with cutaneous and/or respiratory manifestations | History, positive PST and/or serum food-IgE; confirmatory OFC | Variable, food-dependent; milk, soy, egg, and wheat typically outgrown; peanut, tree nuts, seeds, and shellfish typically persistent |
| Oral allergy syndrome (pollen-food allergy syndrome) | Any; most common in young adults (50% of birch pollen adults) | Immediate symptoms on contact of the raw fruit with oral mucosa: pruritus, tingling, erythema or angioedema of the lips, tongue, oropharynx, throat itching/tightness | History, positive prick-prick skin test with raw fruits and vegetables; OFC positive with raw fruit, negative with cooked | Severity of symptoms may vary with pollen season; may be treated with pollen immunotherapy in a subset of patients |
| *IgE and/or cell-mediated* | | | | |
| Allergic eosinophilic esophagitis | Infants, children, adolescents | Chronic/intermittent symptoms of gastroesophageal reflux, emesis, dysphagia, abdominal pain, irritability | History; positive PST and or food-IgE in 50%, but poor correlation with clinical symptoms; patch testing may be of value; elimination diet and OFC; endoscopy, biopsy provides conclusive diagnosis | Variable, not well-established, improvement with elimination diet within 6–8 wk; elemental diet may be required |
| Allergic eosinophilic gastroenteritis | Any | Chronic/intermittent abdominal pain, emesis, irritability, poor appetite, failure to thrive, weight loss, anemia, protein-losing gastroenteropathy | History, positive PST and/or food-IgE in 50%, but poor correlation with clinical symptoms, elimination diet and OFC; endoscopy, biopsy provides conclusive diagnosis | Variable, not well-established, improvement with elimination diet within 6–8 wk; elemental diet may be required |

*Cell-mediated*

| Disorder | Population | Clinical features | Diagnosis | Prognosis |
|---|---|---|---|---|
| Allergic proctocolitis | Young infants (< 6 mo), frequently breast-fed | Blood-streaked stools, otherwise healthy-appearing | History; prompt response (resolution of gross blood in 48 h) to elimination of milk or soy or switching to casein hydrolysate formula; biopsy conclusive but not necessary in vast majority | Majority able to tolerate milk/soy by first year of age |
| Food protein-induced enterocolitis syndrome | Young infants | Chronic emesis, diarrhea, failure to thrive on chronic exposure; upon re-exposure following a period of elimination: subacute, repetitive emesis, dehydration (15% shock), diarrhea; breast-feeding protective | History; response to dietary restriction; OFC | Most resolve in 1–3 y |
| Celiac disease (gluten-sensitive enteropathy) | Any | Chronic diarrhea, malabsorption, abdominal distension, flatulence, failure to thrive or weight loss, may be associated with oral ulcers and/or dermatitits herpetiformis | Biopsy diagnostic: villus atrophy; screening with serum IgA antibodies against tissue transglutaminase and gliadin; resolution of symptoms with gluten avoidance and relapse on oral challenge | Life-long |

---

**Box 3. Patterns of pollen–fruit and vegetable cross-reactivity**

*Birch*
  Apple, peach, plum, nectarine, cherry, almond, hazelnut,
    and carrot
  Celery
  Hazelnut

*Ragweed*
  Melons (watermelon, cantaloupe, and honeyduew)
  Banana
  Tomato

*Grasses*
  Tomato
  Melons
  Kiwi

*Mugwort (weed)*
  Carrot
  Celery
  Spices

---

**Box 4. Key points about food-allergy allergic eosinophilic gastrointestinal disorders**

- Diagnosis of AEE and AEG is established by endoscopy and biopsy.
- Food allergy affects > 50% of patients; > 50% of patients are atopic.
- Food PST and RAST correlate poorly with clinical response to elimination diet; relevant foods may be negative.
- Most common foods implicated in AEE and AEG are milk, soy, egg, and wheat.
- Elimination of the offending food(s) results in improvement in 3 to 6 weeks; repeat biopsy helpful in confirming resolution of eosinophilic inflammation
- Elemental diet based on an amino-acid formula may be necessary for initial improvement, with subsequent gradual introduction of foods, one food every 2 weeks, starting with fruits and vegetables.

have CD are permanently sensitive to gliadin, the alcohol-soluble portion of gluten found in wheat, rye, and barley. Symptoms of CD resolve completely with exclusion of gluten from the diet but recur when gluten is reintroduced. CD is associated with human leukocyte antigen (HLA)-DQ2 and HLA-DQ8 and affects as many as 1% of some white populations. CD is diagnosed by intestinal biopsy showing classic villus atrophy; serologic ELISA tests detecting IgA antibodies to tissue transglutaminase have a sensitivity of 92% to 98% and are a useful screening tool. Biopsy and serologic tests may be falsely negative when taken during gluten elimination; hence testing for CD is only conclusive when the patient ingests gluten on a regular basis for at least several weeks [2–4].

*Respiratory food allergic disorders*

Upper respiratory symptoms (allergic rhinoconjunctivitis) and lower respiratory symptoms (bronchospasm and asthma) have been frequently reported in blinded food challenges, but isolated respiratory symptoms without any cutaneous or gastrointestinal symptoms appear rare [50]. Acute bronchospasm is a feature of severe food-induced anaphylaxis, but airway hyperreactivity and worsening of asthma have been documented in children undergoing oral food challenge and exhibiting milder reactions [51]. Food allergy has been identified as a risk factor for severe asthma requiring intubation in children and adolescents [52]. Inhalation of food particles may induce asthmatic reactions: reactions to exposures to peanut dust on an airplane and vapors or steam from cooking fish have been well documented, as have reactions to occupational exposure to grains and aerosolized egg white in bakery workers [53–56]. In highly allergic individuals, inhalation of trace amounts of food particles may lead to systemic reactions (Table 5) [57].

**Food allergic disorders in adults**

Adult food allergy may represent persistence from childhood (as commonly seen with peanut or tree nuts) or de novo development at an older age. New onset of food allergy has been reported in the setting of heavy occupational exposure by skin contact or inhalation in bakers (wheat, egg), crab processing workers, and harbor workers unloading soybean. In many individuals, reactions are limited to asthma caused by inhalation of food particles, but in some subsequent systemic reactions to ingestion of egg ensue (so-called "egg-egg" syndrome) [58]. Increasingly, adult food allergy is recognized as a consequence of cross-reactivity between respiratory and food allergens. The implicated panallergens are typically highly conserved proteins, such as pathogenesis-related proteins, structural proteins (profilin, tropomyosin), and albumins. Examples include OAS to fresh fruits and vegetables in as many as 50% of pollen-allergic adults, OAS and rare systemic reactions to soy, peanut, and hazelnut in birch pollen–allergic adults, and

Table 5
Respiratory food allergic disorders

| Disorder | Age group | Characteristics | Diagnosis | Prognosis/course |
|---|---|---|---|---|
| *IgE-mediated* | | | | |
| Allergic rhinoconjuctivitis | Any | Ocular pruritis, conjunctival injection and watery discharge, nasal pruritis, congestion, rhinorrhea, sneezing within minutes to 2 h following food ingestion or inhalation; often associated with cutaneous and gastrointestinal manifestations | History, PST, and/or serum food-IgE; OFC | Variable |
| Acute bronchospasm | Any | Cough, wheezing, dyspnea upon ingestion or inhalation of food; may be a risk factor for severe anaphylaxis | History, PST, and/or serum food-IgE; OFC | Variable |
| *IgE- and cell-mediated* | | | | |
| Asthma | Any | Chronic cough, wheezing, dyspnea; food allergy is a risk factor for intubation in children who have asthma | History, PST, and/or serum food-IgE; OFC | Variable |
| *IgG-/cell-mediated (presumed)* | | | | |
| Pulmonary hemosiderosis (Heiner's syndrome) | Infants, children (rare) | Chronic cough, hemoptysis, lung infiltrates, wheezing, anemia; described in cow's milk and buckwheat-allergic infants | History, PST, and serum food-IgE–negative, but milk and buckwheat IgG precipitins positive; lung biopsy with deposits of IgG and IgA | Unknown |

allergy to egg in people exposed to birds (so-called "bird-egg" syndrome) [58]. Immunologic cross-reactivity is also the basis of the allergy to fruits and vegetables (avocado, chestnut, banana, kiwi, papaya, fig, melon, passion fruit, pineapple, peach, and tomato) affecting 35% to 50% of latex-allergic individuals. Exercise and ingestion of alcohol or aspirin have been reported to trigger food allergic reactions in some individuals who otherwise can ingest problematic foods without reactions [59]. Most of these patients are atopic, and some have distant history of a childhood food allergy. Adults receiving antiacid medications have been reported to develop IgE-sensitization and clinical reactions to ingestion of hazelnut [15,16].

Allergic eosinophilic gastroenteropathies such as AEE and AEG are being diagnosed more frequently, in part as a result of increased awareness among adult gastroenterologists that significant mucosal inflammation may occur in the absence of visual endoscopic findings and of the increased frequency with which biopsies are obtained. AEE in particular has become widely accepted as a significant cause of dysphagia in adolescents and adults and should be considered in all patients who present with symptoms of gastroesophageal reflux symptoms unresponsive to antiacids. AEE should also be suspected in any patient with dysphagia and esophageal structures that are recognized as complications of the long-term eosinophilic allergic inflammation. Box 5 summarizes the key points about food allergy in adults.

## Diagnosis of food allergic disorders

Taking a careful medical history is the first step to establishing food allergy diagnosis. However, history needs to be validated by laboratory tests

---

**Box 5. Key points about food allergy in adulthood**

- Estimated prevalence: 2% to 4%
- Most common food allergens: peanut, tree nuts, shellfish, fish, fruits, and vegetables
- Factors predisposing to development of food allergy: heavy occupational exposure, latex allergy, birch pollen allergy; in selected patients, concurrent ingestion of alcohol or aspirin or exercise within 2 to 4 hours following a meal
- Management relies on avoidance; in case of multiple food restrictions, elemental formulas may be necessary.
- Young adults with IgE-mediated allergy to peanut and tree nuts are at high risk for severe anaphylaxis.
- Special considerations in patients with cardiovascular conditions: judicious use of epinephrine of utmost importance because of high risk for stroke or myocardial infarction; diminished efficacy of epinephrine seen in patients treated with β-blockers.
- AEE should be suspected in individuals with gastroesophageal reflux unresponsive to acid blockade and those with dysphagia and esophageal strictures.

and oral food challenges, especially in chronic disorders such as atopic dermatitis and AEG, in which symptoms wax and wane. In such remitting and relapsing disorders, accurate identification of the offending food is particularly difficult and sometimes impossible [3]. A food intake diary may be helpful in tracing the reactions and foods that might have caused them. Dietary elimination of the suspected foods may be helpful. However, it should be followed by reintroduction of the food, because in some patients symptoms improve with dietary restriction and do not recur on reintroduction of the suspected food. A general approach to food allergy diagnosis and management is presented in Fig. 1.

*Prick skin tests*

Well-standardized diagnostic tests are available for IgE-mediated food allergy disorders. PST is a bioassay in which a minuscule amount of food allergen is introduced into the skin by gently disrupting the integrity of the outer skin by scratching, puncturing, or pricking with a special bifurcated needle or lancet or multiprong plastic device. Intradermal skin testing should not be used for diagnosis of food allergy because of the risk of systemic reaction and high rate of false-positive results. In a sensitized individual, food allergen binds to specific IgE antibody present on the surface of the mast cells in the skin and causes degranulation of mast cells. Histamine released from mast cells leads to a flare (erythema) and wheal response within 10 to 15 minutes. PST with commercial food allergen extract has a high negative predictive value (>95%), whereas a positive skin test has only a 30% to 40% positive predictive value. However, in infants and young children, a large PST wheal (mean size 8 to 10 mm) is associated with greater than 95% likelihood of clinical reactivity to cow's milk, egg, and peanut [60]. In patients with OAS caused by raw fruits and vegetables, testing with raw fruit is typically more sensitive than testing with the commercial extract of fruit, because the responsible allergens are very unstable and disintegrate during the allergen extraction process. Prick-prick method involves puncturing the fruit through the peel and then puncturing the skin. PST will become more sophisticated and accurate with the availability of recombinant food allergens. Recombinant allergens of high purity offer superior safety and specificity in allergy testing, although diagnostic sensitivity is generally lower than that of allergen extracts. Recombinant allergens may be of special value in diagnosing allergy to plant foods in subjects who have allergy to pollens.

*Laboratory immune assays for detection of food-IgE antibody*

A number of laboratory immune assays (CAP RAST system) have been developed for the detection of free allergen-specific IgE antibody circulating in the bloodstream. These assays have similar performance to skin tests, in that a negative test (specific IgE antibody < 0.35 kIU/L measured by

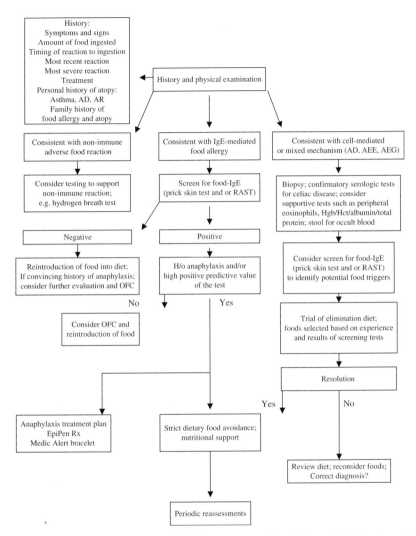

Fig. 1. Schematic approach to diagnosis and management of food allergy. Hgb/Hct, hemoglobin/hematocrit; H/o, history of.

Pharmacia CAP system) has a high negative predictive value (> 95%). The positive predictive value of the CAP system has been evaluated in children undergoing oral food challenges [61,62]. Clinical decision points indicating greater than 95% likelihood of reaction were established for the most common food allergens, including milk, egg, peanut, tree nuts, and fish (Table 6). A child older than 2 years with milk-IgE antibody level of at least 15 kIU/L is highly (> 95%) likely to react during an oral milk challenge, and milk challenge should be deferred unless there is compelling evidence that the child tolerated a significant amount of milk without a reaction. Food-specific IgE

Table 6
Food allergin-specific IgE antibody thresholds of clinical reactivity

| Food | Serum food-IgE (kIU/L) | PPV (%) |
|------|------------------------|---------|
| Milk | 15 | 95 |
|  | 5 if ≤ 1 y | > 95 |
| Eggs | 7 | > 95 |
|  | 2 if ≤ 2 y | > 95 |
| Peanuts | 14 | > 95 |
| Fish | 20 | > 95 |
| Tree nuts | ~15 | > 95 |

*Abbreviation:* PPV, positive predictive value.

antibody levels below the decision points indicate decreasing likelihood of re-action that needs to be determined with oral food challenge.

*Prediction of tolerance development*

Currently available diagnostic methods for food allergy, such as PST and serum food allergen–specific IgE levels, do not distinguish between individuals who will achieve food tolerance and those who will have persistent food allergy. Previous studies aimed at identification of tolerance markers showed that children with long-lasting milk allergy have higher levels of total and milk-specific IgE. Recently, analysis of differences in recognition of allergenic epitopes in peanut-, cow's milk–, and egg-allergic subjects provided new insights into the development of tolerance to these foods. IgE antibodies may be directed at contiguous epitopes composed of sequential amino acids or conformational epitopes composed of amino acid residues from different regions of the allergen brought together by folding of the protein in its native state. Because food allergens are subjected to extensive chemical and proteolytic digestion before absorption and uptake by the cells of the gut-associated lymphoid tissue, it has been suggested that food allergenic epitopes are predominantly sequential in nature. However, it has recently been shown that subjects with transient egg allergy had IgE antibodies predominantly against conformational epitopes of the major egg white allergen, ovomucoid, whereas subjects with persistent allergy developed IgE antibodies against linearized (sequential, reduced, and alkylated) ovomucoid epitopes [63]. Furthermore, cow's milk–, egg-, and peanut-allergic subjects who lacked IgE antibodies against certain sequential epitopes of the major allergens were found to be more likely to achieve tolerance to these foods than subjects whose IgE antibodies were directed against those epitopes. The differences detected in specificity of IgE responses between patients with transient and persistent food allergy may reflect differences in digestion, absorption, or processing of food allergens. Further research focusing on epitope recognition patterns will use microarray technology that allows for automated, cost-effective, and rapid measurements of antibody specificity against multiple epitopes using microliters of patients' sera. The development of markers of persistent food allergy is of tremendous importance because, when therapy for food allergy becomes available, the selection of subjects for therapeutic interventions will be crucial.

## Diagnostic tests for cell-mediated food allergy

PST and measurement of serum food-IgE antibody concentration are not helpful in food allergic disorders with non-IgE, cell-mediated mechanism, such as FPIES, and have limited usefulness in disorders with mixed mechanism, such as AEE and AEG. Recently, patch testing for the diagnosis of food allergy in children who have AD and AEE has been investigated in a number of studies. Patch testing is typically used for diagnosis of delayed contact hypersensitivity reactions in which T cells play a prominent role and involves prolonged contact of the allergenic extract with intact skin under occlusion for 48 hours. The results are evaluated 20 minutes and 72 hours after removing the patch. A positive reaction to patch tests consists of erythema and induration. In children with challenge-proven milk allergy, PST was positive in 67% of cases with acute-onset reactions (under 2 hours) to milk challenge, whereas patch tests tended to be negative [64]. Patch tests were positive in 89% of children with delayed-onset reactions (25–44 hours), although PST was frequently negative. In another study of children with AD, the combination of a positive patch test with evidence of specific IgE or with positive PST had the highest positive predictive value [65]. These results indicate that a combination of patch testing and detection of IgE could enhance the accuracy of diagnosis of food allergy and eliminate the need for oral food challenges. However, before physicians incorporate atopy patch testing into clinical practice, standardization of the reagents, the timing of the results reading, and the scoring system for the interpretation of the results is necessary.

For gastrointestinal food allergy disorders such as AEE and AEG, ultimate diagnosis is established by obtaining a biopsy of the mucosa and finding increased numbers of eosinophils. Noninvasive diagnostic tests are highly desirable, but currently available laboratory techniques offer limited insight into these conditions. Peripheral blood eosinophil numbers may be followed in approximately 50% of subjects with AEE/AEG. Testing stool samples for occult blood may be useful in a subset of patients in whom gastrointestinal inflammation results in microscopic bleeding. Patients who have AEG and protein-losing gastroenteropathy may be followed with serial evaluations of serum albumin, total protein, and immunoglobulins (low IgG with preserved IgM and IgA). Measurements of stool $\alpha$1-antitrypsin may be used to approximate gastrointestinal protein loss.

## Oral food challenges

Oral food challenges (OFC) remain the most accurate method for diagnosing food allergy. OFC may be used for diagnosing IgE-mediated as well as non–IgE-mediated food allergy. OFC may be done to confirm whether the suspected food is indeed causing problems or to determine whether a person with known food allergy might have lost reactivity to food (outgrown food allergy). OFC are particularly useful because IgE antibodies persist after clinical reactivity has cleared. During an oral food challenge for an IgE-mediated food allergy, a premeasured amount of food (typically 8–10 g of dry food or 80–100 mL of liquid food) mixed with a masking food that is well tolerated by the patient is administered in small increments every 10 to 15 minutes over 90 minutes. OFC may be open (ie, both patient and person administering the challenge know which food is administered) or blinded and placebo controlled. In a placebo-controlled challenge, two 90-minute sessions (one with real food, one with placebo food) may be separated by a 90-minute break and completed on a single day, or each session may be done on a separate day. In a single-blind, placebo-controlled food challenge, only the patient is unaware when the real food is administered; in a double-blind, placebo-controlled food challenge, neither the patient nor the person conducting the challenge knows the sequence of real food and placebo. The double-blind, placebo-controlled food challenge is considered the gold standard for diagnosis of food allergy and is preferred in research settings or in patients in whom anxiety may interfere with interpretation of symptoms. Placebo-controlled OFC in which the patient tolerated both sessions without a reaction are always followed by an open challenge, during which a regular portion of food is ingested by the patient over a 30-minute period. OFC are stopped at the first sign of an objective reaction, such as hives, rhinorrhea, sneezing, coughing, or vomiting. Patients are observed for at least 2 hours following completion of an open challenge. In patients who have FPIES, the quantity of food for challenge is calculated as 0.15 to 0.3 g protein per kilogram of body weight (not to exceed 3 g of protein or 10 g of whole food) and administered gradually in three feedings over 45 minutes. If the patient remains symptom-free for 4 hours, a second dose is given, generally a serving amount followed by 2 to 3 hours' observation. OFC are always conducted under physician supervision in a controlled environment with emergency medications (epinephrine, diphenhydramine, methylprednisolone, and volume expanders) immediately available to treat an allergic reaction. Patients who have asthma or a history of severe reactions or who are at higher risk for a positive challenge and all patients with FPIES must have an intravenous line in place before starting a challenge, for immediate vascular access in case of hypotension. Double-blind, placebo-controlled food challenges can be completed during 1 day, or sessions may be conducted on separate days. Patients with AEE or AEG whose food-induced symptoms are delayed and more insidious may require prolonged challenges over several days.

## Management of food allergy

Management of food allergy currently focuses on dietary avoidance of the offending foods, prompt recognition and treatment of food allergic reactions, and nutritional support. Educating patients about how to read food labels is important, because common foods may be labeled using nonintuitive terms. For example, the presence of milk may be indicated as *casein* or *whey*, whereas wheat may be indicated as spelt, bran, farina, or gluten. In addition, *natural flavors* could refer to peanuts, tree nuts, milk, or any other food. Patients commonly make mistakes and are unable correctly to identify the food allergens in store-bought foods; in a recent study, only 7% of parents of children with milk allergy were able correctly to identify products that contained milk, and 22% of parents of children with soy allergy were able correctly to identify products that contained soy [66]. Another impediment faced by food-allergic patients is undisclosed contamination with trace amounts of food resulting from sharing of equipment. Current industry cleaning standards, although stringent, are not sufficient to prevent contamination with trace amounts of food allergens that may trigger severe reactions in highly sensitive food-allergic individuals [67]. This situation is expected to change with the new Food Allergen Labeling and Consumer Protection Law, effective January 1, 2006. The bill requires food manufacturers clearly to state if a product contains any of the eight major food allergens responsible for more than 90% of all allergic reactions: namely, milk, eggs, peanuts, tree nuts, fish, shellfish, wheat, and soy. The new law also requires that the Food and Drug Administration conduct inspections and issue a report within 18 months to ensure that the food manufacturers comply with practices to reduce or eliminate cross-contact of a food with any major food allergens that are not intentional ingredients of the food.

Families of patients with food allergies need information on how to cook foods safely at home and how to handle school, travel, and social situations such as parties and dining. An excellent resource is the Food Allergy and Anaphylaxis Network (www.foodallergy.org), which provides practical advice on dietary avoidance, survival strategies for school, restaurants, and camps, manufacturers' updates, and special support programs for teenagers. The American Partnership for Eosinophilic Disorders Web site (www. apfed.org) contains useful information for patients with eosinophilic gastroenteropathies.

Children who have food allergy, particularly those with multiple food allergies, are at risk for nutritional deficiencies as a result of restricted diets. Nutritional support may be limited to calcium supplementation in children avoiding dairy or may be extensive in children on severely restricted diets. Children allergic to multiple major food allergens are at risk for protein and calorie deficiency and may require a hypoallergenic formula to meet their needs. Hypoallergenic formulas available in the United States are either based on extensively hydrolyzed casein derived from cow's milk (Pregestimil, Nutramigen, Mead Johnson, Alimentum, Ross) or on a mixture of single amino acids (Neocate, SHS, Elecare, Ross). Hypoallergenic formulas are well tolerated by children with IgE-mediated and cell-mediated food allergy [38,40].

In spite of strict avoidance, accidental ingestions and exposures occur, and every food-allergic patient must always be prepared to recognize symptoms and treat food allergic reaction. In children with peanut allergy, 50% reported reactions to peanuts despite avoidance over a 2-year period [68]. Individuals with a history of immediate allergic reactions or anaphylaxis, those with asthma, and those with allergy to foods typically associated with severe reactions (eg, peanut, tree nuts, fish, shellfish) should be prescribed an epinephrine self-injector (EpiPen or EpiPen Jr; Dey, Napa, California). A clear emergency treatment plan indicating symptoms that require treatment with oral antihistamine or epinephrine or both must be provided to the patient by an allergist or primary physician. Templates of anaphylaxis emergency treatment plans may be downloaded from the www.foodallergy.org or www.foodallergyinitiative.org Web sites. Administration of the Epipen should be demonstrated to the patient and the technique reviewed periodically. A single demonstration is not sufficient for most patients [69]. Patients frequently forget to carry their Epipen with them and to check the expiration date. These issues should be reviewed regularly during follow-up visits. Patients must be instructed to seek evaluation in the emergency room following the use of an Epipen. Given the approximately 20% risk of recurrence of allergic symptoms following initial improvement with or without treatment (so-called *biphasic anaphylaxis*), a minimum 4-hour observation period is recommended. Medic Alert bracelets indicating food allergy and specifying the treatment needed in case of a sudden reaction are helpful for older children and adults.

## Future therapy for food allergy

Conventional subcutaneous allergen immunotherapy has been attempted for peanut allergy. In a double-blind, placebo-controlled trial of rush (rapidly increasing doses) peanut immunotherapy, increased tolerance to oral feeding with peanut was observed in four of six patients receiving the active immunotherapy (although two of four could not tolerate maintenance dose) and in none of the six control patients [70]. However, the rate of serious adverse reactions was unacceptably high, even during the maintenance phase of immunotherapy (39%). Birch pollen immunotherapy has been reported to result in resolution or significant diminishment of oral symptoms caused by raw Golden Delicious apple in 49 adult birch-allergic patients in a prospective, nonrandomized, nonblinded clinical trial [71]. Subjects received birch immunotherapy for 12, 24, or 36 months. Forty-one patients (84%) compared with no controls (0%) reported a significant reduction (50% to 95%) or a total clearance (100%) of apple allergy symptoms after immunotherapy (*P* < .001). In a follow-up study, the duration of the effect of birch immunotherapy was evaluated in 30 birch pollen–allergic patients who experienced resolution of apple allergy and loss of skin-test reactivity to fresh apple [72]. More than 50% of patients were still able to tolerate eating apples at the 30-month follow-up visit, although the majority showed evidence of resensitization to apple by PST. These studies strongly suggest that, in a subset of patients with birch pollen AR and oral allergy to apple, birch pollen immunotherapy may produce a long-lasting improvement in OAS.

Recently, a monoclonal IgG antibody against IgE (TNX-901) was tested in subjects older than 12 years who had severe peanut allergy [73]. Following subcutaneous injections of TNX-901, the subjects tolerated significantly greater amounts of peanut protein than those that had provoked symptoms before treatment. Currently, a similar monoclonal anti-IgE antibody, omalizumab, is being evaluated for treatment of peanut anaphylaxis in subjects 6 years and older in a controlled clinical trial. Anti-IgE antibody is the first novel therapy for food allergy undergoing clinical trials in human subjects. Anti-IgE therapy will not cure peanut allergy, but it could protect subjects with extreme peanut allergy who are at risk following the unknowing ingestion of traces of peanut. Other selected approaches to treatment of food allergy are summarized in Table 7.

## Natural history of food allergy

Food allergy to cow's milk and egg is outgrown by most children. Eightyfive percent of milk-allergic children and 66% of egg-allergic children become food tolerant by age 5 years. In contrast, approximately 20% of all children with peanut allergy become peanut tolerant [74]. However, children with peanut-IgE antibody level less than or equal to 5 kIU/L have at least a 50% chance of tolerating peanut [75]. Periodic evaluation should be offered to children with peanut allergy and OFC to peanut should be considered in patients who have not had reactions in the past 1 to 2 years and who have peanut IgE level of less than 5.0 kIU/L. Unlike milk and egg allergy, peanut allergy can recur in children who outgrew it [76]. Risk of recurrence appears to be approximately 10% in children who refuse to eat peanut on a regular basis, compared with no recurrences in children eating peanut regularly [77]. The authors recommend that the possibility of peanut allergy recurrence be discussed before offering OFC to peanut and that patients ingest peanut frequently following a negative OFC. Epipen should be carried until the patient has proved tolerance to multiple ingestions of regular servings of peanut and peanut-containing foods. It appears that tree nuts, seeds, fish, and shellfish are generally not outgrown, similar to peanut. Information regarding the course of food allergy in adults is scarce. In one study, 10 adults with double-blind placebo-controlled food challenge (DBPCFC)-confirmed allergy to 13 foods were followed for 1 to 2 years. On rechallenge, 38% of 13 foods were well tolerated, including milk in two patients and wheat, egg, and tomato in one patient each. The two patients with nut allergy, two patients with milk allergy, and one patient each with potato, garlic, and rice allergy remained reactive [78].

Table 7
Selected promising potential immunomodulatory therapies for food allergy

| Therapy | Mechanism of action | Effects | Comments |
|---|---|---|---|
| Monoclonal anti-IgE antibody | Binds to circulating IgE and prevents IgE deposition on mast cells (blocks mast-cell degranulation and release of the mediators) | Improves symptoms of asthma and allergic rhinitis; possibly protects against food anaphylaxis | Subcutaneous injections at monthly intervals indefinitely; long-term consequences of IgE elimination |
| Anti–IL-5 | Neutralizing antibody against IL-5 | Lowers blood and sputum-eosinophil levels; may lower mucosal eosinophils in EE | In a clinical trial [82] in patients with hypereosinophilic syndrome, anti–IL-5 caused a 10-fold reduction in esophageal eosinophil counts and remarkable clinical improvement in one patient with severe eosinophilic esophagitis |
| Modified peanut immunotherapy | Binding to mast cells eliminated; altered T-cell responses as a result of altering peanut allergenic epitopes by way of site-directed mutagenesis | Protects against peanut anaphylaxis in mice | Improved safety profile compared with conventional immunotherapy; requires identification of IgE binding sites; awaiting FDA approval for stuidies in humans |
| Probiotics | Uknown; possibly increased IgA, IL-10, suppression of TNF-$\alpha$, and inhibition of T-cell activation | Improve severity of atopic dermatitis in infants with milk allergy; prevent development of atopy in at-risk infants | Oral dietary supplement; generally safe and well-tolerated; inexpensive |
| Traditional Chinese medicine | Downregulations of Th2 cytokines (IL-4, IL-5), upregulation of Th1 cytokines (IFN-$\gamma$, IL-12), decreased allergen-IgE | Reverses allergic inflammation in the airways, protects mice from peanut anaphylaxis | Oral; generally safe and well-tolerated; inexpensive |

*Abbreviations:* FDA, US Food and Drug Administration; IFN-$\gamma$, interferon-gamma; IL, interleukin; Th, T-helper cells; TNF-$\alpha$, tumor necrosis factor–alpha.

Food allergy may be viewed as a marker of an atopic predisposition. In many children, food allergy coexists with other atopic conditions, such as AD, asthma, and AR. Sensitization to egg white in children with atopic dermatitis is associated with a 70% risk for respiratory allergic disease (asthma or AR) at age 5 years [79]. Therefore, subjects with past and current food allergy should be considered at high risk for asthma and environmental allergy.

## Prevention of food allergy

Strategies for primary prevention of food allergy have been investigated in a number of studies. Exclusive breastfeeding and introduction of solid foods after 4 to 6 months of age have been associated with decreased risk of AD and cow's milk allergy in infants with an atopic background. If breastfeeding is impossible, formulas with reduced allergenicity, such as extensively hydrolyzed casein formulas or partially hydrolyzed whey formulas, may prevent atopic disease and food allergy [80]. Avoidance of highly allergenic foods (eg, peanut) during pregnancy and breastfeeding has not been shown to have a consistent protective effect. At this time, the American Academy of Pediatrics recommends that in high-risk infants (those with two close relatives—both parents or a parent and a sibling—with atopic disease), breastfeeding or hypoallergenic formula be preferred in the first year of life, solid foods be introduced at age 6 months, and highly allergenic foods, such as peanuts, tree nuts, fish, and shellfish, be delayed until 3 to 4 years of age [81]. Breastfeeding mothers should avoid peanuts and tree nuts in their diets.

## Summary

Food allergy encompasses a variety of immune-mediated adverse reactions to foods. IgE-mediated, cell-mediated, and mixed-mechanism food allergy disorders are recognized. Over the past 2 decades, the prevalence of food allergy doubled and its phenotypic expression increased in Westernized societies. Major food allergens have been identified for many common foods. Laboratory diagnosis of food allergy relies heavily on the detection of food-specific IgE antibodies, but novel approaches include tests for T-cell–mediated disorders and tests for prediction of tolerance. OFC remains the diagnostic standard for food allergy. Management of food allergy focuses on avoidance of the offending foods, nutritional support, and prompt recognition and treatment of acute food allergic reactions. Anti-IgE monoclonal antibody is the first potential therapy for food allergy that is undergoing testing in clinical trials.

## References

[1] Sampson HA. 9. Food allergy. J Allergy Clin Immunol 2003;111(Suppl 2):S540–7.
[2] Munoz-Furlong A, Sampson HA, Sicherer SH. Prevalence of self-reported seafood allergy in the US. J Allergy Clin Immunol 2004;113:S100.

[3] Eigenmann PA, Sicherer SH, Borkowski TA, et al. Prevalence of IgE-mediated food allergy among children with atopic dermatitis. Pediatrics 1998;101(3):E8.

[4] Sicherer SH, Munoz-Furlong A, Sampson HA. Prevalence of peanut and tree nut allergy in the United States determined by means of a random digit dial telephone survey: a 5-year follow-up study. J Allergy Clin Immunol 2003;112(6):1203–7.

[5] Grundy J, Matthews S, Bateman B, et al. Rising prevalence of allergy to peanut in children: data from two sequential cohorts. J Allergy Clin Immunol 2002;110(5):784–9.

[6] Bock SA, Munoz-Furlong A, Sampson HA. Fatalities due to anaphylactic reactions to foods. J Allergy Clin Immunol 2001;107(1):191–3.

[7] Sheikh A, Alves B. Hospital admissions for acute anaphylaxis: time trend study. BMJ 2000; 320(7247):1441.

[8] Rothenberg ME, Mishra A, Collins MH, et al. Pathogenesis and clinical features of eosinophilic esophagitis. J Allergy Clin Immunol 2001;108(6):891–4.

[9] Sampson HA, Anderson JA. Summary and recommendations: classification of gastrointestinal manifestations due to immunologic reactions to foods in infants and young children. J Pediatr Gastroenterol Nutr 2000;30:S87–94.

[10] Salvatore S, Vandenplas Y. Gastroesophageal reflux and cow milk allergy: is there a link? Pediatrics 2002;110(5):972–84.

[11] Sicherer SH, Furlong TJ, Maes HH, et al. Genetics of peanut allergy: a twin study. J Allergy Clin Immunol 2000;106(1 Pt 1):53–6.

[12] Strachan DP. Hay fever, hygiene, and household size. BMJ 1989;299:1259–60.

[13] Lack G, Fox D, Northstone K, et al. Factors associated with the development of peanut allergy in childhood. N Engl J Med 2003;348(11):977–85.

[14] Sampson HA. Clinical practice. Peanut allergy. N Engl J Med 2002;346(17):1294–9.

[15] Untersmayr E, Bakos N, Scholl I, et al. Anti-ulcer drugs promote IgE formation toward dietary antigens in adult patients. FASEB J 2005;19:656–8.

[16] Scholl I, Untersmayr E, Bakos N, et al. Antiulcer drugs promote oral sensitization and hypersensitivity to hazelnut allergens in BALB/c mice and humans. Am J Clin Nutr 2005;81(1): 154–60.

[17] Sampson HA. Food allergy. Part 1: Immunopathogenesis and clinical disorders. J Allergy Clin Immunol 1999;103(5 Pt 1):717–28.

[18] Soothill JF, Stokes CR, Turner MW, et al. Predisposing factors and the development of reaginic allergy in infancy. Clin Allergy 1976;6(4):305–19.

[19] Fergusson DM, Horwood LJ, Shannon FT. Early solid feeding and recurrent childhood eczema: a 10-year longitudinal study. Pediatrics 1990;86(4):541–6.

[20] Husby S. Normal immune responses to ingested foods. J Pediatr Gastroenterol Nutr 2000; 30(Suppl):S13–9.

[21] Husby S, Foged N, Host A, et al. Passage of dietary antigens into the blood of children with coeliac disease. Quantification and size distribution of absorbed antigens. Gut 1987;28(9): 1062–72.

[22] Mayer L. Mucosal immunity and gastrointestinal antigen processing. J Pediatr Gastroenterol Nutr 2000;30(Suppl):S4–S12.

[23] Mayer L, Sperber K, Chan L, et al. Oral tolerance to protein antigens. Allergy 2001;56(Suppl 67):12–5.

[24] Sudo N, Sawamura S, Tanaka K, et al. The requirement of intestinal bacterial flora for the development of an IgE production system fully susceptible to oral tolerance induction. J Immunol 1997;159(4):1739–45.

[25] Sampson HA. Update on food allergy. J Allergy Clin Immunol 2004;113(5):805–19.

[26] Valenta R, Kraft D. Type I allergic reactions to plant-derived food: a consequence of primary sensitization to pollen allergens. J Allergy Clin Immunol 1996;97:895.

[27] Sampson HA. Food anaphylaxis. Br Med Bull 2000;56(4):925–35.

[28] Sampson HA. Food-induced anaphylaxis. Novartis Found Symp 2004;257:161–71.

[29] Palosuo K, Varjonen E, Nurkkala J, et al. Transglutaminase-mediated cross-linking of a peptic fraction of omega-5 gliadin enhances IgE reactivity in wheat-dependent, exercise-induced anaphylaxis. J Allergy Clin Immunol 2003;111(6):1386–92.

[30] Simonte SJ, Ma S, Mofidi S, et al. Relevance of casual contact with peanut butter in children with peanut allergy. J Allergy Clin Immunol 2003;112(1):180–2.

[31] Hallett R, Haapanen LA, Teuber SS. Food allergies and kissing. N Engl J Med 2002;346(23): 1833–4.

[32] Reekers R, Busche M, Wittmann M, et al. Birch pollen–related foods trigger atopic dermatitis in patients with specific cutaneous T-cell responses to birch pollen antigens. J Allergy Clin Immunol 1999;104(2 Pt 1):466–72.

[33] Breuer K, Wulf A, Constien A, et al. Birch pollen–related food as a provocation factor of allergic symptoms in children with atopic eczema/dermatitis syndrome. Allergy 2004;59(9): 988–94.

[34] Sampson HA, McCaskill CC. Food hypersensitivity and atopic dermatitis: evaluation of 113 patients. J Pediatr 1985;107(5):669–75.

[35] Ortolani C, Ispano M, Pastorello E, et al. The oral allergy syndrome. Ann Allergy 1988;61: 47–52.

[36] Ortolani C, Pastorello E, Farioli L, et al. IgE-mediated allergy from vegetable allergens. Ann Allergy 1993;71:470–6.

[37] Rothenberg ME. Eosinophilic gastrointestinal disorders (EGID). J Allergy Clin Immunol 2004;113(1):11–28.

[38] Kelly KJ, Lazenby AJ, Rowe PC, et al. Eosinophilic esophagitis attributed to gastroesophageal reflux: improvement with an amino acid–based formula. Gastroenterology 1995; 109(5):1503–12.

[39] Markowitz JE, Spergel JM, Ruchelli E, et al. Elemental diet is an effective treatment for eosinophilic esophagitis in children and adolescents. Am J Gastroenterol 2003;98(4): 777–82.

[40] Sicherer SH, Noone SA, Koerner CB, et al. Hypoallergenicity and efficacy of an amino acid–based formula in children with cow's milk and multiple food hypersensitivities. J Pediatr 2001;138(5):688–93.

[41] Lake AM, Whitington PF, Hamilton SR. Dietary protein–induced colitis in breast fed infants. J Pediatr 1982;101:906–10.

[42] Powell GK. Milk- and soy- induced enterocolitis of infancy. J Pediatr 1978;93(4):553–60.

[43] Sicherer SH. Food protein–induced enterocolitis syndrome: clinical perspectives. J Pediatr Gastroenterol Nutr 2000;30(Suppl):45–9.

[44] Sicherer SH, Eigenmann PA, Sampson HA. Clinical features of food-protein–induced enterocolitis syndrome. J Pediatr 1998;133(2):214–9.

[45] Nowak-Wegrzyn A, Sampson HA, Wood RA, et al. Food protein–induced enterocolitis syndrome caused by solid food proteins. Pediatrics 2003;111(4 Pt 1):829–35.

[46] Chung HL, Hwang JB, Park JJ, et al. Expression of transforming growth factor beta1, transforming growth factor type I and II receptors, and TNF-alpha in the mucosa of the small intestine in infants with food protein–induced enterocolitis syndrome. J Allergy Clin Immunol 2002;109(1):150–4.

[47] Heyman M, Darmon N, Dupont C, et al. Mononuclear cells from infants allergic to cow's milk secrete tumor necrosis factor alpha, altering intestinal function. Gastroenterology 1994;106:1514–23.

[48] Benlounes N, Candalh C, Matarazzo P, et al. The time-course of milk antigen–induced TNF-alpha secretion differs according to the clinical symptoms in children with cow's milk allergy. J Allergy Clin Immunol 1999;104(4):863–9.

[49] Farrell RJ, Kelly CP. Celiac sprue. N Engl J Med 2002;346(3):180–8.

[50] Perry TT, Matsui EC, Conover-Walker MK, et al. Risk of oral food challenges. J Allergy Clin Immunol 2004;114(5):1164–8.

[51] James JM, Eigenman PA, Sampson HA, et al. Airway reactivity changes in asthmatic patients undergoing blinded food challenges. Am J Respir Crit Care Med 1996;153:597–603.

[52] Roberts G, Patel N, Levi-Schaffer F, et al. Food allergy as a risk factor for life-threatening asthma in childhood: a case-controlled study. J Allergy Clin Immunol 2003;112(1): 168–74.

[53] Sicherer SH, Furlong TJ, DeSimone J, et al. Self-reported allergic reactions to peanut on commercial airliners. J Allergy Clin Immunol 1999;104(1):186–9.

[54] Crespo JF, Pascual C, Dominguez C, et al. Allergic reactions associated with airborne fish particles in IgE-mediated fish hypersensitive patients. Allergy 1995;50(3):257–61.

[55] Baur X, Posch A. Characterized allergens causing bakers' asthma. Allergy 1998;53(6):562–6.

[56] Roberts G, Golder N, Lack G. Bronchial challenges with aerosolized food in asthmatic, food-allergic children. Allergy 2002;57(8):713–7.

[57] Nowak-Wegrzyn A, Shapiro GG, Beyer K, et al. Contamination of dry powder inhalers for asthma with milk proteins containing lactose. J Allergy Clin Immunol 2004;113(3):558–60.

[58] Crespo JF, Rodriguez J. Food allergy in adulthood. Allergy 2003;58(2):98–113.

[59] Sicherer SH. Food allergy. Lancet 2002;360(9334):701–10.

[60] Sporik R, Hill DJ, Hosking CS. Specificity of allergen skin testing in predicting positive open food challenges to milk, egg, and peanut in children. Clin Exp Allergy 2000;30:1540–6.

[61] Sampson HA, Ho DG. Relationship between food-specific IgE concentrations and the risk of positive food challenges in children and adolescents. J Allergy Clin Immunol 1997;100:444–51.

[62] Sampson HA. Utility of food-specific IgE concentrations in predicting symptomatic food allergy. J Allergy Clin Immunol 2001;107:891–6.

[63] Cooke SK, Sampson HA. Allergenic properties of ovomucoid in man. J Immunol 1997; 159(4):2026–32.

[64] Isolauri E, Turnjanmaa K. Combined skin prick and patch testing enhances identification of food allergy in infants with atopic dermatitis. J Allergy Clin Immunol 1996;97:9–15.

[65] Roehr CC, Reibel S, Ziegert M, et al. Atopy patch test, together with determination of specific IgE levels, reduces the need for oral food challenges in children with atopic dermatitis. J Allergy Clin Immunol 2001;107:548–53.

[66] Joshi P, Mofidi S, Sicherer SH. Interpretation of commercial food ingredient labels by parents of food-allergic children. J Allergy Clin Immunol 2002;109(6):1019–21.

[67] Gern JE, Yang E, Evrard HM, et al. Allergic reactions to milk-contaminated "nondairy" products. N Engl J Med 1991;324(14):976–9.

[68] Bock SA. Prospective appraisal of complaints of adverse reactions to foods in children during the first 3 years of life. Pediatrics 1987;79(5):683–8.

[69] Sicherer SH, Forman JA, Noone SA. Use assessment of self-administered epinephrine among food-allergic children and pediatricians. Pediatrics 2000;105(2):359–62.

[70] Nelson HS, Lahr J, Rule R, et al. Treatment of anaphylactic sensitivity to peanuts by immunotherapy with injections of aqueous peanut extract. J Allergy Clin Immunol 1997;99(6 Pt 1): 744–51.

[71] Asero R. Effects of birch pollen–specific immunotherapy on apple allergy in birch pollen–hypersensitive patients. Clin Exp Allergy 1998;28:1368–73.

[72] Asero R. How long does the effect of birch pollen injection SIT on apple allergy last? Allergy 2003;58(5):435–8.

[73] Leung DY, Sampson HA, Yunginger JW, et al. Effect of anti-IgE therapy in patients with peanut allergy. N Engl J Med 2003;348(11):986–93.

[74] Skolnick HS, Conover-Walker MK, Koerner CB, et al. The natural history of peanut allergy. J Allergy Clin Immunol 2001;107(2):367–74.

[75] Fleischer DM, Conover-Walker MK, Christie L, et al. The natural progression of peanut allergy: resolution and the possibility of recurrence. J Allergy Clin Immunol 2003;112(1): 183–9.

[76] Busse PJ, Nowak-Wegrzyn AH, Noone SA, et al. Recurrent peanut allergy. N Engl J Med 2002;347(19):1535–6.

[77] Fleischer DM, Conover-Walker MK, Christie L, et al. Peanut allergy: recurrence and its management. J Allergy Clin Immunol 2004;114(5):1195–201.

[78] Pastorello EA, Stocchi L, Pravettoni V, et al. Role of the elimination diet in adults with food allergy. J Allergy Clin Immunol 1989;84(4 Pt 1):475–83.

[79] Nickel R, Lau S, Niggemann B, et al. Comparison of bronchial responsiveness to histamine in asthma, allergic rhinitis and allergic sensitization at the age of 7 years. Clin Exp Allergy 2002;32(9):1274–7.

[80] Von Berg A, Koletzko S, Grubl A, et al. The effect of hydrolyzed cow's milk formula for allergy prevention in the first year of life: the German Infant Nutritional Intervention Study, a randomized double-blind trial. J Allergy Clin Immunol 2003;111(3):533–40.

[81] American Academy of Pediatrics. Committee on Nutrition. Hypoallergenic infant formulas. Pediatrics 2000;106(2):346–9.

[82] Garrett GK, Jameson SC, Thompson B, et al. Anti-interleukin-5 (mepolizumab) therapy for hypereosinophilic syndromes. J Allergy Clin Immunol 2004;113:115–9.

ELSEVIER
SAUNDERS

THE MEDICAL
CLINICS
OF NORTH AMERICA

Med Clin N Am 90 (2006) 129–148

# Allergic Diseases of the Eye

## Leonard Bielory, MD*

*New Jersey Medical School, University of Medicine and Dentistry
of New Jersey, Newark, NJ, USA*

Physicians in all specialties frequently encounter various forms of allergic diseases of the eye that present as red eyes in their general practice. However, the eye is rarely the only target for an immediate allergic-type response. Typically, patients have other atopic manifestations, such as rhinoconjunctivitis, rhinosinusitis, asthma, urticaria, or eczema. However, ocular signs and symptoms may be the initial and the most prominent feature of the entire allergic response that patients present to their physician.

The prevalence of allergies ranges as high as 30% to 50% of the United States population. Industrialized countries report greater allergy prevalence, correlating with the original reports of vernal catarrh in Great Britain after the Industrial Revolution. Many theories abound about the increasing prevalence of allergies in the United States, such as increased industrialization, pollution, urbanization, and the hygiene theory. The combination of allergic nasal and ocular symptoms (rhinoconjunctivitis) is extremely common (double the prevalence of allergic rhinitis symptoms alone), but it is not clear whether the two are equal (ie, whether rhinitis is more common than conjunctivitis or vice versa). In studies of allergic rhinitis, allergic conjunctivitis is reported in more than 75% of patients, whereas asthma is reported in the range of 10% to 20% [1]. However, in some studies that report a high prevalence of seasonal allergic rhinitis in the United States, the ratio of ocular to nasal symptoms appears clearly to double throughout all sections of the country [2].

The eye is probably the most common site for the development of allergic inflammatory disorders, because it has no mechanical barrier to prevent impact of allergens such as pollen on its surface. Allergic inflammatory disorders are commonly found in conjunction with allergic rhinitis, which is considered the most common allergic disorder. Although the nasal and

---

* New Jersey Medical School, University of Medicine and Dentistry of New Jersey, 90 Bergen Street, DOC Suite 4700, Newark, NJ 07103.

*E-mail address:* bielory@umdnj.edu

0025-7125/06/$ - see front matter © 2005 Elsevier Inc. All rights reserved.
doi:10.1016/j.mcna.2005.08.013     *medical.theclinics.com*

ocular symptoms more appropriately called *conjunctivorhinitis* may be perceived as a mere nuisance, their consequences can profoundly affect the patient's quality of life. Seasonal allergic rhinitis and conjunctivitis have been associated with headache and fatigue, impaired concentration and learning, loss of sleep, and reduced productivity [3,4]. Patients may also suffer from somnolence, functional impairment, and increased occupational risks for accidents or injuries secondary to sedating oral antihistamine therapy. In 70% of seasonal allergy patients, conjunctivitis symptoms are at least as severe as rhinitis symptoms [5].

## The ocular surface

Allergens and other ocular irritants are easily deposited directly on the surface of the eye. Many agents that are systemically absorbed can be also concentrated and secreted in tears, causing allergic conjunctivitis or an irritant form of conjunctivitis [6]. The overuse of vasoconstrictive agents may lead to a form of conjunctivitis medicamentosa in some patients [7]. Other causes of the red eye may include intraocular conditions associated with systemic autoimmune disorders, such as uveitis or scleritis [8]. In addition, allergic inflammatory disorders can have effects on the local ocular tissue, such as those that may affect surrounding skin, mucosa, or even sinuses and release various mediators of inflammation, including histamine, leukotrienes, and neuropeptides [9].

## Clinical examination

The clinical examination of the eyes for signs of ocular allergy requires an evaluation of the periorbital tissue and the eye itself. The eyelids and eyelashes are examined for the presence of erythema on the lid margin, telangiectasias, scaling, thickening, swelling, collarettes of debris at the base of the eyelashes, periorbital discoloration, blepharospasm, and ptoses that are seen in blepharoconjunctivitis and dermatoconjunctivitis. Next, the conjunctivae are examined for hyperemia (injection), cicatrization (scarring), and chemosis (clear swelling). The presence or absence of discharge from the eye is noted, as are its amount, duration, location, and color. The difference between scleral injection (scleritis) and conjunctival injection is that scleritis tends to develop over several days and is associated with moderate or severe ocular pain on motion, whereas conjunctivitis is associated with discomfort but not pain. Scleritis commonly develops in patients with autoimmune disorders, such as systemic lupus erythematosus, rheumatoid arthritis, and Wegener's granulomatosis, but it has been known to occur in the absence of any other obvious clinical disorders [10–12]. Another form of ocular injection is described as a ring of erythema around the limbal junction of the cornea (ciliary flush) that is a clinical sign for intraocular inflammation such as uveitis. The conjunctival surface should also be closely examined for the presence of inflammatory follicles or papillae involving the bulbar and tarsal conjunctivae. Follicles may be distinguished as grayish, clear, or yellow bumps, varying in size from pinpoint to 2 mm in diameter with conjunctival vessels on their surface, whereas papillae contain a centrally located tuft of blood vessels [13]. The cornea is rarely involved in acute forms of allergic conjunctivitis, whereas in the chronic forms of ocular allergy, such as vernal keratoconjunctivitis and atopic keratoconjunctivitis, the *kerato-* reflects the common involvement of the cornea.

The optimum examination of the cornea is with the slit-lamp biomiocroscope, although many important clinical features may be seen with the naked eye or a hand-held direct ophthalmoscope. The direct ophthalmoscope can provide the desired magnification by "plus" (convex) and "minus" (concave) lenses. The cobalt blue filter on the new hand-held ophthalmoscopic heads assists in highlighting anatomic anomalies affecting the cornea or the conjunctiva, which has been stained with fluorescein. The cornea should be perfectly smooth and transparent. Mucus adhering to the corneal or conjunctival surfaces is considered pathologic. Dusting of the cornea may indicate punctate epithelial keratitis. A localized corneal defect may develop into erosion or a larger ulcer. A corneal plaque may be present if the surface appears dry and white or yellow. The limbus is the zone immediately surrounding the cornea and is normally invisible to the naked eye, but when inflamed this area becomes visible as a pale or pink swelling. Some case reports of limbal allergy exist [14]. Discrete swellings with small white dots (Trantas-Horner's dots) are indicative of degenerating cellular debris, which is commonly seen in chronic forms of conjunctivitis. In addition, because the eye has thin layers of tissue surrounding it, there is an increased tendency to develop secondary infections that can further complicate the clinical presentation [15,16].

## Immunopathophysiology of ocular allergy

Allergic diseases affecting the eyes constitute a heterogeneous group of clinicopathologic conditions with a vast array of clinical manifestations that range from simple intermittent symptoms of itching, tearing, or redness to severe sight-threatening corneal impairment (Table 1). These conditions may be considered part of an immunologic spectrum that affects the anterior surface of the eye with a variety of disorders that may overlap and include seasonal and perennial allergic conjunctivitis, vernal and atopic keratoconjunctivitis (VKC, AKC), and giant papillary conjunctivitis (GPC). In addition, tear film dysfunction, otherwise known as dry eye syndrome, commonly complicates ocular allergy and its treatments, especially as the age of the patient increases. This condition is also included to reflect the spectrum from IgE–mast cell hypersensitivity conditions to mixtures of mast cell– and cell-mediated disorders that involve quite different

Table 1
Differential diagnosis of conjunctival inflammatory disorders

| Criteria | AC | VKC | AKC | GPC | DCS | BACT | VIR | CHLMD | DES | BC |
|---|---|---|---|---|---|---|---|---|---|---|
| *Signs* | | | | | | | | | | |
| Predominant cell types | MC/eos | L/eos | L/eos | L/eos | L | PMN | PMN/M/L | M/L | M/L | M/L |
| Chemosis | + | +/- | +/- | +/- | - | +/- | +/- | +/- | - | +/- |
| Lymph node | - | - | - | - | - | + | ++ | +/- | - | - |
| Cobblestoning | - | ++ | ++ | ++ | - | - | +/- | + | - | - |
| Discharge | Clear mucoid | Stringy mucoid | Stringy mucoid | Clear white | +/- | ++ mucopurulent | Clear mucoid | ++ mucopurulent | +/- mucoid | ++ mucopurulent |
| Lid involvement | - | + | + | - | ++ | + (glue lids) | - | - | - | ++ |
| *Symptoms* | | | | | | | | | | |
| Pruritus | + | ++ | ++ | ++ | + | - | - | - | - | + |
| Burning | - | - | - | - | - | - | ++ | + | + | - |
| Gritty sensation | +/- | +/- | +/- | + | - | + | + | + | +++ | ++ |
| Seasonal variation | + | + | +/- | +/- | - | +/- | +/- | +/- | - | - |

The differential diagnosis of the red eye includes various inflammatory conditions that involves the outside and the inside of the eye. The list below focuses on the signs and symptoms of external causes of the red eye which include the predominant cell type found in the conjunctival scraping; the presence or absence of chemosis, lymph node involvement, cobblestoning of the conjunctival surface, discharge, lid involvement, pruritus, gritty sensation and seasonal variation.

*Abbreviations:* AC, allergic conjunctivitis; AKC, atopic keratoconjunctivitis; BACT, bacterial; BC, blepharoconjunctivitis; CHLMD, chlamydial infection; DCS, dermatoconjunctivitis; DES, dry-eye syndrome; eos, eosinophil; GPC, giant papillary conjunctivitis; L, lymphocyte; M, monocyte; MC, mast cell; PMN, polymorphonuclear cell; VC, vernal conjunctivitis; VIR, viral; VKC, vernal keratoconjunctivitis.

mechanisms, cytokines, and cellular populations [17–19]. For example, mast cell degranulation [20–22], histamine release [23–27], and eosinophils [28–30] play key roles in the common forms of seasonal and perennial conjunctivitis. By contrast, AKC and VKC are characterized by more chronic inflammatory cellular infiltrates, primarily composed of Th2 lymphocytes with a minimal interplay with mast cells. Tear film dysfunction, a Th1-mediated disorder, commonly complicates ocular allergy syndromes [31–33].

Mast cell mediators, such as histamine, tryptase, leukotrienes, and prostaglandins in the tear fluid, have diverse and overlapping biologic effects [34–36], all of which contribute to the characteristic itching, redness, watering, and mucous discharge associated with both acute and chronic allergic eye disease. Histamine alone has been shown to be involved in regulation of vascular permeability, smooth muscle contraction, mucus secretion, inflammatory cell migration, cellular activation, and modulation of T cell function. Histamine is a principal mediator involved in ocular allergy and inflammation [23,26]. In fact, it is estimated that human conjunctival tissue contains about 10,000 mast cells per cubic millimeter [17,33]. Large amounts of histamine are present in several mammalian ocular structures, including the retina, choroid, and optic nerve. Histamine receptors have been found on the conjunctiva, cornea, and ophthalmic arteries. Two separate histamine receptors, H1 and H2, have been identified in the conjunctiva [37–40]. Most ocular allergic reactions are mediated through the effects of histamine on H1-receptors. Histamine concentration in tears of patients who have allergic conjunctivitis can reach values greater than 100 ng/mL, as compared with values of 5 to 15 ng/mL in controls. Histamine can induce changes in the eye similar to those seen in other parts of the body. These include capillary dilatation leading to conjunctival redness, increased vascular permeability leading to chemosis, and smooth-muscle contraction.

In the more severe chronic allergy-related conditions, T cells are the key cellular players in ocular surface impairment. Two predominant inflammatory pathways are differentiated by the Th1 and Th2 cell markers, which involve different cytokines and are crudely considered as antagonistic of each other when activated. In previous reports based on conjunctival biopsies in allergic patients, cytokine profiling displayed that Th2 activation occurred in VKC, whereas both Th1 and Th2 activation were found in AKC [33, 41–44]. In addition, it is not rare for a patient treated for typical seasonal allergic conjunctivitis also to develop dry eye, tear film disturbance, meibomian dysfunction, adverse effects from the repeated use of toxic preservative-containing topical drugs, or contact cell-mediated conjunctival or eyelid hypersensitivity, conditions linked to the Th1 cascade [31,45–47].

*Acute allergic conjunctivitis*

The eye may actually be the most common target organ of the IgE/mast cell hypersensitivity–mediated reactions. Allergic conjunctivitis (AC) is due to the direct exposure of the ocular mucosal surfaces to environmental allergens, such as pollens from trees, grasses, and weeds, which interact with the pollen-specific IgE found on the mast cells of the eye. Of all the various pollens, ragweed has been identified as the most common cause of *conjunctivo-rhinitis* in the United States, approaching 75% of all cases of hay fever, with prevalence varying among different age groups in various regions of the world [2,48–50]. In the earliest studies of allergy testing, timothy grass was identified as one of the most potent ocular allergy–inducing allergens [51]. Common conjunctival symptoms are itching, tearing, and perhaps burning. Involvement of the cornea is rare, with blurring of vision being the most common corneal symptom [13,52]. Clinical signs include a milky or pale pink conjunctiva with vascular congestion that may progress to conjunctival swelling (chemosis). A white exudate may form during the acute state, becoming stringy in the chronic form. Although ocular signs are typically mild, the conjunctiva frequently takes on a pale, boggy appearance that evolves into diffuse areas of papillae (small vascularized nodules). These papillae tend to be most prominent on the superior palpebral conjunctiva. Occasionally, dark circles beneath the eyes (allergic shiners) are present as a result of localized venous congestion [53]. Perennial AC, like perennial allergic rhinitis, exhibits the classic IgE/mast cell–mediated hypersensitivity to airborne allergens. Patients who have this condition tend to be sensitive to common perennial household allergens such as dust mites, molds, and animal dander, rather than to grass or weed pollens as in patients with seasonal AC [54–58]. The ocular reaction seen in both seasonal AC and perennial AC often resolves quickly once the offending allergen is removed. Obtaining a detailed history from the patient may expedite the diagnosis of these disorders. Both eyes are typically affected simultaneously, and often a family history of hay fever or atopy is elicited.

## Vernal keratoconjunctivitis

Vernal conjunctivitis is a chronic mast cell/lymphocyte–mediated allergic disorder of the conjunctiva that appears more often in males before pubescence, after which it is equally distributed among the sexes and commonly burns out approximately 10 years later (ie, in the third decade of life). As the name implies, vernal keratoconjunctivitis (VKC) is seasonally recurrent in the spring (*vernal*), with symptoms that include intense pruritus induced by nonspecific stimuli, such as exposure to wind, dust, bright light, hot weather, or physical exertion associated with sweating [32]. Although VKC is considered a form of ocular allergy, more than 50% of patients have negative skin tests or radioallergosorbent tests to allergens [59]. As in other chronic ocular allergy conditions, conjunctival biopsies reveal increased numbers of eosinophils, basophils, and mast cells, as well as plasma cells and lymphocytes that result from increased corneal involvement, with photophobia, foreign body sensation, and lacrimation [33,60]. The most remarkable physical finding is giant papillae on the tarsal conjunctiva, reaching 7 to 8 mm in diameter of the upper tarsal plate, which can result in the cobblestone appearance on examination [61]. In addition, patients may develop a thin, copious, milk-white fibrinous secretion, limbal or conjunctival yellowish-white points (Horner's points and Trantas' dots), an extra lower eyelid crease (Dennie's line), corneal ulcers, or a pseudomembrane formation of the upper lid when everted and exposed to heat (Maxwell-Lyons' sign) [53]. The effects of vernal conjunctivitis may be so severe that blindness results, affecting one eye more than the other in approximately 5% of patients [60,62]. Diffuse areas of punctate corneal epithelial defects may occur in some cases. These defects are best appreciated with a cobalt blue light after the instillation of topical fluorescein dye [63]. In severe cases, these superficial punctate defects may progress to shield ulcers; these are areas of desquamation of epithelial cells, resulting from the release of major basic protein from infiltrating eosinophils [64,65].

*Atopic keratoconjunctivitis*

AKC is a chronic inflammatory process. It is a chronic mast cell/lymphocyte–mediated allergic disorder of the conjunctiva of the eye as periorbital tissue that is associated with a familial history for atopy, such as eczema and asthma [66,67]. Primary care physicians should expect to see approximately 25% of their elderly patients who have eczema develop some components of AKC. Although AKC is commonly seen in individuals older than 50 years, onset occurs as early as the late teens in certain individuals. AKC is an eye disorder with disabling symptoms; when it involves the cornea, it can lead to blindness [60]. Ocular symptoms of AKC are similar to the cutaneous symptoms of eczema and include intense pruritus and edematous, coarse, and thickened eyelids. Severe AKC is associated with complications such as blepharoconjunctivitis, cataract, corneal disease, and ocular herpes simplex [68,69]. The symptoms of AKC commonly include itching, burning, and tearing that are more severe than those in AC or perennial AC and tend to be present throughout the year. Seasonal exacerbations are reported in many patients, especially in the winter or summer months, as is exacerbation from exposure to animal dander, dust, and certain foods [32,63,70]. Ocular disease activity has been shown to correlate with exacerbations and remissions of the dermatitis. AKC-associated cataracts occur in approximately 10% of patients with the severe forms of atopic dermatitis but are especially prone to occur in young adults approximately 10 years after the onset of the atopic dermatitis. A unique feature of AKC cataracts is that they predominantly involve the anterior portion of the lens and may evolve rapidly into complete opacification within 6 months, whereas AKC patients may also develop posterior polar type cataracts due to the prolonged use of topical or oral corticosteroid therapy [71–75]. Keratoconus occurs in a small percentage of patients with atopic dermatitis. Retinal detachment appears to be increased in patients with AKC, although it is also increased in patients with atopic dermatitis in general. The association with specific micro-organisms, such as *Staphylococcus aureus,* is presently under investigation [15,76,77]. Treatment involves corticosteroids, antihistamines, mast cell stabilizers, and treatment of systemic features of atopic dermatitis. Heightened concern exists regarding the use of antihistamines in older patients with this condition, because they may increase drying of the conjunctival surface.

*Giant papillary conjunctivitis*

GPC is not truly an ocular allergy, but many of its features mimic those of other ocular hypersensitivity syndromes, such as an increase in symptoms during the spring pollen season and pruritus. Thus, it is important to include it in the differential diagnosis of ocular allergy [78,79]. GPC has been increasingly common with the advent of extended-wear soft contact lenses and other foreign bodies, such as suture materials and ocular prosthetics. Signs include a white or clear exudate on awakening, which chronically becomes thick and stringy. The patient may develop papillary hypertrophy (cobblestoning), especially in the tarsal conjunctiva of the upper lid, which is more common in wearers of soft ($\sim$5%–10%) than hard ($\sim$4%) contact lenses. The contact lens polymer, preservatives such as thimerosal, and proteinaceous deposits on the surface of the lens have all been implicated in causing GPC, but these theories remain controversial [80–83]. Common symptoms include intense itching, decreased tolerance to contact lens wear, blurred vision, conjunctival injection, and increased mucus production. Treatment involves corticosteroids, antihistamines, mast cell stabilizers, and frequent enzymatic cleaning of the lenses or changing of the lens polymers. Disposable contact lenses have been proposed as an alternative treatment for GPC. It usually resolves when the patient stops wearing contact lenses or when the foreign body is removed.

*Dry-eye syndrome (tear film dysfunction)*

Dry-eye syndrome (DES), also known as tear film dysfunction, develops from decreased tear production, increased tear evaporation, or an abnormality in specific components of the aqueous, lipid, or mucin layers that compose the tear film [84,85]. Symptoms of dry eye are typically vague and include foreign body sensation, easily fatigued eyes, dryness, burning, ocular pain, photophobia, and blurry vision. Patients initially complain of a mildly injected eye with excessive mucus production and gritty sensation, as compared with the itching and burning feeling many patients report with histamine release onto conjunctiva. Symptoms tend to be worse late in the day, after prolonged use of the eyes or exposure to adverse environmental conditions.

Although dry eye may occur as a distinct disorder resulting from intrinsic tear pathology, it is more frequently associated with other ocular and systemic disorders, including ocular allergy, chronic blepharitis, fifth or seventh nerve palsies, vitamin A deficiency, pemphigoid, and trauma [86]. DES is a frequent confounding disorder that may complicate ocular allergic disease with several overlapping signs and symptoms, such as tearing, injection, and exacerbation [87,88]. As the cornea becomes involved, a more scratchy and painful sensation as well as photophobia may appear. DES and ocular allergy conditions are not exclusive; as patients age, the likelihood of tear film dysfunction's complicating ocular allergy increases [89]. A more systemic form of DES, associated with systemic immune diseases such as Sjögren's syndrome, rheumatoid arthritis, and HIV infection [90], is commonly known as keratoconjunctivitis sicca and can be a symptom in post-menopausal women [91].

The most common cause of DES is associated not with an autoimmune disorder but with the use of medications with anticholinergic properties that decrease lacrimation. Drugs with antimuscarinic properties include the first-generation antihistamines and even newer agents, such as loratadine and cetirizine [92], phenothiazines, tricyclic antidepressants, atropine, and scopolamine. Other agents that are associated with a sicca syndrome include the retinoids, beta-blockers, and chemotherapeutic agents. Tear film dysfunction is also associated with several pharmacologic agents, including antihistamines, anticholinergics, and some psychotropic agents [93]. Exacerbation of symptoms occurs in the winter months when heating systems decrease the relative humidity in the household to less than 25%. Diagnostic evaluation commonly uses the Schirmer's test, which typically demonstrates decreased tearing (0–1 mm of wetting at 1 minute and 2–3 mm at 5 minutes). Normal values for the Schirmer test are more than 4 mm at 1 minute and 10 mm at 5 minutes. Treatment includes addressing the underlying pathology, discontinuing the offending drug (if possible), and making generous use of artificial tears or ocular lubricants. Topical cyclosporine (Restasis) has recently been approved by the US Food and Drug Administration for the treatment of DES [31,94]. For severe symptoms, insertion of punctal plugs may be indicated [95].

*Contact dermatitis of the eyelids*

In contradistinction to ocular allergy, with its predominant activation of the IgE-mast cell, contact dermatoconjunctivitis is primarily a delayed type of lymphocytic hypersensitivity reaction involving the eyelids and the conjunctiva [96–98]. The eyelid skin is extremely thin, soft, and pliable and is capable of developing significant swelling and redness with minor degrees of inflammation. As a result, the patient frequently seeks medical attention for a cutaneous reaction that elsewhere on the skin would normally be less of concern. Two principal forms of contact dermatitis are attributed to eye area cosmetics: contact dermatoconjunctivitis and irritant (toxic) contact dermatitis. Contact dermatoconjunctivitis is commonly associated with cosmetics applied to the hair, face, or fingernails (eg, hair dye, nail polish) or with topical ocular medications (eg, neomycin) [99,100]. Preservatives such as thimerosal (found in contact lens cleaning solutions) and benzalkonium chloride (found in many topical ocular therapeutic agents) have been shown by patch tests to be major culprits, as have the active drugs themselves [101–109]. Stinging and burning of the eyes and itching of the lids are the most common complaints. These subjective symptoms are usually transitory and unaccompanied by objective signs of irritation. The patch test can assist in pinpointing the causative antigen, but interpretation of patch-test results may be difficult, and the likelihood of irritant false-positive reactions must be borne in mind [110–112].

*Blepharoconjunctivitis*

Blepharitis is a primary inflammation of the eyelid margins that is most often misdiagnosed as an ocular allergy, because it commonly causes conjunctivitis in a secondary fashion [101,113–115]. The primary causes are various infections and seborrhea. In general, as in patients with atopic dermatitis, the most common organism isolated from the lid margin is *S aureus*. It has been suggested that the antigenic products play the primary role in the induction of chronic eczema of the eyelid margins [15,116–119]. The symptoms include persistent burning, itching, tearing, and a feeling of dryness. Patients commonly complain of more symptoms in the morning than in the evening. By contrast, patients who have DES complain of more symptoms in the evening than in the morning, because the tear film dries out during the day. The crusted exudate that develops in these patients may cause the eye to be glued shut when they awaken in the morning. The signs of staphylococcal blepharitis include dilated blood vessels, erythema, scales, collarettes of exudative material around the eyelash bases, and foamy exudates in the tear film. Blepharitis may be controlled with improved eyelid hygiene using detergents (eg, nonstinging baby shampoos) and steroid ointments applied to the lid margin with a cotton tip applicator that loosens the exudate and scales.

## Ocular allergy treatment

A variety of treatment approaches have been used to manage allergic symptoms, foremost among them the avoidance of triggering allergens. In addition, pharmacotherapies with antihistamines, decongestants, nasal corticosteroids, mast cell stabilizers, and anticholinergics have all proved effective, as has immunotherapy [120,121].

Primary treatment of any allergy, including ocular allergy, focuses on the avoidance of allergens. This strategy primarily involves the use of environmental interventions, from removal of the offending allergen source to a change of occupational venue. Lubrication is a form of avoidance, in that it has a dilutional effect on allergens and released mediators that interact with the conjunctival surface. Cold compresses provide considerable symptomatic relief, especially from ocular pruritus. All ocular medications should be refrigerated to provide additional subjective relief when applied to the conjunctival surface.

Secondary treatment regimens include the symptomatic use of topical agents, as well as oral decongestants, antihistamines, mast cell stabilizing agents, and anti-inflammatory agents. Topical decongestants primarily act as vasoconstrictors, which are highly effective in reducing the erythema and are widely used in combination with topical antihistamines [122]. Adverse effects of topical vasoconstrictors include burning and stinging on instillation, mydriasis, especially in patients with lighter irides, and rebound hyperemia or conjunctivitis medicamentosa with chronic use [7]. In the conjunctiva, H1 stimulation principally mediates the symptom of pruritus, as seen in various binding studies, whereas the H2 receptor has been inferred to be clinically involved in the vasodilatation of the ocular allergic response [40]. Although topical antihistamines may be used alone to treat AC, combined use of an antihistamine and a vasoconstricting agent is more effective than either agent alone [122].

As monotherapy, oral or systemic antihistamines are an excellent choice when one is attempting to control multiple early-phase and some late-phase allergic symptoms in the eyes, nose, and pharynx. Despite their efficacy in relief of allergic symptoms, systemic antihistamines may result in unwanted side effects, such as drowsiness and dry mouth. Newer, second-generation antihistamines are preferred to avoid the sedative and anticholinergic effects associated with first-generation agents.

When the allergic symptom or complaint is isolated, such as ocular pruritus, focused therapy with topical antihistaminic agents is often efficacious and clearly superior, either as monotherapy or in conjunction with an oral or nasal agent. Topical antihistaminic agents provide faster and better relief than do systemic antihistamines. Topical antihistaminic agents also have a longer duration of action than other classes. However, their duration of action may not be as long as that of systemic agents. Some of these agents have been found to have merits as topical multiple-action agents possessing unique properties, including H1-receptor antagonism, low antimuscarinic properties, and H2-receptor antagonism; these maximize the symptomatic treatment of seasonal AC and are now widely used as first-line pharmacotherapy for ocular allergy (Table 2) [123]. Many of the selective H1-receptor antagonists have also demonstrated several anti-inflammatory components that may have an impact on the ocular late-phase reaction seen in more than 50% of patients and may explain the persistent qualities of the acute allergic ocular reaction. For example, some of these newer antihistamines can block intercellular adhesion molecule (ICAM)-1 expression in epithelial cells, effectively reducing inflammatory cell mucosal infiltration.

Table 2
Topical (ophthalmic) multiple-action antihistaminic agents for allergic conjunctivitis

| Multiple-action antihistamine agent generic (trade) name | Dosage | Most common side effects |
|---|---|---|
| Olopatadine (Patanol) | ≥ 3 y: 1–2 drops twice daily in 6–8-h intervals | Headache (7%) |
| Ketotifen (Zaditor) | ≥ 3 y: 1 drop twice daily in 8–12-h intervals | Conjunctival injection, headache, rhinitis (10%–25%) |
| Azelastine (Optivar) | ≥ 3 y: 1 drop twice daily | Ocular burning (∼30%), headache (∼15%), bitter taste (∼10%) |
| Epinastine (Elestat) | ≥ 3 y: 1 drop twice daily | Upper respiratory infection/cold symptoms (10%) |

The use of mast cell stabilizers such as cromolyn was originally approved for more severe forms of conjunctivitis (GPC, AKC, VKC), but many physicians have used it for the treatment of acute seasonal and perennial AC with an excellent safety record. Some of the studies reflecting its clinical efficacy for seasonal and perennial AC found marginal efficacy when compared with placebo in clinical settings [124,125] and some animal models [126]. After many years of clinical use, the mechanisms of cromolyn are still unclear.

Ketorolac is a nonsteroidal anti-inflammatory drug (NSAID) that inhibits the prostaglandin production involved in mediating ocular allergy. Clinical studies have shown that topical NSAIDs significantly diminish the ocular itching and conjunctival hyperemia associated with seasonal antigen-induced AC [127] and VKC [128]. These agents, unlike topical corticosteroids, do not mask ocular infections, affect wound healing, increase intraocular pressure, or contribute to cataract formation. Some of the studies reflecting their clinical efficacy for seasonal and perennial AC showed marginal efficacy when compared with placebo in clinical settings [124,125] and in some animal models [126,129].

Tertiary treatment of ocular allergy using more potent immunomodulatory properties may be considered when topically administered medications, such as antihistamines, vasoconstrictors, or cromolyn sodium, are ineffective. However, the local administration of topical steroids may be associated with localized ocular complications, including increased intraocular pressure, viral infections, and cataract formation. Two modified steroids, rimexolone and loteprednol, have recently been investigated for their efficacy in AC. Rimexolone is a derivative of prednisolone that is quickly inactivated in the anterior chamber. Loteprednol is another modified corticosteroid that is highly effective in the acute and prophylactic treatment of AC [130–137].

Immunotherapy has been used for the primary treatment of allergies, once known as spring *catarrh*, since before the discovery of antihistamines and other pharmacologic agents. In fact, in the original report on allergy immunotherapy in the early 1900s, it was used to "measure the patient's resistance during experiments with pollen extracts to excite a conjunctival reaction" [51]. Immunotherapy involves the application of the suspected proteins in various formulations to the mucosa of the conjunctiva, gastrointestinal tract, and nose.

Although initial studies of allergen immunotherapy did not specifically address ocular symptoms [138], more recent clinical studies have started to identify improvement in ocular signs and symptoms in a separate domain of assessment outcomes [139–141]. Additional physiologic studies have demonstrated a logarithmic increase (10–100 fold) in the tolerance to the allergen in the conjunctival provocation test [142,143] or improvement of ocular symptoms [144,145]. Interestingly, when specific allergen immunotherapy was instituted in adults and children with multiple allergies, the treatment was both effective and specific to the allergens in their season [143,146–149]. Subcutaneous administrations of allergen solutions are not convenient for all patients.

Experimentally, AC has been suppressed by the oral administration of the offending allergen in animal models, with the concomitant decrease in the development of allergen-specific IgE [150]. Recent experimental studies on the use of sublingual immunotherapy have also shown statistical improvement in the nasal and ocular symptom scores, which are also associated with an increase in the threshold dose for the conjunctival allergen provocation tests [151,152]. Experimental topical application of allergen [153] or immunostimulatory sequence oligodeoxynucleotides [154] has predominantly shown a decrease in the late-phase response. Alternative forms of immunotherapy, such as sublingual-swallow therapy, have also been attempted in the treatment of seasonal and perennial rhinitis with a statistical decrease in ocular symptoms [155,156]. Some produce no changes in the rhinitis symptoms, suggesting that ocular symptoms may be more sensitive to treatment with allergen immunotherapy [151].

## Summary

The prevalence of ocular allergy is clearly underappreciated; it has been an underdiagnosed and undertreated area in primary care medicine. The ocular symptoms associated with the most common ocular allergy conditions, such as seasonal and perennial AC, are twice as likely to affect the allergy sufferer as nasal symptoms alone. The emergence of new medications for the specific treatment of ocular symptoms over the course of the past 15 years offers a new field for improved patient care by the primary and subspecialty health care providers.

## Acknowledgments

The author would like to acknowledge Ms. Lynn Baltimore and the staff of the University of Medicine and Dentistry of New Jersey George F. Smith Library for their assistance in the development of this manuscript.

# References

[1] Bousquet J, Knani J, Hejjaoui A, et al. Heterogeneity of atopy. I. Clinical and immunologic characteristics of patients allergic to cypress pollen. Allergy 1993;48(3):183–8.

[2] Nathan H, Meltzer EO, Selner JC, et al. Prevalence of allergic rhinitis in the United States. J Allergy Clin Immunol 1999;99(6):S808–14.

[3] Juniper EF, Howland WC, Roberts NB, et al. Measuring quality of life in children with rhinoconjunctivitis. J Allergy Clin Immunol 1998;101(2 Pt 1):163–70.

[4] Juniper EF, Thompson AK, Ferrie PJ, et al. Validation of the standardized version of the Rhinoconjunctivitis Quality of Life Questionnaire. J Allergy Clin Immunol 1999; 104(2 Pt 1):364–9.

[5] Wuthrich B, Brignoli M, Canevascini M, et al. Epidemiological survey in hay fever patients: symptom prevalence and severity and influence on patient management. Schweiz Med Wochenschr 1998;128(5):139–43.

[6] Palmer RM, Kaufman HE. Tear film, pharmacology of eye drops, and toxicity. Curr Opin Ophthalmol 1995;6(4):11–6.

[7] Spector SL, Raizman MB. Conjunctivitis medicamentosa. J Allergy Clin Immunol 1994; 94(1):134–6.

[8] Zierhut M, Schlote T, Tomida I, et al. Immunology of uveitis and ocular allergy. Acta Ophthalmol Scand 2000;78(Suppl 230):22–5.

[9] Udell IJ, Abelson MB. Chemical mediators of inflammation. Int Ophthalmol Clin 1983; 23(1):15–26.

[10] Dinowitz K, Aldave AJ, Lisse JR, et al. Ocular manifestations of immunologic and rheumatologic inflammatory disorders. Curr Opin Ophthalmol 1994;5(6):91–8.

[11] Haynes BF, Fishman ML, Fauci AS, et al. The ocular manifestations of Wegener's granulomatosis. Fifteen years' experience and review of the literature. Am J Med 1977;63(1): 131–41.

[12] Bistner S. Allergic- and immunologic-mediated diseases of the eye and adnexae. Vet Clin North Am Small Anim Pract 1994;24(4):711–34.

[13] Dinowitz M, Rescigno R, Bielory L. Ocular allergic diseases: differential diagnosis, examination techniques, and testing. Clin Allergy Immunol 2000;15:127–50.

[14] Butrus SI, Abelson MB. Importance of limbal examination in ocular allergic disease. Ann Ophthalmol 1988;20(3):101–4.

[15] Tuft SJ, Ramakrishnan M, Seal DV, et al. Role of *Staphylococcus aureus* in chronic allergic conjunctivitis. Ophthalmology 1992;99(2):180–4.

[16] Cvenkel B, Globocnik M. Conjunctival scrapings and impression cytology in chronic conjunctivitis. Correlation with microbiology. Eur J Ophthalmol 1997;7(1):19–23.

[17] Allansmith MR, Ross RN. Ocular allergy. Clin Allergy 1988;18(1):1–13.

[18] Rothenberg ME, Owen WF Jr, Stevens RL. Ocular allergy. Mast cells and eosinophils. Int Ophthalmol Clin 1988;28(4):267–74.

[19] Leonardi A. The central role of conjunctival mast cells in the pathogenesis of ocular allergy. Curr Allergy Asthma Rep 2002;2(4):325–31.

[20] Udell IJ, Kenyon KR, Hannien LA, et al. Time course of human conjunctival mast cell degranulation in response to compound 48/80. Acta Ophthalmol Suppl 1989;192:154–61.

[21] Li Q, Luyo D, Hikita N, et al. Compound 48/80–induced conjunctivitis in the mouse: kinetics, susceptibility, and mechanism. Int Arch Allergy Immunol 1996;109(3):277–85.

[22] Woodward DF, Ledgard SE, Nieves AL. Conjunctival immediate hypersensitivity: reevaluation of histamine involvement in the vasopermeability response. Invest Ophthalmol Vis Sci 1986;27(1):57–63.

[23] Bachert C. Histamine—a major role in allergy? Clin Exp Allergy 1998;28(Suppl 6):15–9.

[24] Leonardi AA, Smith LM, Fregona IA, et al. Tear histamine and histaminase during the early (EPR) and late (LPR) phases of the allergic reaction and the effects of lodoxamide. Eur J Ophthalmol 1996;6(2):106–12.

[25] Lightman S. Therapeutic considerations: symptoms, cells and mediators. Allergy 1995; 50(21 Suppl):10–38.

[26] Struck HG, Wicht A, Ponicke K, et al. [Histamine in tears in allergic rhinoconjunctivitis.] Ophthalmologe 1998;95(4):241–6 [in German].

[27] Kari O, Salo OP, Halmepuro L, et al. Tear histamine during allergic conjunctivitis challenge. Graefes Arch Clin Exp Ophthalmol 1985;223(2):60–2.

[28] Trocme SD, Aldave AJ. The eye and the eosinophil. Surv Ophthalmol 1994;39(3):241–52.

[29] Hingorani M, Calder V, Jolly G, et al. Eosinophil surface antigen expression and cytokine production vary in different ocular allergic diseases. J Allergy Clin Immunol 1998;102(5): 821–30.

[30] Leonardi A, Borghesan F, Avarello A, et al. Effect of lodoxamide and disodium cromoglycate on tear eosinophil cationic protein in vernal keratoconjunctivitis. Br J Ophthalmol 1997;81(1):23–6.

[31] Bielory L. Ocular allergy and dry eye syndrome. Curr Opin Allergy Clin Immunol 2004; 4(5):421–4.

[32] Bielory L. Allergic and immunologic disorders of the eye. Part II: ocular allergy. J Allergy Clin Immunol 2000;106(6):1019–32.

[33] Bielory L. Allergic and immunologic disorders of the eye. Part I: immunology of the eye. J Allergy Clin Immunol 2000;106(5):805–16.

[34] Gary RK Jr, Woodward DF, Nieves AL, et al. Characterization of the conjunctival vasopermeability response to leukotrienes and their involvement in immediate hypersensitivity. Invest Ophthalmol Vis Sci 1988;29(1):119–26.

[35] Woodward DF, Nieves AL, Williams LS, et al. Interactive effects of peptidoleukotrienes and histamine on microvascular permeability and their involvement in experimental cutaneous and conjunctival immediate hypersensitivity. Eur J Pharmacol 1989;164(2):323–33.

[36] Simons FE. H1-receptor antagonists: does a dose-response relationship exist? Ann Allergy 1993;71(6):592–7.

[37] Umemoto M, Tanaka H, Miichi H, et al. Histamine receptors on rat ocular surface. Ophthalmic Res 1987;19(4):200–4.

[38] Cook EB, Stahl JL, Barney NP, et al. Mechanisms of antihistamines and mast cell stabilizers in ocular allergic inflammation. Curr Drug Targets Inflamm Allergy 2002;1(2):167–80.

[39] Bielory L, Ghafoor S. Histamine rectors in the conjunctiva. Curr Opin Allergy Clin Immunol 2005;5(5):437–40.

[40] Abelson MB, Udell IJ. H2-receptors in the human ocular surface. Arch Ophthalmol 1981; 99(2):302–4.

[41] McGill J. Conjunctival cytokines in ocular allergy. Clin Exp Allergy 2000;30(10):1355–7.

[42] Foster CS. The pathophysiology of ocular allergy: current thinking. Allergy 1995; 50(21 Suppl):6–9 [discussion: 34–8].

[43] Bonini S. IgE and non-IgE mechanisms in ocular allergy. Ann Allergy 1993;71(3):296–9.

[44] Metz DP, Bacon AS, Holgate S, et al. Phenotypic characterization of T cells infiltrating the conjunctiva in chronic allergic eye disease. J Allergy Clin Immunol 1996;98(3):686–96.

[45] Dursun D, Wang M, Monroy D, et al. Experimentally induced dry eye produces ocular surface inflammation and epithelial disease. Adv Exp Med Biol 2002;506(Pt A):647–55.

[46] Stern ME, Gao J, Siemasko KF, et al. The role of the lacrimal functional unit in the pathophysiology of dry eye. Exp Eye Res 2004;78(3):409–16.

[47] Gao J, Morgan G, Tieu D, et al. ICAM-1 expression predisposes ocular tissues to immune-based inflammation in dry eye patients and Sjögrens syndrome–like MRL/lpr mice. Exp Eye Res 2004;78(4):823–35.

[48] Nowak D, Wichmann HE, Magnusson H. Asthma and atopy in Western and Eastern communities—current status and open questions. Clin Exp Allergy 1998;28(9): 1043–6.

[49] Sly RM. Changing prevalence of allergic rhinitis and asthma. Ann Allergy Asthma Immunol 1999;82(3):233–48 [quiz: 248–52].

[50] Strachan D, Sibbald B, Weiland S, et al. Worldwide variations in prevalence of symptoms of allergic rhinoconjunctivitis in children: the International Study of Asthma and Allergies in Childhood (ISAAC). Pediatr Allergy Immunol 1997;8(4):161–76.

[51] Noon L, Cantab BO. Prophylactic inoculation against hay fever. Lancet 1911:1572–3.

[52] Friedlaender MH. Management of ocular allergy. Ann Allergy Asthma Immunol 1995; 75(3):212–22 [quiz: 223–4].

[53] Bielory L. Allergic and immunologic disoders of the eye. In: Adelman DC, Corren J, Casale TB, editors. Manual of allergy and immunology. 4th edition. Lippincott: Williams & Wilkins; 2003. p. 75–92.

[54] Dart JK, Buckley RJ, Monnickendan M, et al. Perennial allergic conjunctivitis: definition, clinical characteristics and prevalence. A comparison with seasonal allergic conjunctivitis. Trans Ophthalmol Soc U K 1986;105(5):513–20.

[55] Boquete M, Carballada F, Armisen M, et al. Factors influencing the clinical picture and the differential sensitization to house dust mites and storage mites. J Investig Allergol Clin Immunol 2000;10(4):229–34.

[56] Valdivieso R, Acosta ME, Estupinan M. Dust mites but not grass pollen are important sensitizers in asthmatic children in the Ecuadorian Andes. J Investig Allergol Clin Immunol 1999;9(5):288–92.

[57] Bertel F, Mortemousque B, Sicard H, et al. [Conjunctival provocation test with *Dermatophagoides pteronyssinus* in the diagnosis of allergic conjunctivitis from house mites.] J Fr Ophtalmol 2001;24(6):581–9 [in French].

[58] van Hage-Hamsten M, Johansson SG, Zetterstrom O. Predominance of mite allergy over allergy to pollens and animal danders in a farming population. Clin Allergy 1987;17(5): 417–23.

[59] Montan PG, Ekstrom K, Hedlin G, et al. Vernal keratoconjunctivitis in a Stockholm ophthalmic centre—epidemiological, functional, and immunologic investigations. Acta Ophthalmol Scand 1999;77(5):559–63.

[60] Tanaka M, Dogru M, Takano Y, et al. The relation of conjunctival and corneal findings in severe ocular allergies. Cornea 2004;23(5):464–7.

[61] Bonini S, Lambiase A, Marchi S, et al. Vernal keratoconjunctivitis revisited: a case series of 195 patients with long-term followup. Ophthalmology 2000;107(6):1157–63.

[62] Rehany U, Rumelt S. Corneal hydrops associated with vernal conjunctivitis as a presenting sign of keratoconus in children. Ophthalmology 1995;102(12):2046–9.

[63] Bielory L, Dinowitz M, Rescigno R. Ocular allergic diseases: differential diagnosis, examination techniques and testing. J Toxicol Cutaneous Ocul Toxicol 2002;21:329–51.

[64] Giuri S. [Corneal ulcerative lesions in type-I immediate hypersensitivity.] Oftalmologia 1998;44(3):20–6 [in Romanian].

[65] Tabbara KF. Ocular complications of vernal keratoconjunctivitis. Can J Ophthalmol 1999; 34(2):88–92.

[66] Casey R, Abelson MB. Atopic keratoconjunctivitis. Int Ophthalmol Clin 1997;37(2):111–7.

[67] Tuft SJ, Kemeny DM, Dart JK, et al. Clinical features of atopic keratoconjunctivitis. Ophthalmology 1991;98(2):150–8.

[68] Bonini S, Lambiase A, Matricardi P, et al. Atopic and vernal keratoconjunctivitis: a model for studying atopic disease. Curr Probl Dermatol 1999;28:88–94.

[69] Power WJ, Tugal-Tutkun I, Foster CS. Long-term follow-up of patients with atopic keratoconjunctivitis. Ophthalmology 1998;105(4):637–42.

[70] Bielory L, Goodman PE, Fisher EM. Allergic ocular disease. A review of pathophysiology and clinical presentations. Clin Rev Allergy Immunol 2001;20(2):183–200.

[71] Norris PG, Rivers JK. Screening for cataracts in patients with severe atopic eczema. Clin Exp Dermatol 1987;12(1):21–2.

[72] Ibarra-Duran MG, Mena-Cedillos CA, Rodriguez-Almaraz M. [Cataracts and atopic dermatitis in children. A study of 68 patients.] Bol Med Hosp Infant Mex 1992;49(12):851–5 [in Spanish].

[73] Beltrani VS, Barsanti FA, Bielory L. Effects of glucocorticosteroids on the skin and eye. Immunol Allergy Clin North Am 2005;25(3):557–80.

[74] Hutnik CM, Nichols BD. Cataracts in systemic diseases and syndromes. Curr Opin Ophthalmol 1999;10(1):22–8.

[75] Castrow FF 2nd. Atopic cataracts versus steroid cataracts. J Am Acad Dermatol 1981;5(1): 64–6.

[76] Chan LS, Robinson N, Xu L. Expression of interleukin-4 in the epidermis of transgenic mice results in a pruritic inflammatory skin disease: an experimental animal model to study atopic dermatitis. J Invest Dermatol 2001;117(4):977–83.

[77] Nivenius E, Montan PG, Chryssanthou E, et al. No apparent association between periocular and ocular microcolonization and the degree of inflammation in patients with atopic keratoconjunctivitis. Clin Exp Allergy 2004;34(5):725–30.

[78] Katelaris CH. Giant papillary conjunctivitis—a review. Acta Ophthalmol Scand Suppl 1999;228:17–20.

[79] Calonge M. Classification of ocular atopic/allergic disorders and conditions: an unsolved problem. Acta Ophthalmol Scand Suppl 1999;228:10–3.

[80] Palmisano PC, Ehlers WH, Donshik PC. Causative factors in unilateral giant papillary conjunctivitis. CLAO J 1993;19(2):103–7.

[81] Mondino BJ, Salamon SM, Zaidman GW. Allergic and toxic reactions of soft contact lens wearers. Surv Ophthalmol 1982;26(6):337–44.

[82] Meisler DM, Krachmer JH, Goeken JA. An immunopathologic study of giant papillary conjunctivitis associated with an ocular prosthesis. Am J Ophthalmol 1981;92(3): 368–71.

[83] Ballow M, Donshik PC, Rapacz P, et al. Immune responses in monkeys to lenses from patients with contact lens induced giant papillary conjunctivitis. CLAO J 1989;15(1):64–70.

[84] Berdy GJ, Hedqvist B. Ocular allergic disorders and dry eye disease: associations, diagnostic dilemmas, and management. Acta Ophthalmol Scand Suppl 2000;230:32–7.

[85] Stern ME, Beuerman RW, Fox RI, et al. The pathology of dry eye: the interaction between the ocular surface and lacrimal glands. Cornea 1998;17(6):584–9.

[86] Pflugfelder SC. Differential diagnosis of dry eye conditions. Adv Dent Res 1996;10(1):9–12.

[87] Michelson PE. Red eye unresponsive to treatment. West J Med 1997;166(2):145–7.

[88] Fujishima H, Toda I, Shimazaki J, et al. Allergic conjunctivitis and dry eye. Br J Ophthalmol 1996;80(11):994–7.

[89] Moss SE, Klein R, Klein BE. Incidence of dry eye in an older population. Arch Ophthalmol 2004;122(3):369–73.

[90] Chronister CL. Review of external ocular disease associated with AIDS and HIV infection. Optom Vis Sci 1996;73(4):225–30.

[91] Pflugfelder SC. Hormonal deficiencies and dry eye. Arch Ophthalmol 2004;122(2):273–4.

[92] Ousler GW, Wilcox KA, Gupta G, et al. An evaluation of the ocular drying effects of 2 systemic antihistamines: loratadine and cetirizine hydrochloride. Ann Allergy Asthma Immunol 2004;93(5):460–4.

[93] Burstein NL. The effects of topical drugs and preservatives on the tears and corneal epithelium in dry eye. Trans Ophthalmol Soc U K 1985;104(4):402–9.

[94] Pflugfelder SC. Antiinflammatory therapy for dry eye. Am J Ophthalmol 2004;137(2): 337–42.

[95] Calonge M. The treatment of dry eye. Surv Ophthalmol 2001;45(Suppl 2):S227–39.

[96] Calonge M. Ocular allergies: association with immune dermatitis. Acta Ophthalmol Scand Suppl 2000;230:69–75.

[97] Zug KA, Palay DA, Rock B. Dermatologic diagnosis and treatment of itchy red eyelids. Surv Ophthalmol 1996;40(4):293–306.

[98] Bielory L, Wagner RS. Allergic and immunologic pediatric disorders of the eye. J Investig Allergol Clin Immunol 1995;5(6):309–17.

[99] Gurwood AS, Altenderfer DS. Contact dermatitis. Optometry 2001;72(1):36–44.

[100] Anibarro B, Barranco P, Ojeda JA. Allergic contact blepharoconjunctivitis caused by phenylephrine eyedrops. Contact Dermatitis 1991;25(5):323–4.

[101] Rafael M, Pereira F, Faria MA. Allergic contact blepharoconjunctivitis caused by phenylephrine, associated with persistent patch test reaction. Contact Dermatitis 1998;39(3): 143–4.

[102] Wilson FM 2nd. Adverse external ocular effects of topical ophthalmic medications. Surv Ophthalmol 1979;24(2):57–88.

[103] de Groot AC, Beverdam EG, Ayong CT, et al. The role of contact allergy in the spectrum of adverse effects caused by cosmetics and toiletries. Contact Dermatitis 1988;19(3):195–201.

[104] Estlander T, Kanerva L, Kari O, et al. Occupational conjunctivitis associated with type IV allergy to methacrylates. Allergy 1996;51(1):56–9.

[105] Estlander T, Kari O, Jolanki R, et al. Occupational allergic contact dermatitis and blepharoconjunctivitis caused by gold. Contact Dermatitis 1998;38(1):40–1.

[106] Fisher AA. Allergic contact dermatitis and conjunctivitis from benzalkonium chloride. Cutis 1987;39(5):381–3.

[107] Fuchs T, Meinart A, Aberer W, et al. [Benzalkonium chloride—a relevant contact allergen or irritant? Results of a multicenter study of the German Contact Allergy Group.] Hautarzt 1993;44(11):699–702 [in German].

[108] Stern GA, Killingsworth DW. Complications of topical antimicrobial agents. Int Ophthalmol Clin 1989;29(3):137–42.

[109] Tosti A, Tosti G. Thimerosal: a hidden allergen in ophthalmology. Contact Dermatitis 1988;18(5):268–73.

[110] Gaspari AA. Contact allergy to ophthalmic dipivalyl epinephrine hydrochloride: demonstration by patch testing. Contact Dermatitis 1993;28(1):35–7.

[111] Marsh RJ, Towns S, Evans KF. Patch testing in ocular drug allergies. Trans Ophthalmol Soc U K 1978;98(2):278–80.

[112] Villarreal O. Reliability of diagnostic tests for contact allergy to mydriatic eyedrops. Contact Dermatitis 1998;38(3):150–4.

[113] Mannis MJ. Allergic blepharoconjunctivitis. Avoiding misdiagnosis and mismanagement. Postgrad Med 1989;86(4):123–9.

[114] Resano A, Esteve C, Fernandez Benitez M. Allergic contact blepharoconjunctivitis due to phenylephrine eye drops. J Investig Allergol Clin Immunol 1999;9(1):55–7.

[115] Kaiserman I. Severe allergic blepharoconjunctivitis induced by a dye for eyelashes and eyebrows. Ocul Immunol Inflamm 2003;11(2):149–51.

[116] O'Callaghan RJ. Role of exoproteins in bacterial keratitis: the Fourth Annual Thygeson Lecture, presented at the Ocular Microbiology and Immunology Group Meeting, November 7, 1998. Cornea 1999;18(5):532–7.

[117] Leung DY, Meissner HC, Fulton DR, et al. Toxic shock syndrome toxin–secreting *Staphylococcus aureus* in Kawasaki syndrome. Lancet 1993;342(8884):1385–8.

[118] Marrack P, Kappler J. The staphylococcal enterotoxins and their relatives. Science 1990; 248(4959):1066.

[119] Seal DV, McGill JI, Jacobs P, et al. Microbial and immunological investigations of chronic non-ulcerative blepharitis and meibomianitis. Br J Ophthalmol 1985;69(8):604–11.

[120] Bielory L. Ocular allergy guidelines: a practical treatment algorithm. Drugs 2002;62(11): 1611–34.

[121] Bielory L. Update on ocular allergy treatment. Expert Opin Pharmacother 2002;3(5):541–53.

[122] Abelson MB, Paradis A, George MA, et al. Effects of Vasocon-A in the allergen challenge model of acute allergic conjunctivitis. Arch Ophthalmol 1990;108(4):520–4.

[123] Bielory L, Lien KW, Bigelsen S. Efficacy and tolerability of newer antihistamines in the treatment of allergic conjunctivitis. Drugs 2005;65(2):215–28.

[124] Sorkin EM, Ward A. Ocular sodium cromoglycate. An overview of its therapeutic efficacy in allergic eye disease. Drugs 1986;31(2):131–48.

[125] Azevedo M, Castel-Branco MG, Oliviera JF, et al. Double-blind comparison of levocabastine eye drops with sodium cromoglycate and placebo in the treatment of seasonal allergic conjunctivitis. Clin Exp Allergy 1991;21(6):689–94.

[126] Kamei C, Izushi K, Tasaka K. Inhibitory effect of levocabastine on experimental allergic conjunctivitis in guinea pigs. J Pharmacobiodyn 1991;14(8):467–73.

[127] Ballas Z, Blumenthal M, Tinkelman DG, et al. Clinical evaluation of ketorolac tromethamine 0.5% ophthalmic solution for the treatment of seasonal allergic conjunctivitis. Surv Ophthalmol 1993;38(Suppl):141–8.

[128] Sharma A, Gupta R, Ram J, et al. Topical ketorolac 0.5% solution for the treatment of vernal keratoconjunctivitis. Indian J Ophthalmol 1997;45(3):177–80.

[129] Groneberg DA, Bielory L, Fischer A, et al. Animal models of allergic and inflammatory conjunctivitis. Allergy 2003;58(11):1101–13.

[130] Dell SJ, Shulman DG, Lowry GM, et al. A controlled evaluation of the efficacy and safety of loteprednol etabonate in the prophylactic treatment of seasonal allergic conjunctivitis. Loteprednol Allergic Conjunctivitis Study Group. Am J Ophthalmol 1997; 123(6):791–7.

[131] Dell SJ, Lowry GM, Northcutt JA, et al. A randomized, double-masked, placebo-controlled parallel study of 0.2% loteprednol etabonate in patients with seasonal allergic conjunctivitis. J Allergy Clin Immunol 1998;102(2):251–5.

[132] Howes JF. Loteprednol etabonate: a review of ophthalmic clinical studies. Pharmazie 2000; 55(3):178–83.

[133] Shulman DG, Lothringer LL, Rubin JM, et al. A randomized, double-masked, placebo-controlled parallel study of loteprednol etabonate 0.2% in patients with seasonal allergic conjunctivitis. Ophthalmology 1999;106(2):362–9.

[134] Abelson M, Howes J, George M. The conjunctival provocation test model of ocular allergy: utility for assessment of an ocular corticosteroid, loteprednol etabonate. J Ocul Pharmacol Ther 1998;14(6):533–42.

[135] Friedlaender MH, Howes J. A double-masked, placebo-controlled evaluation of the efficacy and safety of loteprednol etabonate in the treatment of giant papillary conjunctivitis. The Loteprednol Etabonate Giant Papillary Conjunctivitis Study Group I. Am J Ophthalmol 1997;123(4):455–64.

[136] Howes JF, Baru H, Vered M, et al. Loteprednol etabonate: comparison with other steroids in two models of intraocular inflammation. J Ocul Pharmacol Ther 1994;10(1):289–93.

[137] Hochhaus G, Chen LS, Ratka A, et al. Pharmacokinetic characterization and tissue distribution of the new glucocorticoid soft drug loteprednol etabonate in rats and dogs. J Pharm Sci 1992;81(12):1210–5.

[138] Lowell F, Franklin W. A double-blind study of the effectiveness and specificity of injection therapy in ragweed hay fever. N Engl J Med 1965;273(13):675–9.

[139] Gaglani B, Borish L, Bartleson BL, et al. Nasal immunotherapy in weed-induced allergic rhinitis. Ann Allergy Asthma Immunol 1997;79(3):259–65.

[140] Del Prete A, Loffredo C, Carderopoli A, et al. Local specific immunotherapy in allergic conjunctivitis. Acta Ophthalmol (Copenh) 1994;72(5):631–4.

[141] Juniper EF, Kline PA, Ramsdale EH, et al. Comparison of the efficacy and side effects of aqueous steroid nasal spray (budesonide) and allergen-injection therapy (Pollinex-R) in the treatment of seasonal allergic rhinoconjunctivitis. J Allergy Clin Immunol 1990;85(3): 606–11.

[142] Horak F, Stubner P, Berger UE, et al. Immunotherapy with sublingual birch pollen extract. A short-term double-blind placebo study. J Investig Allergol Clin Immunol 1998;8(3): 165–71.

[143] Dreborg S, Agrell B, Foucard T, et al. A double-blind, multicenter immunotherapy trial in children, using a purified and standardized *Cladosporium herbarum* preparation. I. Clinical results. Allergy 1986;41(2):131–40.

[144] Balda BR, Wolf H, Baumgarten C, et al. Tree-pollen allergy is efficiently treated by short-term immunotherapy (STI) with seven preseasonal injections of molecular standardized allergens. Allergy 1998;53(8):740–8.

[145] Bielory L, Mongia A. Current opinion of immunotherapy for ocular allergy. Curr Opin Allergy Clin Immunol 2002;2(5):447–52.

[146] Olsen OT, Frolund L, Heinig J, et al. A double-blind, randomized study investigating the efficacy and specificity of immunotherapy with *Artemisia vulgaris* or *Phleum pratense/Betula verrucosa*. Allergol Immunopathol (Madr) 1995;23(2):73–8.

[147] Winther L, Malling HJ, Moseholm L, et al. Allergen-specific immunotherapy in birch- and grass-pollen–allergic rhinitis. I. Efficacy estimated by a model reducing the bias of annual differences in pollen counts. Allergy 2000;55(9):818–26.

[148] Ito Y, Takahashi Y, Fujita T, et al. Clinical effects of immunotherapy on Japanese cedar pollinosis in the season of cedar and cypress pollination. Auris Nasus Larynx 1997;24(2):163–70.

[149] Donovan JP, Buckeridge DL, Briscoe MP, et al. Efficacy of immunotherapy to ragweed antigen tested by controlled antigen exposure. Ann Allergy Asthma Immunol 1996;77(1):74–80.

[150] Koizumi T, Abe T. [Induction of oral tolerance to experimental allergic conjunctivitis in rats.] Nippon Ganka Gakkai Zasshi 1995;99(5):515–20 [in Japanese].

[151] Pradalier A, Basset D, Claudel A, et al. Sublingual-swallow immunotherapy (SLIT) with a standardized five-grass-pollen extract (drops and sublingual tablets) versus placebo in seasonal rhinitis. Allergy 1999;54(8):819–28.

[152] La Rosa M, Ranno C, Andre C, et al. Double-blind placebo-controlled evaluation of sublingual-swallow immunotherapy with standardized *Parietaria judaica* extract in children with allergic rhinoconjunctivitis. J Allergy Clin Immunol 1999;104(2 Pt 1):425–32.

[153] Machida H, Nakagami T, Watanabe I. Local ocular immunotherapy for experimental allergic conjunctivitis. Jpn J Ophthalmol 2000;44(6):634–8.

[154] Miyazaki D, Liu G, Clark L, et al. Prevention of acute allergic conjunctivitis and late-phase inflammation with immunostimulatory DNA sequences. Invest Ophthalmol Vis Sci 2000;41(12):3850–5.

[155] Hordijk GJ, Antvelink JB, Luwema RA. Sublingual immunotherapy with a standardised grass pollen extract; a double-blind placebo-controlled study. Allergol Immunopathol (Madr) 1998;26(5):234–40.

[156] Taudorf E, Laursen LC, Lanner A, et al. Oral immunotherapy in birch pollen hay fever. J Allergy Clin Immunol 1987;80(2):153–61.

ELSEVIER
SAUNDERS

Med Clin N Am 90 (2006) 149–167

THE MEDICAL
CLINICS
OF NORTH AMERICA

# Atopic Dermatitis

## Eric L. Simpson, MD, Jon M. Hanifin, MD*

*Department of Dermatology, Oregon Health and Science University, Portland, OR, USA*

Atopic dermatitis (AD) is an eczematous, highly pruritic chronic inflammatory skin disease. It usually begins early in life and often occurs in people with a personal or family history of asthma and allergic rhinitis. The prevalence is high, especially in children, and it has been rising in recent decades, in parallel with asthma prevalence. Although AD is often described as an "allergic" disease, allergic causation is difficult to document, and AD is increasingly viewed as a skin disease that predisposes to allergies. This interpretation, based on clinical, epidemiologic, and animal studies, may greatly influence our approach to therapy and prevention of atopic diseases in the coming years.

### Nomenclature and disease definition

The causation and nomenclature of AD have been realms of confusion, speculation, and misdirection for more than a century. The early term "neurodermatitis," based on Jacquet's erroneous hypothesis that it is "an itch that rashes" [1,2], combined with Freudian psychodynamics, led to a conceptualization of AD as a disease of psychologic instability. Physicians held such ideas for many decades, until systematic studies put the somewhat ridiculous concept to rest [3]. The concept of allergic association and "atopy," developed along with skin test studies in the 1920s [4], led Sulzberger and Wise [5] to the term "atopic dermatitis" in 1933. In modern usage, "atopic dermatitis" and "atopic eczema" are used interchangeably, and both are acceptable. Using "eczema" alone to indicate AD is highly imprecise, because there are many different types and causes within the generic eczema family (Box 1).

---

This article was partially sponsored by a Dermatology Foundation Career Development Award.

* Corresponding author. Department of Dermatology (OP06), Oregon Health and Science University, 3181 SW Sam Jackson Park Road, Portland, OR 97239-3098.

*E-mail address:* hanifinj@ohsu.edu (J.M. Hanifin).

0025-7125/06/$ - see front matter © 2005 Elsevier Inc. All rights reserved.
doi:10.1016/j.mcna.2005.09.002

---

**Box 1. The eczema family**

• Atopic dermatitis
• Seborrheic dermatitis
• Contact dermatitis
  ○ Irritant
  ○ Allergic
• Nummular eczema
• Xerotic (asteatotic) eczema
• Ids (dermatophytids)
• Dyshidrotic eczema (pompholyx)
• Autoeczematization
• Lichen simplex chronicus
• Prelymphomatous

---

In retrospect, the "atopic" appellation was unfortunate, because it resulted in a conceptually misdirected focus on allergy and relative paucity of investigation into the events leading to the spongiotic, pruritic eczematous lesions of AD. Although there is no convincing evidence for an IgE role in the development of eczematous lesions, many investigators have clung to the idea that immediate allergic mechanisms are somehow involved.

Confusion—both conceptual and nomenclatural—has had a recent resurgence because of efforts to split AD into pure versus allergic forms using terms like "intrinsic" versus "extrinsic," "atopiform dermatitis," and the "atopic eczema/dermatitis syndrome" [6]. These exercises highlight the continuing problems in terminology. How can it be "atopic dermatitis" when the patient is not "atopic"? The association with atopy (80%) is very high. The inclusion of AD within the atopic triad was established before the discovery of IgE and before it was recognized that many patients lack IgE reactivity. The confusion is highlighted by a recent assessment of atopy in AD [7]. Perhaps the most basic question to be answered is, What is atopy? No consensus definition exists, and the common connotation of specific IgE reactivity may be too narrow. The most common application is restricted to IgE or immediate allergy—for instance, "presence of IgE specific for one or more allergens" [8]. Not only does this description fail to encompass many common forms of asthma, rhinitis, and AD, but it enfolds myriad people who have chronic *Trichophyton rubrum* infections, insect bites, and parasitosis [9]. Such inconsistencies suggest the need for a more comprehensive definition of atopy: *a genetically predisposed diathesis manifesting as exaggerated responses (eg, bronchoconstriction, IgE production, vasodilatation, pruritus) to a variety of environmental stimuli (irritants, allergens, and microbes).*

Such a definition would obviate the cumbersome attempts currently in vogue to rename AD to conform to the IgE/allergocentric concept of atopic disease. A recent publication on "revised nomenclature" states that "Under the umbrella *dermatitis, eczema* is now the agreed term to replace the transitional term atopic eczema/dermatitis syndrome (AEDS). Atopic eczema is eczema in a person of the atopic constitution" [10]. This statement confounds the question of irritant or allergic contact dermatitis in a "person of the atopic constitution." Does that become atopic eczema? Conversely, is hand eczema in nonatopic individuals to be classified as nonatopic eczema? This revised terminology would greatly undermine systematic clinical research in AD. Clinical, epidemiologic, and genetic studies have long been hampered by the lack of a specific laboratory marker, and the possible AD subtypes are even more difficult to define. An early systematic effort to standardize diagnostic criteria was presented in 1980, motivated by the need to provide homogeneity for clinical research studies [11]. In 1994, Williams and colleagues [12] devised a simplified scheme that could be used by nonphysicians; this has been used and validated for epidemiologic studies, though it lacks the necessary precision for clinical or genetic ascertainment. More recently, a simplified set of criteria encompassing all ages and ethnicities was suggested by an American Academy of Dermatology consensus conference on pediatric AD (Box 2) [13].

## Epidemiology

### Disease prevalence and the hygiene hypothesis

Schultz Larsen and colleagues [14] reported in 1986 that the prevalence of AD in northern Europe had essentially tripled over 4 decades to roughly 10% of infants. A survey study of schoolchildren in northern Europe demonstrated AD prevalence of 15.6%. Using a modification of the same questionnaire, the authors found a prevalence of 17.2% among 7- to 9-year-old Oregon children, with a lower rate of 6.8% when clinical examination and stringent diagnostic criteria were compared with the survey instrument [15,16]. These studies indicate similar prevalence data from northern Europe, the United States, and Asia, where Sugiura and colleagues [17] reported a prevalence of 20% among similarly aged Japanese children.

The prevalence of AD in adults is unknown. Muto and colleagues [18] reported a 3% point prevalence in a highly selected group in Japan, whereas a recent study from the United States found a point prevalence of adult AD to be only 0.8% [19].

Although the prevalence of AD has clearly increased since World War II, particularly in industrialized countries [20,21], this increase appears, at least in Japan, to have leveled off by 1993 [22]. The reason for the increased prevalence of AD and asthma remains uncertain, but the "hygiene hypothesis" has captured considerable interest by suggesting that overzealous hygiene

---

**Box 2. Suggested universal criteria for atopic dermatitis**

A. Essential features; must be present and, if complete, are
   sufficient for diagnosis
   1. Pruritus
   2. Eczematous changes that are acute, subacute, or chronic:
      a. Typical and age-specific patterns
         (i) Facial, neck, and extensor involvement in infants
             and children
         (ii) Current or prior flexural lesions in adults/any age
         (iii) Sparing of groin and axillary regions
      b. Chronic or relapsing course
B. Important features that are seen in most cases, adding support
   to the diagnosis
   1. Early age at onset
   2. Atopy (IgE reactivity)
   3. Xerosis
C. Associated features
   Clinical associations; help in suggesting the diagnosis of AD
      but are too nonspecific to be used for defining or detecting
      AD for research and epidemiologic studies
   1. Keratosis pilaris/Ichthyosis/Palmar hyperlinearity
   2. Atypical vascular responses
   3. Perifollicular accentuation/Lichenification/Prurigo
   4. Ocular/periorbital changes
   5. Perioral/periauricular lesions
D. Exclusions
   Firm diagnosis of AD depends on excluding conditions such
      as scabies, allergic contact dermatitis, seborrheic
      dermatitis, cutaneous lymphoma, ichthyoses, psoriasis,
      and other primary disease entities.

---

*Data from* American Academy of Dermatology. Suggested universal criteria for
atopic dermatitis. American Academy of Dermatology Consensus Conference on
Pediatric Atopic Dermatitis. 2001.

---

may prevent maturation of the child's developing immune system, thereby
skewing immunity toward Th2 responses and allergy development [23,24].
This hypothesis could explain the higher prevalence of AD in industrialized
countries and in urban locales, compared with rural areas where microbial
exposures enhance immune development [20,25]. Not all studies support
the hygiene hypothesis [26,27], and the underlying pathogenic mechanisms
are unknown, though a recent study has uncovered one potential molecular
explanation. McIntire and colleagues [28] reported that exposure to

hepatitis A may protect individuals from atopy if they carry a genetic variant of TIM-1, the gene that codes for the hepatitis A receptor.

*Natural history*

More than 60% of AD cases present before the first year of life, although rarely it can present in adulthood [29]. Early age at onset, respiratory allergy, and urban living predict more severe disease [30]. Disease usually presents in infancy on the face and extensor extremities, moving to flexural areas in childhood, and most commonly manifests as hand eczema in adults. Estimated clearance rates for AD vary greatly, ranging from 40% to 80% [31,32]. Natural history studies, however, suffer from poor definitions of disease (eg, inclusion of seborrheic dermatitis among ethnically predisposed Celtics) and from use of questionnaires that overestimate clearance when subtle features of hand eczema, irritant dermatitis, and xerosis are often retained into adulthood.

*Quality of life and cost of care*

AD negatively affects all aspects of family health and imposes a significant social burden. Caring for a child with moderate-to-severe AD affects a family more than having a child with type I diabetes mellitus [33]. Of all childhood dermatoses, only scabies impacts a child's quality of life more than AD [34]. Symptoms of pruritus and pain have the strongest negative influence on quality of life, and these symptoms often lead to disruptions of sleep, social development, and recreational activity. The economic impact of AD is similar to the costs of other chronic diseases such as emphysema and epilepsy [35]. In 1990 to 1991, the cost of care for AD was estimated at $364 million. Emergency room visits were a substantial expenditure [36]. Better disease education and more frequent follow-up visits may reduce the need for costly emergency room visits.

*Pathogenesis*

Few pathogenic aspects of AD are generally accepted as fact. AD is a strongly familial, multigenic disease, with genetic associations extending to allergic rhinoconjunctivitis, asthma, and atopy. The disease is dependent on and transferred by bone marrow cells [37–39]. It is characterized by increased cutaneous and respiratory inflammatory responsiveness [40].

Beyond these well-accepted generalizations are less certain concepts, the most prominent being that AD has an allergic immunologic basis. That faith was maintained in the past 40 years by the IgE and type 2 immunologic associations. More recently, the breadth of AD research has been expanded by novel and productive studies in keratinocytes, dendritic cells, and neuroinflammatory elements. These developments are helping to increase awareness of elements beyond the immunologic that contribute to inflammation of AD [40–43].

*Genetic aspects*

Genetic aspects of AD have been of interest because of the strong familial associations and the high concordance in monozygotic twin pairs [14]. AD also has higher frequency in families with respiratory allergy, indicating shared genetic determinants, and linkage studies have focused more on IgE/Th2 associations than on AD specifically.

Reports have suggested linkage at the chromosome 5q31-33 cytokine cluster and an association with an interleukin-13 promoter polymorphism [44]. Another northern European study indicated linkage at 3q21, possibly relating to the costimulatory molecules CD80 and 86 [45]. Other studies have demonstrated loci mapped closely to psoriasis and autoimmune susceptibility genes [46,47]. Studies from the United Kingdom and Japan have shown associations of AD and the Netherton disease gene SPINK5, which codes for the LEKTI proteinase inhibitor; this could relate to inflammatory pathways [48,49] via epidermal barrier dysfunction.

*Signaling and regulation*

Fundamental defects in signaling and regulatory pathways might account for the wide variety of abnormalities in AD. This area has been generally overlooked but is beginning to be recognized and approached, especially as new signaling pathways are elucidated. The earliest studies of cell regulation evolved from cyclic nucleotide biochemistry and evidence for reduced intracellular cyclic adenosine monophosphate (cAMP), which inhibits inflammatory cell function, providing a unifying concept to explain the immune and inflammatory hyperactivity so prominent in AD. Subnormal cAMP levels result from increased hydrolysis by cAMP-phosphodiesterase (PDE). PDE inhibitors correct the defect and reduce the overproduction of IgE, interleukin-4, and other cytokines in cell cultures; they have anti-inflammatory effects when applied topically to AD lesions [40].

*The epidermis in atopic dermatitis*

The epidermis in AD is characterized by spongiosis and a severely damaged stratum corneum barrier, leaving viable cells exposed to environmental irritants and antigens. Recently Akdis and colleagues [50] demonstrated that Fas-induced apoptosis precedes the development of spongiosis in biopsy specimens from AD and from allergic contact dermatitis. With in vitro keratinocyte (KC) cultures, they showed that interferon-gamma caused increased expression of Fas receptors on the cells and that Fas ligand from activated T cells initiated the apoptosis. This reaction was Th2- and IgE-independent, and the role of antigen specificity is unclear. The work of these investigators suggests a basic general mechanism for eczematization and barrier disruption in AD and highlights the importance of Th1/KC interaction in the pathogenesis of eczematous lesions. Perhaps most importantly, their system provides a model for study of signaling pathways in AD lesions.

Building on that model system, Iordanov and colleagues [51] have recently confirmed the association of apoptosis and spongiosis and demonstrated in vitro that hyperproliferation, so prominent in AD as lichenification, may be due to generation of epidermal growth factor (EGF) receptor ligands by apoptotic keratinocytes. Studies such as these identify novel molecules that might be therapeutically targeted to treat eczematous diseases like AD.

*The spectrum of immune aberrations*

Immune abnormalities associated with AD include cutaneous immune deficiency and, at the other extreme, systemic immune hyperresponsiveness. The cutaneous immune deficiency in AD is selective, characterized by susceptibility to increased spread of herpes simplex virus, vaccinia, molluscum contagiosum, and warts. Patients also demonstrate mildly reduced capacity for sensitization to chemical contact allergens, such as rhus and dinitrochlorobenzen. The abnormal pathomechanisms underlying these reduced immune responses are uncertain. Studies of AD monocytes and dendritic cells have shown reduced expression of interleukin-12 and increased production of interleukin-10, which enhances Th2 activity and reduces Th1 effects [52]. Another proposed mechanism to account for the cutaneous immune deficit is reduced innate immunity related to production of antimicrobial peptides in the skin [53,54] and the possibility of a toll-like receptor signaling defect skewing toward a Th2 response pattern [55].

At the other end of the spectrum is immune hyperresponsiveness. IgE overproduction and antigen/IgE triggering of mast cells can account for the exaggerated urticarial and respiratory responses that are so common in AD. Activated T cells residing in lesional skin and increased Th2 responses underlie the excessive IgE production evident in approximately 80% of patients. Increased IgE-bearing dendritic cells are also present in AD skin, and as antigen-presenting cells they can amplify the Th2 responses to allergens passing through the disrupted stratum corneum barrier [43]. Recent murine studies have demonstrated that transcutaneous inoculation of antigen can lead to development of asthma and cause 10- to 100-fold increases in IgE production [56,57].

Are the increased Th2 activity and the IgE reactivity relevant to the eczematous skin disease of AD? It is important to remain mindful of the AD dichotomy in which many patients have no IgE reactivity. Clinically, this pure AD is indistinguishable, and certainly no effector role has been demonstrated for IgE, Th2 cells, or eosinophils in eczematization [58]. Classic studies of cutaneous reactions to scabies mites, fleas, and other insects show that, although IgE reactivity eventually develops, the earliest immune response is cell mediated [59,60]. In terms of biologic roles, IgE and eosinophils may represent a back-up antiparasitic immune response that can also cause hives and respiratory disease. This supposition raises the consideration that the low incidence of pure AD is only an evolutionary distortion resulting from increased susceptibility to parasites among individuals genetically unable to generate adequate levels of IgE, eosinophils, and other Th2-related factors for host defense.

*Neuroinflammation*

An important field that has received little attention is that of neurogenic inflammation. Inflammation or itch may result from several neurogenic mechanisms, and recent studies by Steinhoff and colleagues [61] have focused particularly on proteinase-activated receptors (PAR-2). Present on sensory neurons, keratinocytes, mast cells, and endothelial cells, these receptors are activated through cleavage by a variety of trypsin-like serine proteases (eg, trypsin, mast cell tryptase). This process leads to stimulation of signal transduction pathways by means of protein kinases and nuclear factor (NF)κB. PAR-2 agonists recruit leukocytes and cause pruritus and edema. Codeine-induced tryptase release in AD skin increased fourfold over normal controls. Histamine releasability was no different from in normals, but the antihistamine cetirizine abolished itch only in controls. Intradermal injection of a PAR-2 agonist (SLIGKV) caused greater itch in AD skin. Immunohistochemistry showed enhanced PAR-2 staining on AD nerve fibers. The investigators concluded that PAR-2 signaling is an important link between the sensory nervous system and inflammation in AD [62].

*Atopic dermatitis and respiratory atopy: emerging concepts*

The "atopic march" refers to the sequential development of AD, food allergy, asthma, and allergic rhinitis. Longitudinal studies reveal that AD is a risk factor for the future development of allergic airway disease, but the mechanisms behind this connection have not been elucidated. Animal models have revealed that allergen sensitization by way of the skin yields several-fold higher levels of IgE than sensitization by respiratory or intraperitoneal routes [56,59]. Furthermore, inhalational challenge with protein antigen, after cutaneous sensitization, leads to pulmonary inflammation and increased responsiveness to methacholine challenge [56]. These results suggest that disrupted skin, as found in AD, may be the source of antigen sensitization, leading to allergic responses in other organs. As a clinical correlate, a recent study found that the strongest predictor for the development of peanut allergy in children was a history of application of peanut oil to inflamed skin and found no relationship to maternal consumption of peanuts [63].

## Disease management

Optimal management of AD requires a comprehensive approach that addresses both psychosocial and medical issues. Disease severity will determine the appropriate medical therapy, but psychologic and family dynamics affect compliance and force the provider to design individualized strategies that make "cook book" treatment algorithms obsolete.

## Prevention

Given the rising incidence and worldwide distribution of the disease, the primary prevention of AD continues to be an important but elusive goal. Only 7% of clinical studies in AD have addressed disease prevention [64]. No generally accepted primary prevention strategy for AD currently exists, despite many years of research exploration [65,66]. Development of effective prevention strategies hinges on understanding the key pathogenic mechanisms of AD, a difficult task in this immunologically complex disease. Prevention strategies therefore mirror pathogenesis theories, with most research being performed in the field of allergen avoidance.

A Cochrane systematic review updated in 2003 reviewed studies of maternal allergen avoidance as a means of preventing AD [67]. The authors concluded that maternal dietary changes during pregnancy do not show a protective effect against developing AD and may lead to preterm births and reductions in birth weight. Maternal allergen in lactation, by contrast, did show some evidence of a protective effect, but most of the studies had several methodologic shortcomings.

Breastfeeding has been repeatedly evaluated as a means of reducing allergen exposure early in life to prevent AD. Results vary widely, some even showing an increased risk for AD with exclusive breastfeeding. A meta-analysis of 18 studies published in 2001 suggested an overall protective effect of breastfeeding during the first 3 months of life [68]. Many design defects were identified, centered on poor blinding and inadequate randomization (often considered unethical with regard to breastfeeding). The American Association of Dermatology Guidelines Task Force reviewed the subject in 2004 and found no conclusive evidence that breastfeeding or exclusionary diets prevent AD [66]. A recent study found no protective effect after examining a large cohort of Danish children in a retrospective fashion [69].

Infant formulas have been used as another avenue for early allergen avoidance. Hoare and colleagues' [65] technology assessment in 2000 indicated that most trials on this issue suffered from lack of blinding, high drop-out rates, and unclear randomization schemes. Soy milk provided no protective effect over cow's milk formula. Some evidence supported the usefulness of extensively or partially hydrolyzed cow's milk over regular cow's milk in preventing AD in high-risk families. The German Infant Nutritional Intervention study published in 2003 confirmed these results and found extensively hydrolyzed formula protective in high-risk infants [70]. A recent review of dietary prevention of allergic diseases recommends extensively hydrolyzed formula, if needed, until 4 months of age in children with an atopic family history [71]. Using extensively hydrolyzed formula, however, is not likely to be an effective strategy given its high cost, questionable efficacy, and unpalatable taste—demonstrated by high drop-out rates in the intervention groups [72].

Another recently published strategy is derived from the hygiene hypothesis, which has led researchers to focus on the idea that perinatal gut epithelium may be an inhibitor of Th2 responses and that probiotics should reverse intestinal permeability to antigens and promote Th1 responses. Feeding probiotics to pregnant mothers and newborn infants resulted in significantly reduced AD at 2 years (23% in intervention group versus 46% in placebo group) [73]. This protective effect was also seen at a 4-year follow-up study [74]. These are potentially exciting results, but several shortcomings of the study have been identified, such as poor disease definitions, unclear randomization methods, and the absence of intent-to-treat analysis [64].

In conclusion, allergen avoidance prevention strategies have not generated clearly effective interventions. Other potential prevention strategies must begin with a critical look at disease pathogenesis theories. Potential future targets include correcting early skin barrier dysfunction and inhibiting T cell hyperreactivity. These strategies have proved useful in secondary prevention and may even interrupt the development of allergic respiratory disease [75].

*Patient education*

Without detailed patient education, even the most carefully constructed treatment plan will fail. The best method of patient education is by means of a nurse educator. Adding a nurse educator to the management team significantly improves patient outcomes [76]. The three areas of disease management most fraught with confusion and most in need of patient education are bathing, steroid phobia, and food allergy. These areas are reviewed here and have been discussed in more detail previously [77].

*Bathing*

To bathe or not to bathe—the ever-present source of confusion among parents who have seen several pediatricians, allergists, and dermatologists. The best educational approach is to identify why physicians differ on this subject and to communicate that neither approach is wrong. Bathing is beneficial: it provides hydration to the skin, allows improved penetration of topical therapies, and may debride infected eczema. Bathing may also worsen AD: repeated water evaporation dries and disrupts the stratum corneum barrier. Depending on the severity of eczema, the authors recommend daily bathing followed immediately by petrolatum-based moisturizer or topical medication. The emollient must be applied within 3 minutes of getting out of the bath, the time it takes for the water to evaporate from the stratum corneum. When hydration is retained, the skin remains more flexible and medications penetrate more effectively. For severe flares, the authors encourage *twice daily* bathing followed by application of topical medications to affected areas and a thick moisturizer to unaffected skin.

*Topical steroids*

Patients' and families' fears regarding topical steroids interfere with effective management. A study by Charman and colleagues [78] revealed that 72.5% of patients or guardians were worried about using topical corticosteroids. The primary source of information regarding steroid side effects was the patients' primary physician. Although the fear of topical steroids is warranted, it is chronic daily use that can lead to skin atrophy, striae, and hypothalamic-pituitary-adrenal axis suppression. When used in short, 3- to 7-day bursts, even potent topical steroids give little evidence of adverse effects. Conversely, patients, especially children, receiving prolonged topical corticosteroid therapy should be monitored for growth deficits and reduced bone density [66]. Counseling of patients regarding topical steroids should include the following points: (1) Corticosteroids are the best, and sometimes the only, anti-inflammatory therapy for putting the disease in a remission; (2) Mid- to high-potency steroids should be used to improve moderate/ severe disease quickly, eliminating the need for more prolonged exposure to lower-strength preparations; (3) As the dermatitis improves, topical steroids should be tapered to twice weekly ad libitum use in combination with moisturizers for relapse prevention.

*Food allergy*

Many patients and families are convinced that their difficult-to-control eczema is the result of an allergy to something that they have not been able to identify. Usually the specter of food allergy looms largest, causing frustrating therapeutic misdirection and at times malnutrition and even kwashiorkor [79]. No doubt exists that patients who have AD have a higher incidence of immediate food reactions, but controversy centers on whether those foods can exacerbate the eczema. Regardless of whether food allergy is suspected on medical history, the focus of an initial visit should always be on skin care. Redirecting a patient's focus away from food allergy and toward the fundamentals of bathing, moisturizing, and effective anti-inflammatory medication compliance leads to rapid disease control, and food allergy concerns usually wane.

**General therapeutic approach**

AD is characterized by disease flares and remissions. Therefore, the therapeutic approach must change according to the current state of the disease.

In general, disease management may be broken down into three phases: (1) induction of remission, (2) maintenance, and (3) rescue of flares (Box 3). The treatment choice for each phase depends on the severity of disease and complicating medical issues.

*Inducing a remission*

Topical steroids remain the most effective therapy for achieving rapid control of the disease. Medium- to high-potency topical steroid ointment for 5 to 7 days when applied within 3 minutes after twice-daily bathing can achieve excellent results—approaching the efficacy of oral prednisone—in even the most severe of cases. Wet wraps may be useful if a flaring patient refuses or is unable to bathe daily, but in general they place a greater burden on patients and parents.

The topical calcineurin inhibitors, pimecrolimus and tacrolimus, may be used to induce a remission but should only be used in mild flares where topical steroids are contraindicated. The relative potency of these agents is low compared with medium-potency topical steroids, and burning and stinging occur more frequently on acutely inflamed and fissured skin.

*Maintenance therapy*

Emollients are the cornerstone of maintenance therapy and relapse prevention. Despite this, few studies have examined the types of emollient that are best suited for this purpose. Generally speaking, emollients with more lipid concentration provide a more effective barrier than water-based creams and lotions, which may actually dry out the skin on evaporation. Compliance with greasy moisturizers, however, decreases as a result of poor cosmetic acceptance. Recent studies have examined the effectiveness of adding stratum corneum lipids such as ceramides. In one uncontrolled study, a ceramide-dominant emollient added to routine therapy was superior to standard care [80]. The skin barrier is important in the pathogenesis of AD, and current research is directed toward optimizing skin barrier function to improve therapeutic outcomes.

Used alone, topical steroids are most useful for acute control of disease flares, whereas chronic maintenance is limited by adverse effects. Recent controlled trials have presented an alternative approach, demonstrating

---

**Box 3. Objectives in managing atopic dermatitis**

- *Induction:* topical steroids
- *Maintenance:* emollients, topical steroids twice weekly, topical calcineurin inhibitors, ultraviolet (UV) light
- *Rescue:* topical steroids

the safety and efficacy of twice-weekly midpotency topical corticosteroids in preventing disease relapses in AD when applied to healed sites [81,82].

Numerous studies of topical calcineurin inhibitors have demonstrated their usefulness, along with safety for as long as 4 years, for long-term control of even moderate and severe AD [83]. A year-long pediatric study showed that topical pimecrolimus, used at the first signs or symptoms of AD activity, reduced the number of flares and the amount of steroid use [84]. For severe disease, it can be useful to combine twice-weekly topical steroids with topical calcineurin inhibitors 5 days out of the week [85,86]. In early 2005, the US Food and Drug Administration (FDA) issued a Public Health Advisory and recommended adding a warning to the labeling of pimecrolimus and tacrolimus concerning a potential cancer risk with the topical use of these medications. Primates given oral pimecrolimus developed lymphoma when exposed to levels greater than 30 times the highest recorded blood level in a human patient. In clinical studies involving approximately 19,000 subjects, the number of malignancies was actually lower in the pimecrolimus group than in control groups receiving vehicle or topical steroids. This warning was at least partially prompted by a sharp increase in the use of calcineurin inhibitors in children, often as first-line agents, fueled by heavy direct-to-consumer advertising. Moreover, given the minimal systemic absorption of these agents after topical use as measured in clinical studies, even in patients with widespread disease, the likelihood of systemic immunosuppression from the use of topical agents is small. A study of infants revealed that the use of pimecrolimus 1% cream for 2 years did not alter vaccination antibody responses [87]. Providers should discuss these issues with patients, including all the risks and benefits of therapy. Despite the recent FDA warnings, these medications continue to play an important role in the long-term management of AD, especially in situations where prolonged topical steroid use would be damaging.

*Rescue of flares*

When flares occur, they should be treated aggressively with the same approach used for inducing remissions (ie, bathing followed by topical steroids). Additionally, the reason for flaring should be sought. Flare factors include bacterial or viral infections, dry skin, psychologic stress, and noncompliance with maintenance therapy. Failure to recognize trigger factors inhibits rapid control of disease, leading to prolonged exposure to anti-inflammatory therapies.

Recognizing the role of *Staphylococcus aureus* in disease flares deserves special mention. Colonization of AD skin is almost universal and has been found in more than 90% of patients. Limited infections may be controlled with topical antibiotics and appropriate anti-inflammatory therapy, although widespread infection or severe flares are best treated with short, 5-day courses of dicloxicillin or cephalexin. Prolonged oral antibiotics are contraindicated by the increasing frequency of methicillin-resistant *S aureus*. For patients with frequently recurring infections, addition of rifampin for 10 days or a month-long course of tetracycline, along with daily application of topical mupirocin, may reverse the relapsing problem.

*Phototherapy*

Phototherapy, including UVA, UVB, and psoralen UVA (PUVA), has been used successfully in the control of AD. Narrow-band UV-B phototherapy is emerging as the treatment of choice for moderate-to-severe disease that cannot be controlled with topical maintenance therapies [88].

**Systemic therapy**

Oral corticosteroids are reserved for severe flares that are not responding adequately to intensive topical therapy. Oral cyclosporine is the best-studied immunosuppressant medication and has shown good safety and efficacy in the treatment of adult and childhood AD [89,90]. Hypertension and renal toxicity limit its continuous use, and studies have shown rapid disease relapse following discontinuation. Dose levels of 5 mg/kg are usually necessary to induce a remission. Cyclosporine, when no comorbidities preclude its safe use, is the best first-line systemic therapy when both topicals and phototherapy fail to control the disease. Clinical guidelines for its use have been outlined previously [91].

Azathioprine, mycophenolate mofetil, methotrexate, and interferon-gamma have all shown various degrees of efficacy in the treatment of AD [92]. Interferon-gamma given by daily subcutaneous injection can provide rapid and lasting benefit [93]; although expense limits its use, it can be a welcome alternative for severe patients failing cyclosporine. Azathioprine has shown significant improvement compared with placebo in a randomized study, but improvement tends to be slow and moderate at best [94]. Mycophenolate mofetil has not been studied in a controlled manner, but results from a pilot study are encouraging [95]. Although no studies have been published, methotrexate, 2.5 to 5 mg 4 of 7 days each week, can be an effective alternative.

Antihistamines and leukotriene inhibitors are extensively used with no scientific support for efficacy. Two evidence-based reviews of nonsedating antihistamines found no evidence to support their use solely for the treatment of AD [66,96]. Sedating antihistamines, while having no direct effects on AD pruritus and inflammation, may be useful to improve sleep in flaring patients. No controlled studies have demonstrated efficacy for leukotriene receptor antagonists; although some small, industry-encouraged open-label studies have claimed modest improvement over the years. Such inferential reports cannot support the use of expensive, ineffective therapies [97]. A case series in patients with severe AD found no sustained benefit from the addition of these agents to standard care [98].

*Allergen avoidance*

Despite a large volume of literature, a therapeutic role for allergen avoidance in AD management has not been consistently identified. An evidence-based review of food allergy and dust-mite avoidance measures for AD recently concluded that avoidance of foods, with the possible exception of egg in infants, had no therapeutic value in established AD [66]. Many studies have attempted to show benefit from house dust mite (HDM) reduction measures. A study by Tan and colleagues [99] indicated possible benefit in the child group compared with the adult group, but other studies have failed to confirm an effect, and two evidence-based reviews found no conclusive evidence that HDM reduction measures can improve AD [65,66].

*Miscellaneous and adjunctive therapy*

A recent evidence-based review of all published therapies for AD revealed no good evidence to support the use of dietary supplementation with primrose oil, borage oil, fish oil, pyridoxine, vitamin E, or zinc in the management of AD [66]. Some evidence suggests that Chinese herbal remedies may be of benefit, but there is concern about cardio- and hepatotoxicity. A study of topical herbal products revealed the presence of corticosteroids in nearly all [100]. Probiotics provided no significant improvement in objective disease measurements in a controlled study, but patients perceived more improvement in the active group as compared with placebo [101].

## References

[1] Hanifin JM. Atopic dermatitis. J Am Acad Dermatol 1982;6:1–13.

[2] Jacquet L. Prurigos d'Besnier. In: Besnier E, Brocq L, Jacquet J, editors. La pratique dermatologique. Paris: Tome IV; 1904. p. 62.

[3] Crossen J. Psychological assessment and treatment of patients with atopic dermatitis. Dermatol Ther 1996;1:94–103.

[4] Coca AF, Cooke RA. On the classification of the phenomena of hypersensitiveness. J Immunol 1923;6:63.

[5] Wise F, Sulzberger MB. Editorial remarks. In: Year book of dermatology and syphilogy. Chicago: Year Book Medical Publisher; 1933. p. 59.

[6] Hanifin JM. Atopiform dermatitis: do we need another confusing name for atopic dermatitis? Br J Dermatol 2002;147(3):430–2.

[7] Flohr C, Johansson SGO, Wahlgren C-F, et al. How atopic is atopic dermatitis? J Allergy Clin Immunol 2004;114:150–8.

[8] Rocken M, Schallreuter K, Renz H, et al. What exactly is "atopy"? Exp Dermatol 1998; 7(2–3):97–104.

[9] Hanifin JM, Ray LR, Lobitz WC. Immunological reactivity in dermatophytosis. Br J Dermatol 1974;90:1–8.

[10] Johansson SGO, Bieber T, Dahl R, et al. Revised nomenclature for allergy for global use: report of the Nomenclature Review Committee of the World Allergy Organization, October 2003. J Allergy Clin Immunol 2004;113:832–6.

[11] Hanifin JM, Rajka G. Diagnostic features of atopic dermatitis. Acta Derm Venereol Suppl (Stockh) 1980;92:44–7.

[12] Williams HC, Burney PGJ, Hay RJ, et al. The UK working party's diagnostic criteria for atopic dermatitis. I: Derivation of a minimum set of discriminators for atopic dermatitis. Br J Dermatol 1994;131:383–96.

[13] Eichenfield LF, Hanifin JM, Luger TA, et al. Consensus Conference on Pediatric Atopic Dermatitis. J Am Acad Dermatol 2003;49:1088–95.

[14] Schultz Larsen F, Holm NV, Henningsen K. Atopic dermatitis: a genetic-epidemiologic study in a population-based twin sample. J Am Acad Dermatol 1986;15:487–94.

[15] Laughter D, Istvan J, Tofte S, et al. The prevalence of atopic dermatitis in Oregon school-children. J Am Acad Dermatol 2000;43:649–55.

[16] Schultz Larsen F, Diepgen T, Svensson A. The occurrence of atopic dermatitis in North Europe: an international questionnaire study. J Am Acad Dermatol 1996;34: 760–4.

[17] Sugiura H, Umemoto N, Deguchi H, et al. Prevalence of childhood and adolescent atopic dermatitis in a Japanese population: comparison with the disease frequency examined 20 years ago. Acta Derm Venereol Suppl (Stockh) 1998;78:293–4.

[18] Muto T, Hsieh SD, Sakurai Y, et al. Prevalence of atopic dermatitis in Japanese adults. Br J Dermatol 2003;148:117–21.

[19] Naleway AL, Belongia EA, Greenlee RT, et al. Eczematous skin disease and recall of past diagnoses: implications for smallpox vaccination. Ann Intern Med 2003; 139(1):1–7.

[20] Williams HC, Robertson C, Stewart A, et al. Worldwide variation in the prevalence of symptoms of atopic eczema. J Allergy Clin Immunol 1999;103:125–38.

[21] Visscher MO, Hanifin JM, Bowman WJ, et al. Atopic dermatitis and atopy in non-clinical populations. Acta Derm Venereol Suppl (Stockh) 1989;(Suppl 144):34–40.

[22] Yura A, Shimizu T. Trends in the prevalence of atopic dermatitis in school children: longi-tudinal study in Osaka Prefecture, Japan, from 1985 to 1997. Br J Dermatol 2001;145: 966–73.

[23] Strachan DP. Hay fever, hygiene, and household size. BMJ 1989;299:1259–60.

[24] Liu AH, Murphy JR. Hygiene hypothesis: fact or fiction? J Allergy Clin Immunol 2003;111: 471–8.

[25] Gehring U, Bolte G, Borte M, et al. Exposure to endotoxin decreases the risk of atopic eczema in infancy: a cohort study. J Allergy Clin Immunol 2001;108:847–54.

[26] Flohr C, Pascoe D, Williams HC. Atopic dermatitis and the "hygiene hypothesis": too clean to be true? Br J Dermatol 2005;152(2):202–16.

[27] Simpson EL, Hanifin JM. Periodic synopsis on atopic dermatitis. J Am Acad Dermatol 2005;53(1):115–28.

[28] McIntire JJ, Umetsu SE, Macaubas C, et al. Hepatitis A virus link to atopic disease. Nature 2003;425:576.

[29] Kay J, Gawkrodger DJ, Mortimer MJ, et al. The prevalence of childhood atopic eczema in a general population. J Am Acad Dermatol 1994;30:35–9.

[30] Ben-Gashir MA, Seed PT, Hay RJ. Predictors of atopic dermatitis severity over time. J Am Acad Dermatol 2004;50:349–56.

[31] Hanifin JM. Epidemiology of atopic dermatitis. In: Schlumberger H, editor. Monographs in allergy/epidemiology of allergic diseases. Vol. 21. Basel (Switzerland): S. Karger; 1987. p. 116–31.

[32] Williams HC. Atopic dermatitis—the epidemiology, causes and prevention of atopic ec-zema. Cambridge (UK): Cambridge University Press; 2000.

[33] Su JC, Kemp AS, Varigos GA, et al. Atopic eczema: its impact on the family and financial cost. Arch Dis Child 1997;76:159–62.

[34] Lewis-Jones MS, Finlay AY. The Children's Dermatology Life Quality Index (CDLQI): initial validation and practical use. Br J Dermatol 1995;132:942–9.

[35] Ellis CN, Drake LA, Prendergast MM, et al. Cost of atopic dermatitis and eczema in the United States. J Am Acad Dermatol 2002;46:361–70.

[36] Lapidus CS, Schwarz DF, Honig PJ. Atopic dermatitis in children: who cares? who pays? J Am Acad Dermatol 1993;28:699–703.

[37] Parkman R, Rappeport J, Geha R, et al. Complete correction of the Wiskott-Aldrich syndrome by allogeneic bone-marrow transplantation. N Engl J Med 1978;298(17):921–7.

[38] Saurat JH. Eczema in primary immune-deficiencies. Clues to the pathogenesis of atopic dermatitis with special reference to the Wiscott-Aldrich syndrome. Acta Derm Venereol Suppl (Stockh) 1985;(Suppl 114):125–8.

[39] Agosti JM, Sprenger JD, Lum LG, et al. Transfer of allergen-specific IgE-mediated hypersensitivity with allogeneic bone marrow transplantation. N Engl J Med 1988;319: 1623–8.

[40] Nassif A, Chan SC, Storrs FJ, et al. Abnormal skin irritancy in atopic dermatitis and in atopy without dermatitis. Arch Dermatol 1994;130:1402–7.

[41] Girolomoni G, Pastore S. The role of keratinocytes in the pathogenesis of atopic dermatitis. J Am Acad Dermatol 2001;45:S25–8.

[42] Akdis CA, Akdis M, Trautmann A, et al. Immune regulation in atopic dermatitis. Curr Opin Immunol 2000;12:641–6.

[43] Klubal R, Osterhoff B, Wang B, et al. The high-affinity receptor for IgE is the predominant IgE-binding structure in lesional skin of atopic dermatitis patients. J Invest Dermatol 1997; 108(3):336–42.

[44] Hummelshoj T, Bodtger U, Datta P, et al. Association between an interleukin-13 promoter polymorphism and atopy. J Immunogenet 2003;30:355–9.

[45] Lee Y-A, Wahn U, Kehrt R, et al. A major susceptibility locus for atopic dermatitis maps to chromosome 3q21. Nat Genet 2000;26:470–3.

[46] Cookson WOCM, Ubhi B, Lawrence R, et al. Genetic linkage of childhood atopic dermatitis to psoriasis susceptibility loci. Nat Genet 2001;27:372–3.

[47] Becker KG, Barnes KC. Underlying disease specificity of genetic loci in atopic dermatitis. J Invest Dermatol 2001;117:1325–7.

[48] Walley AJ, Chavanas S, Moffatt MF, et al. Gene polymorphism in Netherton and common atopic disease. Nat Genet 2001;29:175–8.

[49] Kato A, Fukai K, Oiso N, et al. Association of SPINK5 gene polymorphisms with atopic dermatitis in the Japanese population. Br J Dermatol 2003;148:655–69.

[50] Akdis CA, Blaser K, Akdis M. Apoptosis in tissue inflammation and allergic disease. Curr Opin Immunol 2004;16(6):717–23.

[51] Iordanov MS, Sundholm AJ, Simpson EL, et al. Cell death-induced activation of epidermal growth factor receptor in keratinocytes: implications for restricting epidermal damage in dermatitis. J Invest Dermatol 2005;125(1):134–42.

[52] Ohmen JD, Hanifin JM, Nickoloff BJ, et al. Overexpression of IL-10 in atopic dermatitis: contrasting cytokine patterns with delayed-type hypersensitivity reactions. J Immunol 1995;154:1956–63.

[53] Ong PY, Ohtake T, Brandt C, et al. Endogenous antimicrobial peptides and skin infections in atopic dermatitis. N Engl J Med 2002;347:1151–60.

[54] Howell MD, Novak N, Bieber T, et al. Interleukin-10 down regulates anti-microbial peptide expression in atopic dermatitis. J Invest Dermatol 2005;125(4):738–45.

[55] Gaspari AA. Multiple pathways driving IgE production and chronic dermatitis in mice: a model for atopic dermatitis? J Invest Dermatol 2005;124(1):xi–xii.

[56] Spergel JM, Mizoguchi E, Brewer JP, et al. Epicutaneous sensitization with protein antigen induces localized allergic dermatitis and hyperresponsiveness to methacholine after single exposure to aerosolized antigen in mice. J Clin Invest 1998;101:1614–22.

[57] Herrick CA, MacLeod H, Glusac E, et al. Th2 responses induced by epicutaneous or inhalational protein exposure are differentially dependent on IL-4. J Clin Invest 2000;105: 765–75.

[58] Wills-Karp M, Karp CL. Eosinophils in asthma: remodeling a tangled tale. Science 2004; 305:1725-6.

[59] Mellanby K. The development of symptoms, parasitic infection, and immunity in human scabies. Parasitology 1944;35:197-206.

[60] Feingold BF, Benjamini E, Michaeli D. The allergic responses to insect bites. Annu Rev Entomol 1968;13:137-58.

[61] Steinhoff M, Stander S, Seeliger S, et al. Modern aspects of cutaneous neurogenic inflammation. Arch Dermatol 2003;139(11):1479-88.

[62] Steinhoff M, Nisius U, Ikoma A, et al. Proteinase-activated receptor-2 mediates itch: a novel pathway for pruritus in human skin. J Neurosci 2003;23:6176-80.

[63] Lack G, Fox D, Northstone K, et al. Factors associated with the development of peanut allergy in childhood. N Engl J Med 2003;348(11):977-85.

[64] Williams HC. Prevention of atopic eczema: a dream not so far away? [editorial]. Arch Dermatol 2002;138(3):391-2.

[65] Hoare C, Li Wan Po A, Williams H. Systematic review of treatments for atopic eczema. Health Technol Assess 2000;4(37):1-191.

[66] Hanifin JM, Cooper KD, Ho VC, et al. Guidelines of care for atopic dermatitis. J Am Acad Dermatol 2004;50:391-404.

[67] Kramer MS, Kakuma R. Maternal dietary antigen avoidance during pregnancy and/or lactation for preventing or treating atopic disease in the child. In: The Cochrane Library. Issue 4. Chichester (UK): John Wiley & Sons; 2004.

[68] Gdalevich M, Mimouni D, David M, et al. Breast-feeding and the onset of atopic dermatitis in childhood: a systematic review and meta-analysis of prospective studies. J Am Acad Dermatol 2001;45(4):520-7.

[69] Benn CS, Wohlfahrt J, Aaby P, et al. Breastfeeding and risk of atopic dermatitis, by parental history of allergy, during the first 18 months of life. Am J Epidemiol 2004;160(3):217-23.

[70] von Berg A, Koletzko S, Grubl A, et al, (for the German Infant Nutritional Intervention Study Group). The effect of hydrolyzed cow's milk formula for allergy prevention in the first year of life: the German Infant Nutritional Intervention Study, a randomized double-blind trial. J Allergy Clin Immunol 2003;111:533-40.

[71] Muraro A, Dreborg S, Halken S, et al. Dietary prevention of allergic diseases in infants and small children. Part III: Critical review of published peer-reviewed observational and interventional studies and final recommendations. Pediatr Allergy Immunol 2004;15: 291-307.

[72] Osborn DA, Sinn J. Formulas containing hydrolysed protein for prevention of allergy and food intolerance in infants. In: The Cochrane Library. Issue 1. Chichester (UK): John Wiley & Sons; 2004.

[73] Kalliomaki M, Salminen S, Arvilommi H, et al. Probiotics in primary prevention of atopic disease: a randomized placebo-controlled trial. Lancet 2001;357:1076-9.

[74] Kalliomaki M, Salminen S, Poussa T, et al. Probiotics and prevention of atopic disease: 4-year follow-up of a randomized placebo-controlled trial. Lancet 2003;361:1869-71.

[75] Spergel JM, Paller AS. Atopic dermatitis and the atopic march. J Allergy Clin Immunol 2003;112(Suppl 6):S118-27.

[76] Broberg A, Kalimo K, Lindblad B, et al. Parental education in the treatment of childhood atopic eczema. Acta Derm Venereol 1990;70(6):495-9.

[77] Hanifin JM, Tofte SJ. Patient education in the long-term management of atopic dermatitis. Dermatol Nurs 1999;11:284-9.

[78] Charman CR, Morris AD, Williams HC. Topical corticosteroid phobia in patients with atopic eczema. Br J Dermatol 2000;142(5):931-6.

[79] Carvalho NF, Kenney RD, Carrington PH, et al. Severe nutritional deficiencies in toddlers resulting from health food milk alternatives. Pediatrics 2001;107(4):E46.

[80] Chamlin SL, Frieden IJ, Fowler A, et al. Ceramide-dominant, barrier-repair lipids improve childhood atopic dermatitis. Arch Dermatol 2001;137(8):1110-2.

[81] Van der Meer JB, Glazenburg EJ, Mulder PGH, et al, on behalf of the Netherlands Adult Atopic Dermatitis Study Group. Management of moderate to severe atopic dermatitis in adults with topical fluticasone propionate. Br J Dermatol 1999;140:1115–21.

[82] Hanifin J, Gupta AK, Rajagopalan R. Intermittent dosing of fluticasone propionate cream for reducing the risk of relapse in atopic dermatitis patients. Br J Dermatol 2002;147: 528–37.

[83] Hanifin JM, Paller A, Eichenfield L, et al. Long-term (up to 4 years) efficacy and safety of tacrolimus ointment in patients with atopic dermatitis. J Am Acad Dermatol 2005; 53(2 Suppl 2):S186–94.

[84] Wahn U, Bos JD, Goodfield M, et al. Flare Reduction in Eczema With Elidel (Children) Multicenter Investigator Study Group. Efficacy and safety of pimecrolimus cream in the long-term management of atopic dermatitis in children. Pediatrics 2002;110(1 Pt 1):e2.

[85] Nakahara T, Koga T, Fukagawa S, et al. Intermittent topical corticosteroid/tacrolimus sequential therapy improves lichenification and chronic papules more efficiently than intermittent topical corticosteroid/emollient sequential therapy in patients with atopic dermatitis. J Dermatol 2004;31(7):524–8.

[86] Furue M, Ogata F, Ootsuki M, et al. Hyperresponsibility to exogeneous interleukin 4 in atopic dermatitis. J Dermatol 1989;16:247–50.

[87] Papp KA, Werfel T, Folster-Holst R, et al. Long-term control of atopic dermatitis with pimecrolimus cream 1% in infants and young children: a two-year study. J Am Acad Dermatol 2005;52:240–6.

[88] Scheinfeld NS, Tutrone WD, Weinberg JM, et al. Phototherapy of atopic dermatitis. Clin Dermatol 2003;21:241–8.

[89] Berth-Jones J, Finlay AY, Zaki I, et al. Cyclosporine in severe childhood atopic dermatitis: a multicenter study. J Am Acad Dermatol 1996;34:1016–21.

[90] Sowden JM, Berth-Jones J, Ross JS, et al. Double-blind, controlled, crossover study of cyclosporine in adults with severe refractory atopic dermatitis. Lancet 1991;338:137–40.

[91] Akhavan A, Rudikoff D. The treatment of atopic dermatitis with systemic immunosuppressive agents. Clin Dermatol 2003;21:225–40.

[92] Sidbury R, Hanifin JM. Systemic therapy of atopic dermatitis. Clin Exp Dermatol 2000;25: 559–66.

[93] Stevens SR, Hanifin JM, Hamilton T, et al. Long-term effectiveness and safety of recombinant human interferon-gamma therapy for atopic dermatitis despite unchanged serum IgE levels. Arch Dermatol 1998;134(7):799–804.

[94] Berth-Jones J, Takwale A, Tan E, et al. Azathioprine in severe adult atopic dermatitis: a double-blind, placebo-controlled, crossover trial. Br J Dermatol 2002;147:324–30.

[95] Grundmann-Kollmann M, Podda M, Ochsendorf F, et al. Mycophenolate mofetil is effective in the treatment of atopic dermatitis. Arch Dermatol 2001;137(7):870–3.

[96] Klein PA, Clark RA. An evidence-based review of the efficacy of antihistamines in relieving pruritus in atopic dermatitis. Arch Dermatol 1999;135(12):1522–5.

[97] Pei AY, Chan HH, Leung TF. Montelukast in the treatment of children with moderate-to-severe atopic dermatitis: a pilot study. Pediatr Allergy Immunol 2001;12(3):154–8.

[98] Silverberg NB, Paller AS. Leukotriene receptor antagonists are ineffective for severe atopic dermatitis [letter]. J Am Acad Dermatol 2004;50(3):485–6.

[99] Tan BB, Weald D, Strickland I, et al. Double-blind controlled trial of effect of housedust-mite allergen avoidance on atopic dermatitis. Lancet 1996;347:15–8.

[100] Keane FM, Munn SE, du Vivier AW, et al. Analysis of Chinese herbal creams prescribed for dermatological conditions. BMJ 1999;318(7183):563–4.

[101] Rosenfeldt V, Benefeldt E, Nielsen SD, et al. Effect of probiotic Lactobaccillus strains in children with atopic dermatitis. J Allergy Clin Immunol 2003;111(2):389–95.

ELSEVIER
SAUNDERS

Med Clin N Am 90 (2006) 169–185

THE MEDICAL
CLINICS
OF NORTH AMERICA

# Allergic Contact Dermatitis

Barry J. Mark, MD*, Raymond G. Slavin, MD

*Division of Allergy and Immunology, Saint Louis University School of Medicine,
St. Louis, MO, USA*

Contact dermatitis, from both allergic and irritant etiologies, is the most common occupational disease in the United States and accounts for 90% of skin disorders acquired in the workplace [1,2]. Of the more than 6 million chemicals in the environment today, nearly 3000 have been known to cause allergic contact dermatitis (ACD) [3,4]. As new chemical sensitizers are introduced into the environment, the morbidity of ACD continues to grow. The occupationally related annual cost of ACD includes $250 million in lost productivity, medical care, and disability payments [5]. Moreover, the chronicity of the disease renders many patients uncomfortable, depressed, and unable to pursue employment or recreation [6].

## Pathophysiology

### Allergic versus irritant contact dermatitis

Distinguishing between allergic and irritant triggers of contact dermatitis by clinical and histologic examination alone can be challenging (Table 1). Irritant contact dermatitis (ICD) is responsible for approximately 80% of all contact dermatitis cases. Although both forms of contact dermatitis involve an inflammatory pathway, the skin reactions of ICD are nonimmunologic and result from direct epidermal keratinocyte damage after contact with a stimulus [3]. Unlike ACD, which affects only genetically susceptible persons who have been previously sensitized by allergen exposure, ICD may affect any person at any time if the concentration of the irritant and the duration of contact with the skin are sufficient [7].

---

* Corresponding author. Division of Allergy and Immunology, Saint Louis University School of Medicine, 1402 South Grand Boulevard, R-209, St. Louis, MO 63104.
*E-mail address:* markbj@slu.edu (B.J. Mark).

0025-7125/06/$ - see front matter © 2005 Elsevier Inc. All rights reserved.
doi:10.1016/j.mcna.2005.08.008 *medical.theclinics.com*

Table 1
Comparisons of irritant and allergic contact dermatitis

| Criteria | Irritant | Allergic |
|---|---|---|
| People at risk | Anyone, especially if repeated exposures | Genetically predisposed and previously sensitized |
| Mechanism | Direct tissue damage; nonimmunologic | Delayed-type hypersensitivity |
| Concentration of agent | Usually high; dose effect | May be low; threshold dose; all or nothing |
| Risk if atopic | Increased | Decreased |
| Histology | Spongiosis; primarily neutrophilic infiltrates | Spongiosis; primarily lymphocytic infiltrates |
| Symptoms | Burning, stinging, soreness | Itching |
| Appearance | Erythemia, edema, desquamation, fissures | Erythemia, edema, vesicles, papules, lichenification |
| Demarcation | Usually sharp | Sometimes sharp |
| Typical onset | Minutes to hours | Hours to days |
| Common agents | Water, soaps, detergents, acids, bases, solvents, saliva, urine, stool | Poison ivy, poison oak, poison sumac, metals, cosmetics, medicines, foods, rubbers, resins, adhesives |
| Diagnostic test | None | Patch test |

Clearly, some chemicals are more common triggers of ACD and ICD than others, because of their ubiquity in the environment and their innate physical properties. Physical conditions, such as heat, cold, repeated frictional exposure, or low humidity, can increase the likelihood and severity of contact dermatitis, particularly ICD. Any prior damage to the skin, whether from dehydration or trauma, compromises the integrity of its epidermal barrier (stratum corneum) and leaves it more vulnerable to irritants [8]. Interestingly, atopic persons as a group (ie, those with a propensity to produce specific IgE antibodies after exposure to allergens), when compared with nonatopic persons, seem to have skin with a greater relative susceptibility to contact irritants rather than to contact allergens [7]. This phenomenon may be caused by the classic "itch-scratch cycle" of atopic dermatitis, which further breaches the skin's barrier and permits increased dose-dependent penetration of irritants (while perhaps not permitting a threshold quantity of allergens to penetrate); and the tendency in atopy to favor pathways of the Th2 subset of T-helper lymphocytes rather than the Th1 pathways of ACD.

*Sensitization (afferent phase)*

Unlike most clinical allergic diseases, which feature an immediate hypersensitivity response involving IgE, ACD is the prototypic delayed (or cell-mediated) hypersensitivity reaction. As such, it depends on previously sensitized T-helper cells to fuel its inflammatory cascade. The contact allergens that initiate the afferent phase of this immune response are typically haptens, which first must covalently bond with tissue proteins to become fully immunogenic. The degree of Th1 sensitization is ultimately proportional to the stability of these hapten-protein couplings [6]. The most chemically reactive haptens are lipid-soluble, low-molecular-weight molecules, which can easily penetrate the stratum corneum and strongly bind carrier proteins [9].

Once within the epidermis, the hapten-protein complexes (now functional allergens) are engulfed by Langerhans cells, the primary antigen-presenting cells of the skin. This ingestion by pinocytosis is followed by degradation of the allergens, and the resulting processed peptides are displayed on the Langerhans cell surface in the context of major histocompatibility complex class II molecules [7]. These Langerhans cells migrate to regional draining lymph nodes where the processed peptides are presented to naïve Th1 cells. The specific T-cell receptors for these new peptides and major histocompatibility complex II molecules are found only on the Th1 cells of susceptible patients (ie, those who have the necessary repertoire of genetically rearranged T-cell receptor variable regions) [10]. Upon successful allergen presentation, interleukin-1 and -2 are secreted by the Langerhans cells and Th1 cells, respectively, thereby initiating the clonal proliferation of the newly sensitized Th1 cells in the paracortical region of the lymph nodes [9]. When this cascade follows a patient's initial contact with an allergen, the number of responding Th1 cells is insufficient to elicit a clinically visible response, although memory Th1 cells are released into the circulation in anticipation of the next exposure [11].

*Elicitation (efferent phase)*

The immune cascade that follows a patient's subsequent exposure to an identical allergen is boosted by the existing supply of circulating specific memory Th1 cells. Allergen presentation by Langerhans cells to this expanded pool of Th1 cells now occurs in the epidermis, dermis, and regional draining lymph nodes, thanks to skin-specific homing receptors on the Th1 cells and further clonal proliferation [3,9]. Once the cloned Th1 cells home to the initial hapten-provoked skin site, they release more inflammatory cytokines, including interferon-$\gamma$ (which is chemotactic for macrophages, cytotoxic T cells, and natural killer cells) and granulocyte-macrophage colony–stimulating factor (which augments the bone marrow's production of lymphocytes, granulocytes, and monocytes) [6,11,12]. These changes culminate in the epidermal spongiosis (intercellular edema) and dermal infiltrate that are characteristic of ACD [6]. The latency period from allergen contact to clinical dermatitis corresponds to the travel time for Langerhans cells to present the allergen to Th1 cells plus the time for Th1 cells to proliferate, secrete cytokines, and home with other inflammatory cells to the site of contact [3]. For many allergens, this latency is typically between 12 to 48 hours in a previously sensitized person [8].

## Clinical features

*History*

A patient's detailed history can uncover potentially hidden sources of contact allergens. Any patient with a skin disease always must be evaluated for an occupational exposure. Industries in which workers are at the highest risk for occupational skin diseases include food production, construction, printing, metal plating, machine tool operation, engine service, leather work, health care, cosmetology, and forestry. The presence of skin diseases in fellow workers, control measures taken in the workplace, and specific chemical agents encountered on the job may reveal the underlying cause. The temporal relationship of days off and return to work should be correlated with symptoms [1]. Although it might be tempting to focus a patient's history on recent exposures, long-term exposures are frequently implicated in ACD [10]. Unlike strong allergens, such as poison ivy, which may exert their effect within several hours to days and after as few as one exposure, many occupational allergens, such as chromate, are weak sensitizers and may require repeated exposures over several months to years to develop skin sensitivity [6]. Exposures outside of the workplace to such items as jewelry, clothing, cosmetics, fragrances, soaps, detergents, household cleaning agents, paints, resins, rubbers, latex, adhesives, and topical medicines may also result in ACD or ICD and must be elucidated from the history. No matter which agent is implicated or how variable the rash may appear, the one uniformly present feature of ACD is pruritus, without which the diagnosis of ACD is virtually excluded.

*Physical examination*

The appearance of the lesion in ACD often corresponds to the stage at which the patient presents. During the acute stage there is marked erythema, edema, and vesicle formation. Edema predominates if areas of loose tissue, such as the eyelids or genitalia, are affected. Vesicles are often multiple and severe and may coalesce into bullae. The vesicles of ACD are filled with a clear, transudative fluid and rupture during the subacute stage, the time when patients typically present to physicians. This rupture may lead to oozing and eroded skin with a characteristic eczematous appearance [6,13]. The vesicular fluid does not contain appreciable amounts of the allergen and so does not spread the eruption to other areas of the body or to other individuals [7]. As the vesicles become less pronounced, they may be replaced by papules (Fig. 1). Crusting and scaling soon become more prominent than the erythema and edema. As the papulovesicular lesions disappear and the ACD enters its chronic stage, lichenification and further scaling predominate. These stages of ACD are classified broadly, and the potential for overlap prohibits a sharp delineation among them [6,13]. Nonetheless, unless a secondary bacterial infection is also suspected,

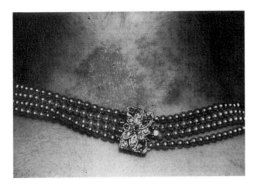

Fig. 1. The classic erythematous, papulovesicular eruption of ACD on the back of this patient's neck is caused by contact from nickel-plated jewelry.

the principles of prevention and treatment of ACD remain similar, regardless of the stage.

*Differential diagnosis*

Near the end of a patient's initial visit, the physician's clinical suspicion of ACD may be quite high. It is paramount, however, to consider other less likely, but potentially more serious, etiologies and mimickers of a patient's dermatitis. Although ICD may be the skin condition most often confused with ACD, atopic dermatitis is another frequent imitator of ACD. Both atopic dermatitis and ACD may appear eczematous, but whereas atopic dermatitis generally has its onset in infancy or early childhood, ACD is uncommon in children younger than 8 years old [6,9]. In addition, the dry skin and pruritus of atopic dermatitis are prominent features before the lesions appear, not afterwards as in ACD. Atopic dermatitis also tends to be symmetrically distributed on extensor surfaces in infancy and on flexural surfaces in childhood and beyond. The lesions of seborrheic dermatitis, meanwhile, have a predilection for the eyebrows, nasal labial folds, and scalp. Unlike ACD, seborrheic dermatitis presents with typically mild pruritus and tends to have a greasy or oily coating with scaly, irregularly shaped erythema [6,14]. More intensely pruritic eruptions include two endogenous dermatoses, described as nummular and dyshidrotic. Nummular dermatitis consists of one or a group of coin-shaped, eczematous patches 2 to 10 cm in diameter that are usually seen on the torso and extremities but not the head. Dyshidrotic dermatitis commonly appears as multiple vesicles 1 to 2 mm in diameter on the palms, soles, and lateral aspects of the fingers and toes [15].

Photocontact dermatitis is caused by the interaction between an exogenous chemical in the skin and the UV component of sunlight. The photosensitive agent may be a recently ingested drug, such as a sulfonamide, fluoroquinolone, tetracycline, oral contraceptive, or nonsteroidal anti-inflammatory drug, or a topically applied substance, such as a cold tar extract

[6,14]. Clinically, only sun-exposed areas, such as the face, arms, and upper chest are affected, whereas the skin under the chin, behind the ears, and on the upper eyelids is noticeably spared [9]. The two forms of photocontact dermatitis, phototoxic reactions and photoallergic reactions, can be thought of as subsets of ICD and ACD, respectively. A phototoxic reaction manifests as a macular and tender erythema, which can resemble severe sunburn. Like ICD, its nonimmunologic mechanism requires no sensitizing period, so symptoms may occur on the first exposure to UV light. With a photoallergic reaction, a delayed hypersensitivity reaction is induced by UV light, which chemically alters the sensitizing allergen in the skin. This reaction may produce a pruritic, papulovesicular, eczematous dermatitis similar to ACD [13,16].

Like photocontact dermatitis, two types of contact urticaria have been recently recognized as subsets of contact dermatitis. In its nonallergic form, the urticaria remains localized to the site of contact and may be caused by direct mast cell mediator release from fragrances, food preservatives, insect stings or hairs, or topical medicines [9,17]. Allergic contact urticaria results from IgE-mediated mast cell stimulation and requires prior exposure to sensitizing allergens, such as foods, metals, animal saliva, latex, industrial products, or topical medicines [9]. Both forms of contact urticaria resemble noncontact urticaria, and their classic wheal and flare response usually appears within 30 minutes of exposure. Although allergic contact urticaria may become generalized and even progress to angioedema or anaphylaxis, most cases of urticaria, angioedema, and anaphylaxis result from ingested or internal causes rather than from contact or physical triggers. Any form of urticaria or angioedema, whether contact or noncontact, can be easily mistaken for ACD, particularly when the eyelids are involved (Fig. 2).

Various skin infections are among the many other masqueraders of ACD and must be strongly considered in immunocompromised patients. Cellulitis presents with erythema and edema, but also with warmth and tenderness. Trauma is a common precipitant of cellulitis, which, unlike ACD, is often accompanied by a fever and leukocytosis. Dermatophytic or tinea infections

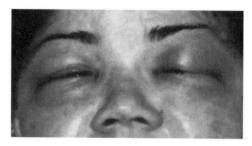

Fig. 2. Marked eyelid swelling may mimic angioedema, but here is caused by contact from the *p*-phenylenediamine allergen in hair dye with the thin skin of the patient's eyelids.

typically appear as dry, scaling erythema with an annular ring and central clearing. This diagnosis is easily made by scraping scales from the lesion onto a glass slide, adding potassium hydroxide solution, and visualizing branching hyphae under light microscopy [18].

Several other infections present primarily with vesicular lesions, including herpes simplex virus, varicella zoster virus, and impetigo. Herpes simplex virus vesicles are tender, may umbilicate, and have a predilection for perioral and genital regions. Patients with primary varicella zoster virus infection (chickenpox) exhibit a 2- to 3-day prodrome of flulike symptoms, followed by erythematous maculopapules that progress to diffuse, pruritic vesicles. Those with reactivated varicella zoster virus (shingles) have few constitutional symptoms, but experience localized pain and paresthesias 2 to 3 days before the eruption of closely grouped vesicles in a dermatomal distribution. Impetigo may affect all age groups, but is usually seen in young children. *Streptococcus pyogenes* or *Staphylococcus aureus* are the usual culprits in impetigo, which generally involves the face, has regional lymphadenopathy, and is self-limited to 2 to 3 weeks. Its vesicles may progress to pustules, which easily rupture, leaving a superficial honey-colored crust [18].

The thick, silver-scaled plaques over bright erythema on the extensor surfaces of patients with psoriasis, and the asymmetric, finely scaled plaques on the trunk and groin of patients with mycosis fungoides (the primary cutaneous T-cell lymphoma) sometimes resemble the lesions of ACD. A biopsy may be warranted to rule out these two recalcitrant conditions. In general, however, a biopsy has low utility in the work-up of ACD, because the histologic finding of spongiosis is not very specific among eczematous dermatoses [14,19].

### Anatomic approach

In addition to the history and appearance of the rash in question, its anatomic distribution may help distinguish ACD from other types of dermatitis [10]. Exposure to the suspect allergen should be congruent with the distribution of the eruption. Because the more exposed areas of skin are more open to allergen encounter, the hands and face are the most common body parts presenting with ACD [3].

### Head and neck

The skin of the scalp tends to be thicker and have greater resistance to ACD than the face, ears, and neck. Hair dyes and shampoos often spare the scalp but involve its nearby landmarks (see Fig. 2) [20]. The thin skin of the eyelids and cheeks are frequently affected by facial cosmetics and also by products applied to the hands, particularly nail polish, which are inadvertently transmitted to the face [21]. Metals from jewelry piercings anywhere on the face and ears and topical antibiotics for the eyes and ears are common triggers of ACD. The neck may be primarily involved through direct contact with cosmetics and fragrances; metals and exotic woods from necklaces (see Fig. 1); and even chemicals and accessories from musical instruments that rest between the neck and shoulder [3].

### Extremities

More than half of all cases of contact dermatitis involve the hands. The list of household and occupational materials that are frequently handled is extensive, but should also include supposed innocuous items, such as foods, moisturizers, musical instruments, and protective gloves. ICD is most common on the fingertips [9]. ACD frequently occurs on the dorsal side of the hands, where, in general, the skin is thinner and the density of Langerhans cells is greater than on the palmar side [5,22]. Bracelets, watches, and rings may lead to both ACD from metal exposure and ICD from soap and detergent accumulation under these accessories [23]. When hand dermatitis is contiguous with the forearms and is associated with a facial dermatitis, a photosensitive process should be suggested. ACD over the dorsal aspect of the feet may be caused by the chrome-tanned leather, glues, and rubber components of shoes [5]. Stasis dermatitis of the lower legs from chronic varicose inflammation of the skin significantly increases the risk of ACD from topically applied products [24]. Metals from keys and coins and even the striking surfaces of match boxes in pants pockets may be the culprits in ACD of the upper legs [20].

### Torso and groin

Fragrances from deodorants may cause ACD involving the entire axillary vault, whereas formaldehyde, detergents, and dyes from clothes may preferentially involve the torso and axillary folds with sparing of the vault [12]. Rubber chemicals in the elastic of undergarments may affect the bra line and waistline. ACD of the periumbilical region is often caused by the metallic fasteners of belts and pants [20]. Incontinent, bed-bound patients frequently develop ICD from urine and stool along a diaper distribution. Contraceptive devices often affect rubber- and latex-sensitive patients. Medicines, douches, and spermicides may cause contact dermatitis in the genital area, principally the vulva and adjacent thighs rather than the vaginal mucosa [3].

### Oral mucosa

Although Langerhans cells are abundant in the epidermal layer of skin, they are sparse at mucosal sites [10]. Nonetheless, the lichenoid plaques and erosions of contact stomatitis (along with other signs of contact gingivitis and cheilitis) may result from various dental metals, such as nickel, palladium, mercury, and gold. One theory for these eruptions is that the saliva in the mouth enhances the leaching of these metals from their dental amalgams [25]. In general, however, saliva has a buffering and diluting effect on the allergen, thereby limiting its potency. The brief duration of surface contact and the rapid dispersal and absorption of the allergen because of extensive vascularity in the mouth also account for the low incidence of contact stomatitis compared with contact dermatitis [6]. Any allergen from metal dental gear or oral piercings or from any foods or medicines that contact the oral mucosa may further predispose a person to a systemic skin reaction.

*Systemic involvement*

Systemic ACD is a form of autoeczematization, also known as an "id reaction." This secondary dermatitis presents rarely in patients who have been sensitized topically to an allergen and are subsequently re-exposed systemically. This re-exposure may occur orally, intravenously, intramuscularly, rectally, vaginally, by inhalation, or after dental or surgical devices have been implanted [5]. The generalized eruption is thought to result from the hematogenous dissemination of stimulated, circulating, antigen-specific Th1 cells and their cytokines from a primary local site to distal ones [10,26].

**Common contact allergens**

*Poison ivy*

Poison ivy is the most ubiquitous of the four species of the *Toxicodendron* genus of the Anacardiaceae plant family, which also includes poison sumac and two species of poison oak. In the United States, these four species of plants are responsible for more cases of ACD than all other contact allergens combined. It is estimated that over 70% of the United States population would acquire ACD if casually exposed to these plants. The strongly sensitizing allergen of *Toxicodendron* plants is urushiol, a catechol derivative found in the plants' sap [27]. Once the sap binds to a patient's skin, it is difficult to wash off, but washing with any soap should still be attempted, ideally within 10 minutes of exposure, to prevent adherence [8]. Poison ivy dermatitis initially appears as a linear streaking of erythema and vesicles. The vesicular fluid is often believed to be contagious, but there is no evidence that the fluid is allergenic. The chronicity and spread of symptoms, however, frequently come from the continued unintentional exposure to urushiol, which may persist on clothing, tools, sports equipment, and the fur of pets [16]. Cross-reactions may occur in patients exposed to catechol derivatives similar to urushiol that are found in other members of the Anacardiaceae family, such as mangoes, cashews, ginkgoes, and Brazilian peppers [27].

*Metals*

Nickel is the most common metal allergen in the United States with an estimated prevalence of 7% to 17%. The prevalence in women is considerably higher because of their increased exposure to jewelry and early sensitization from ear piercings. Other frequent causes of metal allergy include chromium, cobalt, gold, and organic forms of mercury. Cross-reactions among different metals are extremely rare [28]. Sensitivity to aluminum is quite uncommon, and the substitution of aluminum items for sensitizing metal items in the workplace may reduce the incidence of ACD [29]. Among the most commonly used metal alloys for medical devices and implants is stainless steel, which contains both nickel and chromium. Although a true metal implant allergy is very unusual, it may present with persistent localized or generalized eczema and loosening of the implant. Patch testing (discussed later) with the suspect metals has low specificity and only moderate sensitivity in the work-up of a metal implant allergy, but if it is clinically suspected, the implant should be removed [30].

*Medications*

Topical antibiotics, such as neomycin and bacitracin, induce more ACD than any other class of medicines. Patients with sensitivities to these antibiotics may find mupirocin to be a safe alternative [7]. Topical anesthetics of the ester class, such as benzocaine and tetracaine, are frequently implicated in ACD, whereas the amide class of anesthetics, such as lidocaine, dibucaine, and mepivacaine, are rare sensitizers [31]. Topical corticosteroids had previously been dismissed as unlikely allergens based on their inhibition of lymphocyte proliferation. It is now well recognized that the structure of corticosteroids may be altered to induce allergenicity through both metabolism in the skin and degradative reactions within the pharmaceutical preparation [32]. Even topical antihistamines are known to act as sensitizers and may predispose patients to an id reaction after systemic administration of an antihistamine from the same class [33]. Ethylenediamine is a common allergenic preservative found in aminophylline, some antihistamines, and other topical medicines. The preservative with the highest prevalence of positive patch tests, however, is thimerosal, found principally in vaccines and numerous topical medicines for the eyes, ears, and nose [34].

*Latex and rubber chemicals*

Natural rubber latex is created from the latex fluid of the Brazilian rubber tree, *Hevea brasiliensis*. Chemical accelerators and antioxidants are added to natural rubber latex during its vulcanization process to catalyze its compounding. These chemicals, which include thiurams, carbamates, and mercaptobenzothiazole, are the primary sensitizers of ACD in rubber products. Immediate hypersensitivity reactions are mediated by specific IgE against the latex protein itself. The IgE responses manifest as urticaria, rhinitis, conjunctivitis, asthma, and anaphylaxis, usually within minutes of direct contact or airborne exposure to the proteins [35]. Of all the rubber products manufactured, latex gloves are the leading cause of not only these immediate-type reactions, but also of both the delayed-type reactions of ACD and the most frequently seen complication of latex, ICD.

## Formaldehyde and fragrances

Formaldehyde and formaldehyde-releasers, such as quaternium-15, are the most common preservatives responsible for ACD outside of thimerosal [34]. These two preservatives are found in numerous cosmetics, moisturizers, and fabrics. Fragrances are widely used in cosmetics, fabrics, and topical medicines; in flavorings of foods, drinks, spices, and oral hygiene products; and in perfumes and colognes [17]. Balsam of Peru is the fragrance most often implicated in both ACD and nonallergic contact urticaria. In addition to the previously mentioned products, balsam of Peru also is found in sunscreens and shampoos. Both its beneficial actions and its topical side effects may be partly caused by its ability to stimulate capillary beds and increase local circulation [36].

## Patch testing

### Principles

The epicutaneous patch test is considered the gold standard for diagnosing ACD. Its first rudimentary use was in 1895 when Josef Jadassohn suspected a patient's rash was the result of mercury sensitivity [37]. Since then, the patch test has evolved into a refined, albeit simple, means of reproducing a similar ACD with the same or cross-reacting allergen over a small area of a patient's back. Standardized samples of allergens are manufactured within or placed on small delivery vehicles before application on the skin. Because the classic ACD eruption typically appears within 2 to 3 days of sufficient allergen contact, patch testing is performed over at least a 3-day period.

The number of allergens applied on a patient depends on the physician's clinical suspicion of likely culprits. Routine, ready-to-apply, screening panels of 20 to 30 of the most prevalent ACD allergens, however, often are used because of the simplicity of their application. The panels applied perhaps most frequently by physicians are packaged as a thin layer rapid-use epicutaneous test, known as the TRUE Test (Mekos Laboratories A/S, Hillerød, Denmark). The 23 allergens and one negative control of the standard TRUE Test are incorporated into a gel delivery system on two rectangular panels, each less than 3 × 6 in (Table 2) [38]. Each of the 12 samples per panel is just 1 cm$^2$, and they are adequately spaced apart from one another. The standard TRUE Test identifies about 70% of clinically relevant allergens in ACD when compared with the extensive, lesser used, 58-allergen screening series of the North American Contact Dermatitis Group [39]. More tailored panels that include many allergens of one particular category, such as metals, classes of medicines, cosmetics, and fragrances, alternatively may be

Table 2
TRUE Test 24-allegen panel

| Patch test allergen | Conventional products |
|---|---|
| 1. Nickel sulfate | Jewelry, fasteners |
| 2. Wool alcohols (lanolin)[a] | Cosmetics, soaps, skin care creams |
| 3. Neomycin sulfate | Topical antibiotics, eye/ear drops |
| 4. Potassium dichromate | Chrome-tanned leather, cement |
| 5. Caine mix | Topical anesthetics |
| 6. Fragrance mix | Perfumes, toiletries, flavorings |
| 7. Colophony[b] | Adhesives, cosmetics, household cleaners |
| 8. Paraben mix[a] | Cosmetics, sunscreen, skin care creams |
| 9. Negative control | — |
| 10. Balsam of Peru | Perfumes, sunscreen, shampoo, flavorings |
| 11. Ethylenediamine dihydrochloride[a] | Topical antibiotics/fungicides/antihistamines |
| 12. Cobalt Dichloride | Metal-plated objects, paints |
| 13. *p-tert*-Butylphenol formaldehyde[b] | Glue, fabrics |
| 14. Epoxy[b] | Paints, paste, adhesives |
| 15. Carba mix[c] | Pesticides, paints, gloves, adhesives |
| 16. Black rubber mix[c] | Shoes, gloves, tires, hoses |
| 17. Methylchloroisothiazolinone[a] | Cosmetics, shampoo, skin care creams |
| 18. Quaternium-15[a] | Cosmetics, shampoo, skin care creams |
| 19. Mercaptobenzothiazole[c] | Shoes, gloves, clothes, detergents |
| 20. *p*-Phenylenediamine | Hair dyes, cosmetics, printing inks |
| 21. Formaldehyde[a] | Cosmetics, fabrics, plastics |
| 22. Mercapto mix[c] | Shoes, gloves, elastics, pet products |
| 23. Thimerosal[a] | Vaccines, eye/ear/nose drops, cosmetics |
| 24. Thiuram mix[c] | Pesticides, paints, gloves, adhesives |

[a] Preservatives.
[b] Resins.
[c] Rubber chemicals.

used if clinically warranted. Another option uses personally chosen assortments of allergens, individually applied to filter paper in 8-mm aluminum disks known as "Finn Chambers" (Epitest Ltd Oy, Tuusula, Finland) along with a 5-mm ribbon of petrolatum for allergen dispersion [38].

*Techniques*

No matter which type of patch test is performed, the techniques of application and interpretation are the same. For the most reliable results, the allergens are applied together (as a patch) to a hairless region of the upper back between the spine and scapula that has been washed with plain water and gently dried. An adhesive keeps the allergens secured, and its edges are marked with a pen. For the patch to remain in place, patients are instructed not to shower or exercise to the point of perspiring. Although mild pruritus beneath the patch may be expected, severe pruritus or pain should prompt a call to the physician for possible early removal to prevent skin sloughing [40]. Otherwise, patients should return to the physician's office for a second visit 48 to 72 hours after the initial application for patch removal. After waiting 20 to 30 minutes to allow for any nonspecific mechanical irritation from the removed patch to subside, the reactions are graded (Table 3).

Distinguishing ACD from ICD is difficult at this second visit, particularly if the skin reaction is a weak one. For this reason, patients should return for a third visit 24 to 96 hours later. By that time, an ICD reaction would have subsided, whereas an ACD reaction would arrive, persist, or worsen. A 96-hour interval between the second and third visits may be optimal for interpreting patch tests of elderly patients, who tend to take longer mounting an allergic response than younger patients. This also may be the appropriate interval if allergens known to induce late-phase reactions, such as cobalt, neomycin, and topical corticosteroids, are clinically suspected [5,40].

*Precautions*

Patch testing should not be performed in the presence of an acute or widespread contact dermatitis because a positive patch test reaction with the offending allergen may induce a flare-up of the existing ACD or progress to autoeczematization. In addition, the increased reactivity of the skin during active ACD may lead to false-positive patch test results [6]. Any pruritus within minutes of patch test application should raise suspicions of contact urticaria and the remote possibility of subsequent anaphylaxis if the patch is not removed [37].

Physicians who routinely use the standard TRUE Test panels for ACD evaluation should remember that bacitracin and gold, two of the most prevalent ACD allergens in the United States, are not among the 23 included allergens. Poison ivy also is not included in these panels, nor should it be applied separately as a patch test, because urushiol's strong sensitizing potential may cause severe reactions. Judicious use of patch tests may prevent the test allergens themselves from sensitizing a previously nonexposed patient. Repeat patch testing rarely is indicated. Patch tests may need to be delayed if a patient has used potent topical steroids nearby the anticipated test site. Systemic steroids, however, in doses of 20 mg or less of prednisone daily, should not inhibit positive reactions [37].

Table 3
Guide to patch test results

| Score | Reaction | Signs |
| --- | --- | --- |
| − | Negative | None |
| ? | Doubtful | Faint macular, homogenous erythema, no infiltration |
| + | Weak positive | Erythema, infiltration, papules |
| ++ | Strong positive | Erythema, infiltration, papules, discrete vesicles |
| +++ | Extreme positive | Coalescing vesicles, bullous reaction |
| IR | Irritant | Discrete patchy erythema, no infiltration |

## Prevention and treatment

The central tenets of ACD prevention and treatment are to accurately identify the culprit allergen and to institute the necessary avoidance measures. If patch testing fails to incriminate a likely allergen and the diagnosis of contact dermatitis is still strongly considered, a detailed diary of the patient's daily activities may help discover patterns of allergen or irritant exposure. When the appropriate allergen is identified, the patient must be educated about potential sources of exposure and cross-reacting allergens, and offered suggestions for avoidance. If an occupational allergen is implicated, the workplace employer should provide the patient with material safety data sheets, which may uncover hidden sources of exposures in that environment.

When the allergen cannot be avoided, wearing protective barriers is the next best preventive option. Because of the high incidence of dermatitis of the hands and their ability to transfer allergens to other body parts and objects, wearing appropriate gloves may be the most effective means of allergen and irritant protection. The ideal gloves are vinyl, waterproof, and heavy-duty, and can be worn atop cotton gloves for greater comfort. Long-sleeved shirts and pants often are recommended, particularly during outdoor activities with a high risk of poison ivy contact. Nonallergenic barrier creams and emollients may further protect and also soothe and gently hydrate the skin. In addition to these personal barriers, the contacted objects sometimes can be modified to become less allergenic themselves, such as nickel-plated fasteners and jewelry that are painted with a clear polyurethane varnish [7].

Because corticosteroids halt lymphocyte proliferation and decrease cytokine production, they have become the mainstay of ACD therapy [41]. For mild or moderate localized dermatitis, topical corticosteroids applied twice daily are usually effective within a few days and should be continued for 2 weeks. To limit their cutaneous side effects, lower potency agents should be applied to the face and intertriginous areas, with higher potency steroids reserved for the extremities and torso. Steroid creams may have greater cosmetic appeal than steroid ointments. Creams typically contain more potentially allergenic preservatives and fragrances, however, whereas ointments penetrate more deeply into the skin, increasing their potency. Cool water compresses may also facilitate topical steroid absorption. When applied with a smooth cotton cloth, cool water may be soothing and antipruritic, and may also debride vesicular crusts and promote dermal vasoconstriction to reduce inflammation [7].

When the dermatitis is particularly severe or widespread, involves the mucous membranes, or continues to progress beyond initial therapy, systemic corticosteroids should be used [8]. The response to systemic steroids generally is dramatic, with improvement noted within a few hours. A prepackaged steroid prescription, such as a methylprednisolone dose pack tapered over 6 days, is usually inadequate for the treatment of ACD and frequently results in rebound dermatitis. Oral prednisone is most effective when prescribed at 1 mg/kg/d for several days and tapered slowly over at least 2 weeks.

Medications other than corticosteroids remain second-line agents at best. Although the delayed-type reactions of ACD do not involve histamine release from mast cells, oral antihistamines may still provide some antipruritic and soporific effects. Although their benefits may be nominal, any reduction in pruritus and scratching ultimately limits the incidence of secondary bacterial infections. When such superinfections do occur, oral antibiotics against *S aureus* and *S pyogenes* are preferred to topical antibiotics (just as oral antihistamines are preferred to topical ones) because these topical medications are frequent allergic sensitizers. The immunosuppressive effects of topical calcineurin inhibitors, such as tacrolimus and pimecrolimus, do not have the proven use in the treatment of ACD as they have in the treatment of atopic dermatitis [41,42]. Recalcitrant or chronic ACD may require adjuvant, long-term therapy with psoralen and UVA or UVB [13]. Unlike IgE-mediated reactions to aeroallergens, drugs, and insect stings, desensitization protocols (allergy shots) have no role in treating delayed-type hypersensitivities to contact allergens [3].

## Summary

The pathophysiology of ACD follows an intricate design and results in the characteristic, delayed inflammatory response. Although the astute physician may correctly diagnose ACD from its initial, classic history and presentation, alternative diagnoses should be considered and excluded. Patch testing performed with a relevant panel of contact allergens is the ultimate confirmatory test of ACD. Correctly identifying the inciting allergen permits appropriate personal avoidance. Corticosteroids remain the principal treatment options.

## References

[1] Peate WF. Occupational skin disease. Am Fam Physician 2002;66:1025–32.
[2] Burress JW, Christiani DC. Occupational health and disability issues in primary care. In: Noble J, editor. Textbook of primary care medicine, 3rd edition. St. Louis: Mosby; 2001. p. 104–24.
[3] Beltrani VS, Beltrani VP. Contact dermatitis. Ann Allergy Asthma Immunol 1997;78: 160–75.
[4] Cohen DE. Contact dermatitis: a quarter century perspective. J Am Acad Dermatol 2004;51: S60–3.
[5] Belsito DV. The diagnostic evaluation, treatment, and prevention of allergic contact dermatitis in the new millennium. J Allergy Clin Immunol 2000;105:409–20.
[6] Slavin RG. Contact dermatitis. In: Patterson R, Grammer LC, Greenberger PA, editors. Allergic diseases. 5th edition. Philadelphia: Lippincott-Raven; 1997. p. 413–24.

[7] Welch MP. Contact dermatitis. In: Altman LC, Becker JW, Williams PV, editors. Allergy in primary care. Philadelphia: WB Saunders; 2000. p. 241–58.

[8] Halstater B, Usatine RP. Contact dermatitis. In: Milgrom EC, Usatine RP, Tan RA, et al, editors. Practical allergy. Philadelphia: Mosby; 2004. p. 64–77.

[9] Mydlarski PR, Katz AM, Mamelak AJ, et al. Contact dermatitis. In: Adkinson NF Jr, Yunginger JW, Busse WW, et al, editors. Middleton's allergy: principles & practice. 6th edition. Philadelphia: Mosby; 2003. p. 1581–97.

[10] Weston WL, Bruckner A. Allergic contact dermatitis. Pediatr Clin North Am 2000;47: 897–907.

[11] Anderson W. Immunology. Madison (CT): Fence Creek; 1999.

[12] Boguniewicz M, Beltrani VS. Contact dermatitis. In: Leung DYM, Sampson HA, Geha RS, et al, editors. Pediatric allergy: principles and practice. St. Louis: Mosby; 2003. p. 584–94.

[13] Contact dermatitis. In: The allergy report. Volume 3: conditions that may have an allergic component. Milwaukee (WI): American Academy of Allergy, Asthma & Immunology; 2000. p. 33–50.

[14] Beltrani VS. Allergic dermatoses. Med Clin North Am 1998;82:1105–33.

[15] Shaw JC. Overview of dermatitis. In: Rose BD, editor. UpToDate. Wellesley (MA): UpToDate; 2004. Available at: http://www.uptodate.com. Accessed February 12, 2005.

[16] Whitmore SE. Common problems of the skin. In: Barker LR, Burton JR, Zieve PD, editors. Principles of ambulatory medicine. 5th edition. Baltimore: Lippincott Williams & Wilkins; 1999. p. 1499–539.

[17] Katsarou A, Armenaka M, Kalogeromitros D, et al. Contact reactions to fragrances. Ann Allergy Asthma Immunol 1999;82:449–55.

[18] Fleischer AB, Feldman SR, Katz AS, et al. 20 common problems in dermatology. New York: McGraw-Hill; 2000.

[19] Gaspari AA. The role of keratinocytes in the pathophysiology of contact dermatitis. Immunol Allergy Clin North Am 1997;17:377–405.

[20] Rietschel RL, Fowler JF Jr. Regional contact dermatitis. In: Fisher's contact dermatitis. 4th edition. Baltimore: Williams & Wilkins; 1995. p. 66–91.

[21] Leung DYM, Diaz LA, DeLeo V, et al. Allergic and immunologic skin disorders. JAMA 1997;278:1914–23.

[22] Berman B, Chen VL, France DS, et al. Anatomical mapping of epidermal Langerhans cell densities in adults. Br J Dermatol 1983;109:553–8.

[23] Rietschel RL, Fowler JF Jr. Hand dermatitis due to contactants: special considerations. In: Fisher's contact dermatitis. 4th edition. Baltimore: Williams & Wilkins; 1995. p. 330–57.

[24] Shupp DL, Winkelmann RK. The role of patch testing in stasis dermatitis. Cutis 1991;47: 528–9.

[25] Schultz JC, Connelly E, Glesne L, et al. Cutaneous and oral eruption from oral exposure to nickel in dental braces. Dermatitis 2004;15:154–7.

[26] Evans MP, Bronson D. Id reaction (autoeczematization). eMedicine Journal (serial online). 2003. Available at: http://www.emedicine.com/derm/topic193.htm. Accessed February 12, 2005.

[27] Rietschel RL, Fowler JF Jr. Toxicodendron, plants, and spices. In: Fisher's contact dermatitis. 4th edition. Baltimore: Williams & Wilkins; 1995. p. 461–523.

[28] Rietschel RL, Fowler JF Jr. Contact dermatitis and other reactions to metals. In: Fisher's contact dermatitis. 4th edition. Baltimore: Williams & Wilkins; 1995. p. 808–85.

[29] Rietschel RL, Fowler JF Jr. Reactions to selected topical medications. In: Fisher's contact dermatitis. 4th edition. Baltimore: Williams & Wilkins; 1995. p. 141–70.

[30] Rietschel RL, Fowler JF Jr. Dermatitis from medical devices and implants. In: Fisher's contact dermatitis. 4th edition. Baltimore: Williams & Wilkins; 1995. p. 414–47.

[31] Rietschel RL, Fowler JF Jr. Local anesthetics. In: Fisher's contact dermatitis. 4th edition. Baltimore: Williams & Wilkins; 1995. p. 236–48.

[32] Wilkinson SM. Hypersensitivity to topical corticosteroids. Clin Exp Dermatol 1994;19:1–11.

[33] Rietschel RL, Fowler JF Jr. Antihistamine dermatitis. In: Fisher's contact dermatitis. 4th edition. Baltimore: Williams & Wilkins; 1995. p. 226–35.

[34] Marks JG, Belsito DV, DeLeo VA, et al. North American contact dermatitis group patch-test results, 1998 to 2000. Am J Contact Dermat 2003;14:59–62.

[35] Charlesworth EN. Allergic skin disease. In: Slavin RG, Reisman RE, editors. Expert guide to allergy and immunology. Philadelphia: American College of Physicians; 1999. p. 81–103.

[36] Rietschel RL, Fowler JF Jr. Medications from plants. In: Fisher's contact dermatitis. 4th edition. Baltimore: Williams & Wilkins; 1995. p. 171–83.

[37] Adams RM. Patch testing: a recapitulation. J Am Acad Dermatol 1981;5:629–43.

[38] Bernstein IL, Storms WW. Practice parameters for allergy diagnostic testing. Ann Allergy Asthma Immunol 1995;75(6 Part 2):543–625.

[39] Larkin A, Rietschel RL. The utility of patch tests using larger screening series of allergens. Am J Contact Dermat 1998;9:142–5.

[40] Fonacier L. Contact dermatitis & patch testing. Presented at the annual meeting of the Workshops of the American College of Allergy, Asthma, & Immunology. Boston, Massachusetts, November 12–17, 2004.

[41] Weston WL. Contact dermatitis in children. In: Rose BD, editor. UpToDate. Wellesley (MA): UpToDate; 2004. Available at: http://www.uptodate.com. Accessed February 12, 2005.

[42] Amrol D, Keitel D, Hagaman D, et al. Topical pimecrolimus in the treatment of human allergic contact dermatitis. Ann Allergy Asthma Immunol 2003;91:563–6.

ELSEVIER
SAUNDERS

THE MEDICAL
CLINICS
OF NORTH AMERICA

Med Clin N Am 90 (2006) 187–209

# Urticaria: Selected Highlights and Recent Advances

## Donald A. Dibbern, Jr, MD*

*Division of Allergy and Clinical Immunology, Oregon Health and Sciences University, Portland, OR, USA*

Urticaria is a common and ancient malady. Early Chinese medical literature refers to this as "wind-rash-patch," or *Fong-Tzen-Kwai* [1]. This condition was also known to Western medicine by Pliny, Celsus, and Hippocrates [2]. More recently, in the eighteenth century, it was elegantly described by Heberden as, "The little elevations upon the skin in the 'nettle' rash often appear involuntarily, especially if the skin be rubbed, or scrubbed, and seldom stay many hours in the same place, and sometimes not many minutes. There is no body exempt from 'them' and by far the greatest number experience no other evil from it besides the intolerable anguish arising from the itching..." [3]. Comparing one recent review of urticaria [4] with another a half-century prior [5], the similarities are perhaps more remarkable than the differences in the present understanding of this challenging illness. Rather than presenting a comprehensive overview, this article instead highlights selected topics, controversies, and recent advances in the diagnosis, evaluation, and management of this fascinating condition.

## Approaches to evaluation

There are no shortcuts in the evaluation of urticaria. This symptom (when described by the patient) and sign (when observed by the clinician) is notable for the fact that despite numerous possible causes, most cases turn out to be idiopathic in nature [6]. Idiopathic urticaria is a diagnosis of exclusion, however, and should be reached only after a thorough and detailed history and physical examination. Early in the evaluation, a few key

---

Dr. Dibbern is on the Speakers' Bureau for Pfizer.

* Division of Allergy and Clinical Immunology (OP34), Oregon Health and Sciences University, 3181 SW Sam Jackson Park Road, Portland, OR 97239–3098.
*E-mail address:* dibbernd@ohsu.edu

0025-7125/06/$ - see front matter © 2005 Elsevier Inc. All rights reserved.
doi:10.1016/j.mcna.2005.08.003

points should be determined. First, it seems obvious but it is important to establish that this rash is indeed urticarial [7]. Because these lesions are by nature transient, it is common for patients to be entirely free of symptoms at the time of evaluation. Although urticarial lesions have a distinctive typical clinical appearance, easily confirmed by an experienced observer, nonmedical terms, such as "hives" or "welts," may be used by patients for many different types of rashes that may or may not be truly urticarial in nature. The convenience and low cost of digital imaging has recently become popular, and consumer-quality cameras are now widely available (often even as part of cellular telephones). This has made it far easier for patients to document the actual appearance of an intermittently present rash for later review [8].

The duration of symptomatic episodes should next be established. This can be defined as the period of daily, or nearly daily, symptoms. By their nature, individual urticarial lesions are evanescent, but as some lesions resolve, others may appear. Although somewhat arbitrary, most experts agree that 6 weeks is a useful division between acute urticaria and chronic urticaria. This is valuable information in creating a differential diagnosis, because common causes of acute urticaria involve allergic or pseudoallergic reactions (foods, medications, insect stings, blood transfusions, contact allergies) and infections (particularly viral upper respiratory infections), although a significant number remain idiopathic [5,9–11]. Chronic urticaria, however, is far less likely to reveal a specific cause, despite extensive investigation [12]. While following this condition over time, it may be particularly useful to quantitate symptoms and various approaches have been described [13,14]. This can help more objectively to monitor disease progress and assess responses to therapy.

Angioedema commonly accompanies the spectrum of urticarial conditions and is essentially caused by release of the same types of vasoactive mediators into lower, dermal or subcutaneous, layers of the skin [15,16]. Whether manifest in the superficial layers of the skin as urticaria, or deeper as angioedema, the causes and treatments are similar [5]. The presence of angioedema, however, may carry certain prognostic implications, including increased average severity and duration of symptoms [17,18]. It is also important to note that isolated angioedema without urticaria has a very different differential diagnosis (eg, hereditary or acquired angioedema), and is beyond the scope of this article.

Another important historical point to establish early in the evaluation of urticaria is the approximate duration of individual lesions. It is not uncommon for patients to be uncertain of this, although they often have a vague sense of these symptoms lasting "all day." Sometimes this is caused by the large numbers of transient lesions composing their extensive rash that does indeed last all day, although any individual lesion may only last several hours. Occasionally, it may be useful to have patients circle a particular lesion with ink to determine how long a single wheal may last [19]. This is valuable information in excluding the rare, but serious, condition of urticarial vasculitis. Although lesions lasting over 24 hours are often cited as potentially concerning for urticarial vasculitis, typically this condition produces lesions lasting well over 36 to 48 hours. An even more suggestive finding is urticarial lesions that leave prolonged pigmentary changes (inflammatory lesions) or, especially, palpable purpura (presumptive evidence of intradermal vasculitis) [20]. Diascopy, or the more sophisticated but similar technique of dermoscopy (skin surface microscopy), can sometimes be helpful in this regard, to confirm that lesions blanch with pressure and help exclude vasculitis [21,22]. Vasculitic lesions may also be rather less pruritic than typical common urticaria; instead, patients may be more likely to complain of lesions in terms of burning, soreness, or tenderness [20]. Ultimately, a skin biopsy is usually definitive in confirming or excluding the presence of vasculitis.

Having established the condition as either acute or chronic urticaria, and excluded urticarial vasculitis by history or biopsy, a thorough history is crucial to consider systematically the differential diagnosis as extensively (although not exhaustively) outlined in Box 1 [23]. Of note, most cases are autoimmune or idiopathic, which are largely diagnoses of exclusion. Although questionnaires or similar forms may be useful to help focus or guide the history-taking, there is no adequate substitute for the time-consuming process of detailed personal questioning of the patient by a health professional familiar with urticarial illness. Various expert approaches have been recently published [4,12,14,24–27] and are not reviewed further here. Instead, a few notable highlights of unsuspected or occult causes or contributors to urticarial symptoms are discussed further.

Certain medications are well known as causing or exacerbating urticarial and angioedematous symptoms, such as nonsteroidal anti-inflammatory drugs (NSAID) [28], opiates and narcotics [16], angiotensin-converting enzyme inhibitors [29], and β-blockers [30]. Many patients, however, do not volunteer information about certain medications unless asked directly and specifically about their use. Most common relevant items omitted from patients' medication lists include over-the-counter analgesics; β-blocker eye drops; hormonal treatments (eg, contraceptives or hormone-replacement therapy); herbal products; complementary and alternative medicine treatments; vitamin supplementation; and recent vaccinations (unpublished observations, 2005). Although many lay individuals assume "natural" herbal products (including complementary and alternative medicine) are safe and unlikely to cause side-effects, allergic reactions to a wide variety of these products have been extensively documented in an Australian adverse drug reaction database. Specifically, urticaria or angioedema has been associated with cranberry, *Echinacea*, feverfew and willow, garlic, ginger, glucosamine, horseradish, *Hypericum*, phytoestrogen, propolis, royal jelly, and valerian, among others [31]. Also of note, allergy patients maintained on chronic allergen immunotherapy may well warrant a trial of discontinuation.

**Box 1. A current nosology of urticaria, with examples**

*Ordinary urticaria*
Allergic (foods, medications, herbs, insect bites and stings)
Pseudoallergic
    Direct mast-cell releasers (opiates, vancomycin)
    Indirect (presumed metabolic or vascular) reactions
        Aspirin, nonsteroidal anti-inflammatory drugs,
            cyclooxygenase-2 inhibitors
        Angiotensin-converting enzyme inhibitors, angiotensin
            receptor blockers
        β-Blockers
Other different or unknown mechanisms
    Radiocontrast media (presumed osmotic shock)
    Certain foods (eg, berries, tomatoes, and so forth)
    Ingested vasoactive amines (eg, scombroid fish poisoning)
Infection-associated (viral, parasitic, bacterial, fungal)
Autoimmune (anti-FcεRIα, anti-IgE, urticaria associated with
    rheumatic disease)
Idiopathic (persistent, recurrent)

*Physical urticaria*
Dermatographic
Cholinergic
Cold
Delayed-pressure, vibratory
Other rare types (solar, aquagenic, other variants)

*Contact urticaria (latex, cosmetics, chemicals)*

*Transfusion reactions (of various mechanisms)*

*Endocrinologic*
Thyroid disease (hyperthyroid, hypothyroid, autoimmune)
Pruritic urticarial papules and plaques of pregnancy
Autoimmune progesterone dermatitis

*Primary mast cell disease*
Urticaria pigmentosa
Systemic mastocytosis

*Paraneoplastic (rare, various)*

*Rare syndromes*
Food-dependent exercise-induced urticaria or anaphylaxis
Urticarial vasculitis
Schnitzler's syndrome
Muckle-Wells syndrome

Topical products need to be assessed in detail in patients with urticaria. The recent popularity of herbal handmade or craft soaps is particularly notable. Many of these may contain plant-derived essential oils for color or fragrance, which may cause contact rash [32,33]. Occasionally, distribution of symptoms may suggest cosmetics, hair, or nail products as contact allergens [34]. Various medicaments used to treat the skin may paradoxically contribute to worsening symptoms. Melaleuca, or tea-tree oil, is worth special mention because it is considered a natural skin remedy, yet has been associated with cutaneous allergy [35]. Conventional topical treatments can also be associated with contact dermatitis or urticaria, such as topical anesthetics and antipruritics [36–40], even topical steroids [41]. Occasionally, latex exposure in a sensitized individual [42,43] or allergy to tattoo pigment [44] may be responsible for urticaria, yet initially overlooked as a cause.

A significant proportion of chronic urticaria is triggered through particular physical stimuli. Most common among these physical urticarias is dermatographism [17,45–47], in which mast cell degranulation is caused by minor skin trauma (eg, simple scratching). Cold-induced urticaria is another relatively common form of chronic physical urticaria. In this condition, contact with cold acts through unclear mechanisms to trigger the mast cells to degranulate [48]. Cholinergic urticaria is an uncommon clinical entity with rather characteristic small monomorphic urticaria occurring on exertion to the point of sweating, also notable for especially intense pruritus and erythematous flaring [49]. Although often categorized with the physical urticarias, it is probably more properly considered a neuroimmunogenic form of chronic urticaria. Careful questioning, confirmed by relevant forms of challenge testing, is key to diagnosing these distinctive clinical syndromes [47]. Rare forms of physical urticaria include delayed pressure urticaria and angioedema, and solar urticaria; even an aquagenic urticaria, associated with water exposure, has been reported [47]. Finally, questions regarding cutaneous vasodilators (eg, alcohol, exercise, hot tubs, emotion) are relevant, because these may increase dissemination of urticarial mediators and increase symptoms [50].

After obtaining an extensive history and physical examination, the clinician is next confronted by decisions on testing. Any medical conditions or abnormalities identified and possibly relevant to urticaria should be thoroughly investigated, although most cases lack any obvious cause at this point. Issues regarding appropriate screening tests, in the absence of indications other than the chronic urticaria itself, remain controversial at present and are discussed in detail next.

### Testing issues

For many years, most patients with chronic urticaria were subjected to exhaustive and even invasive testing to identify any specific cause of these symptoms. As experts in the field became familiar with the typically fruitless outcome of nondirected testing, fewer and fewer tests remained as part of a standard evaluation for this condition. Several large studies of the value of certain tests in identifying otherwise unsuspected or occult causes of these symptoms have been published [9,24,51]. Recently a comprehensive meta-analysis of 29 large studies (including a total of 6462 patients) emphatically showed the overall futility of this approach [12]. Although various guidelines have been published and experts' approaches do vary somewhat [4,11,14,25–27], virtually all standard testing is of overall quite low (although not zero) yield. In the meta-analysis by Kozel and coworkers [12], screening laboratory testing revealed only 1.6% unsuspected internal diseases thought to be the cause of urticaria. A few simple and inexpensive tests may be reasonable and prudent, particularly if symptoms are persistent or severe. Note particularly that this only applies in the absence of any suspected contributing factor or disease. Anything relevant identified on history or physical should be thoroughly investigated. This especially applies to any suspicion of a specific physical urticaria, which should be confirmed with appropriate challenge testing [47]. Most patients should be routinely tested for dermatographism at the time of physical examination.

For the usual situation, apparently idiopathic urticaria in otherwise healthy patients, my general approach is to defer further testing and simply start symptomatic treatment for 6 to 12 weeks. Often, patients have already had extensive testing done and I ask to review all outside records and test results in detail. If symptoms persist, or are particularly severe, I obtain a complete blood count with differential, erythrocyte sedimentation rate, and thyroid testing (including sensitive thyroid-stimulating hormone level and thyroid autoantibody panel). Any suspicion of renal or hepatic disease prompts the addition of a metabolic and hepatic panel, whereas any suspicion of autoimmune or rheumatic disease adds an antinuclear antibody titer and complement studies. If urticarial vasculitis is a possibility, a skin biopsy is also indicated. Skin biopsy may also be useful in excluding atypical urticarial presentations of other primary dermatologic diseases [52], particularly in prolonged or severe disease. Some experts think that variations found in the dermatopathology of chronic urticaria may relate to differential prognosis and response to therapy [7,53,54].

These few simple, and relatively inexpensive, tests can largely rule out most diseases associated with urticaria (including thyroid illness, infections and parasitic infestation, hematologic and oncologic conditions, and rheumatologic and other inflammatory disorders). The role of chronic infections and parasites in the etiology of chronic urticaria has probably been overemphasized. Studies of intestinal infestation in tropical India have shown that, although commonly coexistent, treatment and eradication of parasitosis rarely results in clearing of urticaria [55]. One large study of over 2000 cases of urticaria documents infection as a clear cause in only 1% [2]. Issues of testing and treatment of asymptomatic enteric *Helicobacter pylori* remain particularly controversial at present [56–59]. Although symptomatic infection clearly warrants therapy, it is not at present my routine practice to screen (nor treat) for *H pylori* colonization in otherwise healthy urticaria patients without gastrointestinal complaints.

Allergy testing for foods is another controversial area for chronic urticaria. It is well-established that food allergies are common causes of acute urticaria and the particular culprit foods are usually strongly suspected from the clinical history [5,60,61]. Indeed, often this is so obvious to patients themselves that they may not even present for medical evaluation, but simply begin to avoid the offending food entirely. Although virtually any food can act as a food allergen, it is remarkable that most type I (IgE-mediated) food allergies are caused by a rather limited number of food categories. Specifically, milk (dairy), egg, wheat, legume (including peanut, soybean, and pea), tree nut, and seafood (fish, crustacean, and mollusk) accounted for more than 95% of all food allergies documented with double-blinded placebo-controlled food challenges in 480 children [62]. It is also distinctly uncommon for individuals to be allergic to more than one or two particular food types [62].

Given most patients' familiarity with the association between acute urticarial symptoms and food allergies, it is not surprising that many assume foods to be the cause of their chronic urticaria. One prospective study of 220 patients demonstrated a typical overestimation of the role of food allergies in chronic urticaria, where 31% of patients themselves and 20% of the evaluating dermatologists suspected an adverse food reaction as causative, yet serum food allergy testing and expert review confirmed relevant allergies in less than 7% [24]. Another recent study in 54 children with urticaria revealed that, despite 28 (52%) of these patients' and their families suspecting foods or food additives as causing these symptoms, skin testing and open challenge confirmed only three (less than 6%) with this etiology [63]. Champion's 1988 update of his and coworkers' landmark prior work [17] summarized all cases of urticaria referred to a single dermatology department over 32 years (2310 cases), and identified allergy to ingested food in 53 (2.3%), although there were a few additional cases caused by inhaled or contact food allergens [2]. In the absence of any particular suspected foods, despite detailed questioning, it seems to be uncommon to uncover an unsuspected food allergen as the cause of chronic urticaria [9]. Some allergists advocate various screening panels of food allergy testing, either skin prick testing or serum radioallergosorbent testing. I find nondirected testing unhelpful in this situation, however, because it is significantly limited by weak positive predictive values. Although correctly performed tests are relatively sensitive, potentially useful for ruling-out certain foods as causative, they are poorly specific and false-positive results caused by irritant skin responses are frequent, especially in the setting of the dermatographism common to this patient population. Obviously, appropriate positive (histamine) and negative (saline) controls for skin testing are crucial to enable proper test interpretation. Potentially misleading results also carry some risk of patients convincing themselves of false allergies and unnecessarily eliminating foods from their diet, which may be entirely unrelated to this condition. Occasionally, this may become a focus of serious psychologic concern, and patients may pursue markedly abnormal and unhealthy dietary patterns [64–66].

My recommended approach is to perform selected and directed food allergy testing only if a clearly suspected specific food (or limited number of foods) is identified on history. The time course of IgE-mediated food allergies is particularly relevant to review: a survey of 122 children with peanut and tree nut allergy identified allergy symptom onset (eg, urticaria) within a relatively short range of time, from less than 1 minute to 45 minutes [67]. Although 95% of episodes had symptom onset within 20 minutes, the median time of onset was at just 2 to 3 minutes from exposure [67]. If patients have only a vague sense of foods as a cause, after a discussion of common food allergens and their usual time course, they are encouraged to keep a written food and symptom diary. Occasionally, this clarifies matters by identifying limited foods for later testing, which may then be more useful. More commonly, however, no particular foods clearly correlate with symptom occurrence. Note also that skin testing and radioallergosorbent testing evaluate only IgE-mediated allergic sensitization. Non–IgE-mediated food allergy mechanisms are also possible, although presently practical identification of these is only possible through a food and symptom diary (and trials of exclusion and challenge).

There is also substantial discussion and controversy with regard to so-called "pseudoallergens" in the medical literature of chronic urticaria. Broadly speaking, these may include direct mast-cell–releasing agents of various types (eg, opiates and radiocontrast media); presumed nonallergic (nonspecific) immunologic mechanisms (eg, certain peptides in strawberries); and certain foods and additives often clinically associated with urticaria that apparently act through unknown mechanisms [68]. The latter group often includes tomatoes, food dyes, artificial flavorings and sweeteners, and preservatives (including tartrazines, nitrates, nitrites, sulfites, monosodium glutamate, aspartame, parabens-benzoates, butylated hydroxyanisole and butylated hydroxytoluene, and others) [11,69–71]. A detailed review of multiple studies in this area, including an excellent discussion of the challenges and limitations of study design, was published in 2000 [72]. Scombroid poisoning is caused by improperly stored fish; bacterial contamination may convert the amino acid histidine (found in high levels in the protein of certain species) to histamine, thereby causing urticarial, even anaphylactoid, symptoms [73]. Other foods may also contain various vasoactive amines [74]. Although various reports have suggested improvement on special urticaria diets to avoid pseudoallergens, challenge testing results have been quite variable [11,72,75–79]. Of particular note, unlike IgE-mediated immediate-type hypersensitivity reactions to foods, improvement is often rather slow on these diets (taking weeks, instead of days, after avoidance). These issues remain unresolved, although research on possible mechanisms is ongoing [80]. Interestingly, there have also been a few reports implicating caffeine [81–84], alcohol [85], and nicotine [86] as directly causative of urticaria in a few patients.

Experimental studies using autologous serum skin testing (ASST) helped lead to the discovery that approximately one third to one half of patients with chronic urticaria has autoantibodies to IgE or the IgE receptor [87]. This procedure involves intradermal skin testing in patients with chronic urticaria, analogous to standard allergy skin tests, but using a centrifuged sample of their own serum with appropriate controls [88]. The ASST provides a functional in vivo assay for these autoantibodies. Although this testing is not yet routinely performed in chronic urticaria patients, relatively standardized protocols have been developed, and its sensitivity (approximately 70%) and specificity (approximately 80%) for autoimmune urticaria have been established [87,89]. It is not clear why a positive ASST seems to persist well beyond resolution of urticarial symptoms in many patients but, interestingly, this may correlate with thyroid abnormalities [90]. Progress on development of a reliable in vitro binding assay for these autoantibodies is ongoing, but has been technically challenging to date [91–93].

## Pathophysiology and recent research

Early work on mechanisms of vascular response to skin injury focused on the pathophysiology of the urticarial triple response described by Lewis [94]. This consists of an initial erythematous flush from vasodilation; with a spreading flare caused by a neuronal axon reflex; and finally development of a wheal (localized edema) from increased vascular permeability. These effects are now known to be associated with the release of vasoactive mediators, primarily histamine, from dermal mast cells [95,96]. Ongoing investigation has revealed much about the importance of many other secondary mediators, some secreted preformed like histamine, and others rapidly synthesized on mast cell activation [68,95]. Other research has identified the composition of the perivascular cell infiltrate seen in biopsies of urticaria [97], and has elucidated many of the detailed molecular mechanisms of cell degranulation [98]. The triggering of mast cells in most types of acute allergic urticaria is relatively straightforward, by crosslinking of IgE (bound to the mast cell surface at the Fcε receptor) with specific immunologic recognition of a hapten from the relevant food or drug allergen. There are also a number of types of acute urticarial drug reactions (eg, those involving vancomycin, opiates, and others) that seem to trigger direct mast cell degranulation in nonimmunologic fashion, through effects on the cell membrane or other mechanisms [68,99]. Recent insight into possible metabolic pathways responsible for the association between NSAIDs and urticaria are discussed in detail later.

Until recently, mechanisms accounting for chronic (nonallergic) urticaria had been far less well understood than that of acute allergic urticaria. It had long been recognized that many patients with chronic urticaria could be found to have antithyroid autoantibodies of uncertain significance [100,101]. This led investigators to postulate possible autoimmunity as a direct cause of chronic urticaria. One of the most important advances in this area was the identification of autoimmune antibodies, with specific pathogenic significance, in the sera of a substantial number of patients with chronic presumed idiopathic urticaria [88,102,103]. A recent review of multiple studies approximates that 35% to 40% of these cases are caused by an IgG antibody recognizing a particular portion of the cell surface high-affinity IgE receptor (Fc$\epsilon$RI$\alpha$), and an additional 5% to 10% are caused by an IgG antibody binding directly to IgE itself [93]. Similar rates of autoimmune urticaria also have recently been found in pediatric chronic urticaria [89]. By directly cross-linking the IgE receptors themselves (or the bound IgE in nonspecific fashion, in the less-common case of IgG anti-IgE), these autoantibodies can thereby result in chronic recurrent mast cell degranulation without exposure to exogenous allergen. Further data demonstrating the inhibition of autoimmune histamine release, after preincubation with IgE myeloma protein, suggest that the anti-Fc$\epsilon$RI$\alpha$ cross-linking primarily involves unoccupied receptors [93,104]. Experimental reduction in autoantibodies through plasmapheresis has resulted in symptomatic improvement in patients with severe autoimmune urticaria [105].

Recent laboratory studies also implicate the complement system, particularly C5a, as involved in a significant pathogenic role in chronic urticaria [104,106]. This may account for the lack of pulmonary symptoms in chronic urticaria, because the C5a receptor (CD88) is present on cutaneous but not pulmonary mast cells [107]. Preliminary work has identified certain HLA class II associations (HLA-DR4 and -DQ8) of the major histocompatibility complex in patients with chronic autoimmune urticaria [108,109]. Research into differential expression of adhesion molecules [110] and cytokines [111] in chronic urticaria is also ongoing.

**Treatment**

Obviously, if a specific cause for either acute or chronic urticaria can be identified, avoidance of this trigger or effective treatment of the underlying condition is paramount. Unfortunately, this situation is only sometimes present in acute urticaria and disappointingly infrequent in chronic cases. Occasionally, the urticaria is of a type caused by something that cannot be avoided entirely (eg, cold, pressure, and similar physical triggers), yet limiting these exposures through practical interventions may still be quite useful in minimizing symptoms. For example, warm and protective clothing to avoid contact with cold objects (for cold urticaria), padded gloves and properly fitting supportive shoes (for delayed pressure urticaria), and other similar measures are logical and often quite helpful [112,113]. Minimizing or avoiding relatively nonspecific exacerbations associated with heat, alcohol, NSAIDs, and similar agents is also important. Still, most cases ultimately require medication management for adequate symptomatic control.

Since the development of the first antihistamines in the 1930s and 1940s [114], these medications have played a key role in the treatment of urticaria [115–118]. As one of the major vasoactive mediators released by the mast cell [99], blockade of the action of histamine is crucial in attempting to achieve adequate symptomatic control. Many medications of this large pharmacologic class have been developed and various differences in pharmacodynamics (dose-response), pharmacokinetics (duration of action), and side effect profile have emerged [119–121]. The ideal agent to treat urticaria would have a rapid onset of action; stay conveniently long-acting (with once-daily dosing); bind to both $H_1$ and $H_2$ histamine receptors in a highly potent manner; be entirely nonsedating and free of other unwanted side effects; and remain safe even at higher than usual doses. This has not yet been achieved, so different antihistamines are often selected, tried, and combined as tolerated and as effective, to maximize symptom control while minimizing adverse reactions. Unfortunately, the more sedating agents tend to be more effective at suppressing symptoms, perhaps even through their effects on perception [5,122]. Often, one of the more troublesome complaints from patients is difficulty in sleeping, because of pruritus that is often found to be more bothersome at night. One common combination is the use of a nonsedating antihistamine (eg, fexofenadine or loratadine) each morning, with a sedating or semisedating antihistamine (eg, hydroxyzine, cetirizine, or diphenhydramine) each night before bed [27,68].

It has long been known that blood vessels in the skin have both $H_1$ and $H_2$ histamine receptors [123]. One technique to maximize effectiveness of antihistamine therapy in urticaria is to block both $H_1$ and $H_2$ receptors [124–126]. This can be achieved either through the use of separate agents, or by using a tricyclic antidepressant (eg, doxepin), which has potent binding to both types of receptors [127–130]. Also, patients should be advised to use these medications on a regularly scheduled maintenance basis, not simply as needed. Recent research has suggested that antihistamines are not, strictly speaking, receptor antagonists. Instead they are inverse agonists, binding to an inactive conformation of the receptor and stabilizing it in that form; they may also have some anti-inflammatory properties independent of their effects on histamine [131]. They are expected to be more effective when already available and bound to receptors, before release of the histamine agonist, as opposed to having subsequently to compete with released histamine [119]. This seems to correlate well with long-appreciated clinical observations [7,68]. Although some physicians use multiple antihistamines of different classes, dosing well above recommended labeling, or rotation of these agents in some scheduled manner, I have found these techniques typically less efficacious and more problematic than sequentially adding agents of other complementary pharmacologic classes as outlined later.

The concept of urticaria combination therapy tends to maximize benefit and minimize side effects (Table 1), just as with this approach to medication management in the treatment of other medical conditions as varied as asthma and cancer. Beyond ensuring adequate blockade of both $H_1$ and $H_2$ histamine receptors, the addition of an antileukotriene may be helpful [132–134]. It does seem to be important that these medications are used in addition to antihistamines, as opposed to as monotherapy [135–137]. At the time of this writing, in the United States, drugs of this class are now limited to leukotriene receptor antagonists (eg, montelukast), because production and availability of zileuton (a 5-lipoxygenase inhibitor) had ceased. Some anecdotal reports had suggested, however, that zileuton might be more effective at symptomatic control than the leukotriene receptor antagonists [138,139].

The interactions of nonselective NSAIDs and urticaria have long been appreciated, with these medications commonly known to cause or exacerbate symptoms in many cases [28,68]. NSAIDs are cyclooxygenase inhibitors and the theoretical basis for this may involve the fact that these enzymes are responsible for the synthesis of both proinflammatory ($PGD_2$) and anti-inflammatory ($PGE_2$) prostaglandins. $PGE_2$ down-regulates leukotriene synthesis ($LTB_4$); blocking $PGE_2$ production could increase leukotriene production and their associated symptoms [140]. This is further confounded by the fact that arachidonic acid is the common eicosanoid precursor substrate for both lipoxygenase and cyclooxygenase pathways, and can be converted into vasoactive leukotrienes ($LTC_4$, $LTD_4$) or prostaglandins, respectively [141]. Nonspecific blockade of the cyclooxygenase pathway might also metabolically shunt toward the lipoxygenase pathway, again with resulting overproduction of leukotrienes and worsening symptoms. Interestingly, however, cyclooxygenase-2–specific inhibitors are a new class of medications that may hold significant promise in treatment of urticaria. Of note, cyclooxygenase-2–specific blockade may preferentially block more proinflammatory prostaglandins than anti-inflammatory prostaglandins [28], and might be particularly useful as add-on therapy for patients already treated with antileukotrienes. Two reports of small trials of cyclooxygenase-2 therapy in urticaria were recently published [142,143], but it was not clear if patients who improved were also on concurrent antileukotriene therapy. Unfortunately, these medications have been associated with an increased risk of thrombotic vascular events, such as heart attack and stroke, perhaps through alterations of prostacyclin ($PGI_2$) and thromboxane ($TXA_2$) balance, and two have recently been withdrawn from the market (rofecoxib and valdecoxib) [144,145]. It is not presently clear if this is a class effect and applies to other cyclooxygenase-2 agents still available (eg, celecoxib), but exercising caution in this regard seems prudent

Table 1
Therapeutics for urticaria

| Drug | Comments | Caution |
|------|----------|---------|
| $H_1$-antihistamines[a] | • Mainstay of therapy<br>• Use on scheduled maintenance basis, not as needed<br>• Sedating agents may be more effective, but less well-tolerated | — |
| $H_2$-antihistamines | • May provide small but significant additional benefit to $H_1$-antihistamines<br>• Usually well-tolerated | — |
| Antileukotrienes | • May provide additional benefit, in combination with antihistamines<br>• Usually well-tolerated | — |
| Tricyclic antidepressants | • Potent antihistamine properties, but often poorly tolerated | • Note potential adverse drug interaction with adrenergics |
| COX-2 inhibitors | • May enhance effectiveness of antileukotrienes<br>• May worsen symptoms without concurrent anti-leukotriene therapy | • Caution regarding possible prothrombotic (cardiac, cerebral) vascular effects |
| Adrenergics | • Oral adrenergics occasionally useful in refractory cases<br>• Parenteral epinephrine important in cases with significant airway angioedema/anaphylaxis | • Caution regarding cardiovascular effects<br>• Note potential adverse drug interaction with tricyclics |
| Steroids | • Avoid if possible, unless for potentially serious angioedema/anaphylaxis<br>• Use brief courses, moderate doses, and appropriate taper<br>• Remain aware of possible post-steroid flaring of symptoms | — |
| Cyclosporine | • Steroid-sparing, but potentially significant side-effect profile | — |
| Others | • Includes hydroxychloroquine, dapsone, colchicine, sulfasalazine, thyroxine, calcium channel blockers, methotrexate, tacrolimus, IV immunoglobulin, plasmapheresis, among others with anecdotal support (but little randomized/blinded/controlled clinical trial data) | — |

[a] Note these are the only drugs with US FDA-approval for urticaria.

[145]. Although all of these agents are much more selective than traditional NSAIDs, it is important to note that different cyclooxygenase-2 drugs do vary somewhat in their selectivity, and this may be relevant in terms of treatment and possible side effects [28,146]. There are other drugs in development, with combined lipoxygenase and cyclooxygenase inhibitory activity, which might be of significant interest to study in chronic urticaria [147,148].

Adrenergics are one category of medications previously used extensively to treat urticaria, but now little used routinely [61]. Most familiar is the use of epinephrine for life-threatening allergic angioedema or anaphylaxis, but β-agonists, such as terbutaline, have been used in chronic urticaria. They still remain occasionally useful in difficult cases and I have treated a few patients who seemed to demonstrate dramatic response to these agents. Caution is particularly warranted, however, in patients at risk of hypertension or other cardiovascular diseases. Large randomized placebo-controlled trials of these agents are not available, but there are some small trials and reports published in the urticaria literature [60,149].

Many, although not all, patients with chronic urticaria improve on systemic steroids [9,60,113]. These medications do not inhibit mast cell histamine release, but suppress multiple facets of the cellular and humoral immune system and thereby attenuate their involvement in this condition [68,150]. Steroids also exert significant anti-inflammatory activity through extensive blockade of arachidonate metabolism at the level of cytosolic phospholipase $A_2$, thereby preventing formation of both the leukotrienes and the prostaglandins [148]. Unfortunately, there are several significant concerns with the use of medications of this class. In addition to the numerous and well-known side effects of steroids, I routinely ask patients about poststeroid flaring of their urticarial symptoms after taper and discontinuation of these medications and have found this to be rather commonly reported (unpublished data, 2005). This can lead to a seesaw effect on symptoms through the course of this condition. Often, increasingly frequent bursts of steroids follow, sometimes even maintenance of long courses of treatment, with their expected untoward long-term effects. I recommend that the use of systemic steroids be largely avoided, if possible, apart from their use for specific clearly defined goals (treatment of acute severe angioedema, a brief burst and taper for initial control of severe refractory symptoms, and similar situations). In these instances, reasonable doses should be used; in particular, it is rare that urticaria and angioedema unresponsive to 0.5 to 1 mg/kg/d doses of prednisone or prednisolone will respond significantly better to substantially higher doses. Interestingly, there seems to be marked differences in the use of medications of different classes among types of specialists who treat urticaria. A recent review of a large database of ambulatory medical care surveys revealed that, whereas $H_1$-antihistamines were the most prescribed agents by all categories of physicians in this condition, internists prescribed steroids at far higher rates (29% of visits) than allergists (6% of visits), and allergists were the most likely to use off-label medications [151].

Most recently, studies have increasingly demonstrated the effectiveness of cyclosporine in treating chronic urticaria [152–154]. Patients with severe refractory disease often experienced significant side effects from chronic use of systemic steroids, and cyclosporine A was initially tried as a steroid-sparing immunosuppressant. New data show, however, that much of the symptom control of this agent may come from other properties distinctly different than those of steroids. In particular, cyclosporine A seems directly to inhibit mast cell degranulation [155], unlike steroids, which do not have this effect [156]. Unfortunately, cyclosporine also has potentially serious side effects and requires careful monitoring [152,157]. Tacrolimus (FK506) is another medication that has immunosuppressant and anti-inflammatory properties similar to cyclosporine, with a different side effect profile. A pilot study of tacrolimus treatment in 19 patients with severe chronic urticaria has recently been published, which demonstrated an approximately 70% clinical response, although 2 of the 19 did not complete the study because of side effects [158].

There are a wide variety of other medications that have been used to treat chronic urticaria of various types (see Table 1). Most have only limited experimental or anecdotal support, and discussion of these is beyond the scope of this article; these have been reviewed in detail elsewhere [113,159–161]. The recent development of a novel allergy medication, omalizumab (humanized murine monoclonal anti-IgE), presents interesting possibilities as an agent to be tested in chronic autoimmune or idiopathic urticaria. Because most autoimmune urticaria is thought to be the result of anti-FcεRIα antibodies, and cell surface expression of the Fcε receptor is known to be feedback-regulated by the level of free serum IgE [162], this medication might theoretically provide a mechanism for addressing this condition [163].

## Course and prognosis

The course of illness in urticarial conditions is fundamentally dependent on the specific diagnosis. Acute urticaria, by definition, lasts less than 6 weeks. In the event that a particular cause (often allergic) can be identified, symptoms resolve rapidly after avoidance and do not recur without further exposure. It is also common for acute symptoms to have no obvious cause and spontaneously resolve over the course of a few weeks. Much of the understanding of the natural history of chronic urticaria is from large descriptive studies published many years ago [2,9,17], before autoimmune forms could be reliably distinguished from otherwise idiopathic chronic urticaria. Autoimmune and idiopathic chronic urticaria are conditions that usually remain symptomatic for months to years, although this is quite variable [164]; some patients may experience periodic remissions and relapses. Some more recent studies suggest that patients with detectable relevant autoantibodies (eg, anti-FcεRIα antibody, positive ASST) may have more severe or prolonged disease [18,165–167]. Physical urticarias, too, seem to run a more persistent course [168]. Early studies of the self-assessed quality of life of patients with significant chronic urticaria indicated substantial impairment, similar to that of patients with severe coronary artery disease awaiting bypass grafting [169]. These findings have been further corroborated by other studies in different patient populations and control groups [170].

## Summary

Urticaria has been called a vexing problem [5] and remains so today. The most important part of the diagnostic evaluation remains a comprehensive and detailed history and physical examination, supplemented with limited laboratory testing. Although acute urticaria has been relatively well understood for some time, significant and important recent advances in understanding the pathogenesis of chronic urticaria are beginning to provide insight in this challenging field, notably the identification of many of these patients with an autoimmune etiology. Antihistamines of various types continue to represent the keystone of symptomatic treatment, with adjunctive support from medications of other classes, such as antileukotrienes, adrenergics, and immunosuppressive and anti-inflammatory agents (including steroids and cyclosporine). Although some progress has been made at improving symptomatic control of urticaria, further research and discovery are necessary before there can yet be an effective impact on the underlying course and natural history of this condition.

## References

[1] Sun SM. Qian-jin-yao-fang. 3rd edition. Taipei (Taiwan): Freedom Publishers; 1982 [in Chinese].
[2] Champion RH. Urticaria: then and now. Br J Dermatol 1988;119:427–36.
[3] Heberden W. Of the nettle rash. In: Medical transactions, vol. 2. 1772. p. 173.
[4] Dibbern DA, Dreskin SC. Urticaria and angioedema: an overview. Immunol Allergy Clin North Am 2004;24:141–62.
[5] Sheldon JM, Mathews KP, Lovell RG. The vexing urticaria problem: present concepts of etiology and management. J Allergy 1954;25:525–60.
[6] Stafford CT. Urticaria as a sign of systemic disease. Ann Allergy 1990;64:264–70.
[7] Charlesworth EN. The spectrum of urticaria: all that urticates may not be urticaria. Immunol Allergy Clin North Am 1995;15:641–57.
[8] Armstrong DJ. The mobile phone as an imaging tool in SLE. Rheumatology (Oxford) 2004; 43:1195.
[9] Quaranta J, Rohr AS, Rachelefsky GS, et al. The natural history and response to therapy of chronic urticaria and angioedema. Ann Allergy 1989;62:421–4.
[10] Zuberbier T, Ifflander J, Semmler C, et al. Acute urticaria: clinical aspects and therapeutic responsiveness. Acta Derm Venereol 1996;76:295–7.
[11] Zuberbier T. Urticaria. Allergy 2003;58:1224–34.
[12] Kozel MMA, Bossuyt PMM, Mekkes JR, et al. Laboratory tests and identified diagnoses in patients with physical and chronic urticaria and angioedema: a systematic review. J Am Acad Dermatol 2003;48:409–16.

[13] Greaves MW. Antihistamine treatment: a patient self-assessment method in chronic urticaria. BMJ 1981;283:1435–6.

[14] Zuberbier T, Greaves MW, Juhlin L, et al. Definition, classification, and routine diagnosis of urticaria: a consensus report. J Invest Dermatol Symp Proc 2001;6:123–7.

[15] Fox RW. Chronic urticaria: mechanisms and treatment. Allergy Asthma Proc 2001;22: 97–100.

[16] Grattan CE. The urticaria spectrum: recognition of clinical patterns can help management. Clin Exp Dermatol 2004;29:217–21.

[17] Champion RH, Roberts SOB, Carpenter RG, et al. Urticaria and angio-oedema: a review of 554 patients. Br J Dermatol 1969;81:588–97.

[18] Toubi E, Kessel A, Avshovich N, et al. Clinical and laboratory parameters in predicting chronic urticaria duration: a prospective study of 139 patients. Allergy 2004;59:869–73.

[19] Kulp-Shorten CL, Callen JP. Urticaria, angioedema, and rheumatologic disease. Rheum Dis Clin North Am 1996;22:95–115.

[20] Davis MDP, Brewer JD. Urticarial vasculitis and hypocomplementemic urticarial vasculitis syndrome. Immunol Allergy Clin North Am 2004;24:183–213.

[21] Dahl MV. Clinical pearl: diascopy helps diagnose urticarial vasculitis. J Am Acad Dermatol 1994;30:481–2.

[22] Vazquez-Lopez F, Maldonado-Seral C, Soler-Sanchez T, et al. Surface microscopy for discriminating between common urticaria and urticarial vasculitis. Rheumatology (Oxford) 2003;42:1–4.

[23] Grattan CEH. Autoimmune urticaria. Immunol Allergy Clin North Am 2004;24:163–81.

[24] Kozel MM, Mekkes JR, Bossuyt PM, et al. The effectiveness of a history-based diagnostic approach in chronic urticaria and angioedema. Arch Dermatol 1998;134:1575–80.

[25] Joint Task Force on Practice Parameters. The diagnosis and management of urticaria: a practice parameter. Ann Allergy Asthma Immunol 2000;85(6 Pt 2):521–44.

[26] Bindslev-Lensen C, Finzi A, Greaves M, et al. Chronic urticaria: diagnostic recommendations. J Eur Acad Dermatol Venereol 2000;14:175–80.

[27] Grattan C, Powell S, Humphreys F, et al. Management and diagnostic guidelines for urticaria and angio-oedema. Br J Dermatol 2001;144:708–14.

[28] Sanchez-Borges M, Capriles-Hulett A, Caballero-Fonseca F. Cutaneous reactions to aspirin and nonsteroidal antiinflammatory drugs. Clin Rev Allergy Immunol 2003;24: 125–36.

[29] Bhalla M, Thami GP. Delayed diagnosis of angiotensin-converting enzyme (ACE) inhibitor induced angioedema and urticaria. Clin Exp Dermatol 2003;28:333–4.

[30] Howard PJ, Lee MR. Beware beta-adrenergic blockers in patients with severe urticaria! Scott Med J 1988;33:344–5.

[31] Mullins RJ, Heddle R. Adverse reactions associated with Echinacea: the Australian experience. Ann Allergy Asthma Immunol 2002;88:42–51.

[32] Sugiura M, Hayakawa R, Kato Y, et al. Results of patch testing with lavender oil in Japan. Contact Dermatitis 2000;43:157–60.

[33] Bleasel N, Tate B, Rademaker M. Allergic contact dermatitis following exposure to essential oils. Australas J Dermatol 2002;43:211–3.

[34] Niinimaki A, Niinimaki M, Makinen-Kiljunen S, et al. Contact urticaria from protein hydrolysates in hair conditioners. Allergy 1998;53:1078–82.

[35] Knight TE, Hausen BM. Melaleuca oil (tea tree oil) dermatitis. J Am Acad Dermatol 1994; 30:423–7.

[36] Waton J, Boulanger A, Trechot PH, et al. Contact urticaria from Emla cream. Contact Dermatitis 2004;51:284–7.

[37] Hayashi K, Kawachi S, Saida T. Allergic contact dermatitis due to both chlorpheriramine maleate and dibucaine hydrochloride in an over-the-counter medicament. Contact Dermatitis 2001;44:38–9.

[38] Heine A. Diphenhydramine: a forgotten allergen? Contact Dermatitis 1996;35:311–2.

[39] Taylor JS, Praditsuwan P, Handel D, et al. Allergic contact dermatitis from doxepin cream: one-year patch test clinic experience. Arch Dermatol 1996;132:515–8.

[40] Coskey RJ. Contact dermatitis caused by diphenhydramine hydrochloride. J Am Acad Dermatol 1983;8:204–6.

[41] Bircher AJ, Levy F, Langauer S, et al. Contact allergy to topical corticosteroids and systemic contact dermatitis from prednisolone with tolerance of triamcinolone. Acta Derm Venereol 1995;75:490–3.

[42] Pecquet C, Leynadier F, Dry J. Contact urticaria and anaphylaxis to natural latex. J Am Acad Dermatol 1990;22:631–3.

[43] Wrangsjo K, Wahlberg JE, Axelsson IG. IgE-mediated allergy to natural rubber in 30 patients with contact urticaria. Contact Dermatitis 1988;19:264–71.

[44] Bagnato GF, DePasquale R, Giacobbe O, et al. Urticaria in a tattooed patient. Allergol Immunopathol (Madr) 1999;27:32–3.

[45] Wong RC, Fairley JA, Ellis CN. Dermographism: a review. J Am Acad Dermatol 1984;11: 643–52.

[46] Humphreys F, Hunter JAA. The characteristics of urticaria in 390 patients. Br J Dermatol 1998;138:635–8.

[47] Dice JP. Physical urticaria. Immunol Allergy Clin North Am 2004;24:225–46.

[48] Wanderer AA, Hoffman HM. The spectrum of acquired and familial cold-induced urticaria/urticaria-like syndromes. Immunol Allergy Clin North Am 2004;24:259–86.

[49] Hirshmann JV, Lawlor F, English JSC, et al. Cholinergic urticaria: a clinical and histologic study. Arch Dermatol 1987;123:462–7.

[50] Mathews KP. A current view of urticaria. Med Clin North Am 1974;58:185–205.

[51] Jacobson KW, Branch LB, Nelson HS. Laboratory tests in chronic urticaria. JAMA 1980; 243:1644–6.

[52] Stewart GE. Histopathology of chronic urticaria. Clin Rev Allergy Immunol 2002;23: 195–200.

[53] Zavadak D, Tharp MD. Chronic urticaria as a manifestation of the late phase reaction Immunol Allergy Clin North Am 1995;15:745–59.

[54] Tharp MD. Chronic urticaria: pathophysiology and treatment approaches. J Allergy Clin Immunol 1996;98:S325–30.

[55] Pasricha JS, Pasricha A, Prakash OM. Role of gastro-intestinal parasites in urticaria. Ann Allergy 1972;30:348–51.

[56] Hook-Nikanne J, Varjonen E, Harvima RJ, et al. Is Helicobacter pylori infection associated with chronic urticaria? Acta Derm Venereol 2000;80:425–6.

[57] Federman DG, Kirsner RS, Moriarty JP, et al. The effect of antibiotic therapy for patients infected with Helicobacter pylori who have chronic urticaria. J Am Acad Dermatol 2003;49: 861–4.

[58] Moreira A, Rodrigues J, Delgado L, et al. Is Helicobacter pylori infection associated with chronic idiopathic urticaria? Allergol Immunopathol (Madr) 2003;31:209–14.

[59] Fukuda S, Shimoyama T, Umegaki N, et al. Effect of Helicobacter pylori eradication in the treatment of Japanese patients with chronic idiopathic urticaria. J Gastroenterol 2004;39: 827–30.

[60] Green GR, Koelsche GA, Kierland RR. Etiology and pathogenesis of chronic urticaria. Ann Allergy 1965;23:30–6.

[61] Nizami RM, Baboo MT. Office management of patients with urticaria: an analysis of 215 patients. Ann Allergy 1974;33:78–85.

[62] Bock SA, Atkins FM. Patterns of food hypersensitivity during sixteen years of double-blind, placebo-controlled food challenges. J Pediatr 1990;117:561–7.

[63] Sackesen C, Sekerel BE, Orhan F, et al. The etiology of different forms of urticaria in childhood. Pediatr Dermatol 2004;21:102–8.

[64] Warner JO, Hathaway MJ. Allergic form of Meadow's syndrome (Munchausen by proxy). Arch Dis Child 1984;59:151–6.

[65] Roesler TA, Barry PC, Bock SA. Factitious food allergy and failure to thrive. Arch Pediatr Adolesc Med 1994;148:1150–5.

[66] Bethune CA, Gompels MM, Spickett GP. Physiological effects of starvation interpreted as food allergy. BMJ 1999;319:304–5.

[67] Sicherer SH, Burks AW, Sampson HA. Clinical features of acute allergic reactions to peanut and tree nuts in children. Pediatrics 1998;102:e6.

[68] Beltrani VS. Urticaria and angioedema. Dermatol Clin 1996;14:171–98.

[69] Goodman DL, McDonnell JT, Nelson HS, et al. Chronic urticaria exacerbated by the antioxidant food preservatives, butylated hydroxyanisole (BHA) and butylated hydroxytoluene (BHT). J Allergy Clin Immunol 1990;86(4 Pt 1):570–5.

[70] Ehlers I, Niggemann B, Binder C, et al. Role of nonallergic hypersensitivity reactions in children with chronic urticaria. Allergy 1998;53:1074–7.

[71] Zuberbier T, Pfrommer C, Specht K, et al. Aromatic components of food as novel eliciting factors of pseudoallergic reactions in chronic urticaria. J Allergy Clin Immunol 2002;109: 343–8.

[72] Simon RA. Additive-induced urticaria: experience with monosodium glutamate (MSG). J Nutr 2000;130:1063S–6S.

[73] Predy G, Honish L, Hohn W, et al. Was it something she ate? Case report and discussion of scombroid fish poisoning. CMAJ 2003;168:587–8.

[74] Bodmer S, Imark C, Kneubuhl M. Biogenic amines in foods: histamine and food processing. Inflamm Res 1999;48:296–300.

[75] Supramaniam G, Warner JO. Artificial food additive intolerance in patients with angiooedema and urticaria. Lancet 1986;2:907–9.

[76] Malanin G, Kalimo K. The results of skin testing with food additives and the effect of an elimination diet in chronic and recurrent urticaria and recurrent angioedema. Clin Exp Allergy 1989;19:539–43.

[77] Zuberbier T, Chantraine-Hess S, Hartmann K, et al. Pseudoallergen-free diet in the treatment of chronic urticaria: a prospective study. Acta Derm Venereol 1995;75:484–7.

[78] Nettis E, Colanardi MC, Ferrannini A, et al. Suspected tartrazine-induced acute urticaria/ angioedema is only rarely reproducible by oral rechallenge. Clin Exp Allergy 2003;33: 1725–9.

[79] Nettis E, Colanardi MC, Ferrannini A, et al. Sodium benzoate-induced repeated episodes of acute urticaria/angio-oedema: randomized controlled trial. Br J Dermatol 2004;151: 898–902.

[80] Buhner S, Reese I, Kuehl F, et al. Pseudoallergic reactions in chronic urticaria are associated with altered gastroduodenal permeability. Allergy 2004;59:1118–23.

[81] Gancedo SQ, Freire P, Rivas MF, et al. Urticaria from caffeine. J Allergy Clin Immunol 1991;88:680–1.

[82] Fernandez-Nieto M, Sastre J, Quirce S. Urticaria caused by cola drink. Allergy 2002;57: 967–8.

[83] Hinrichs R, Hunzelmann N, Ritzkowsky A, et al. Caffeine hypersensitivity. Allergy 2002; 57:859–60.

[84] Infante S, Baeza ML, Calvo M, et al. Anaphylaxis due to caffeine. Allergy 2003;58: 681–2.

[85] Sticherling M, Brasch J, Bruning H, et al. Urticarial and anaphylactoid reactions following ethanol intake. Br J Dermatol 1995;132:464–7.

[86] Lee IW, Ahn SK, Choi EH, et al. Urticarial reaction following the inhalation of nicotine in tobacco smoke. Br J Dermatol 1998;138:486–8.

[87] Sabroe RA, Grattan CE, Francis DM, et al. The autologous serum skin test: a screening test for autoantibodies in chronic idiopathic urticaria. Br J Dermatol 1999;140:446–52.

[88] Grattan CE, Francis DM, Hide M, et al. Detection of circulating histamine releasing autoantibodies with functional properties of anti-IgE in chronic urticaria. Clin Exp Allergy 1991;21:695–704.

[89] Brunetti L, Francavilla R, Miniello VL, et al. High prevalence of autoimmune urticaria in children with chronic urticaria. J Allergy Clin Immunol 2004;114:922–7.

[90] Fusari A, Colangelo C, Bonifazi F, et al. The autologous serum skin test in the follow-up of patients with chronic urticaria. Allergy 2005;60:256–8.

[91] Fiebinger E, Maurer D, Holub H, et al. Serum IgG autoantibodies directed against the alpha chain of Fc epsilon RI: a selective marker and pathogenic factor for a distinct subset of chronic urticaria patients? J Clin Invest 1995;96:2606–12.

[92] Ferrer M, Kinet JP, Kaplan AP. Comparative studies of functional and binding assays for IgG anti-Fc(epsilon)RIalpha (alpha-subunit) in chronic urticaria. J Allergy Clin Immunol 1998;101:672–6.

[93] Kaplan AP. Chronic urticaria: Pathogenesis and treatment. J Allergy Clin Immunol 2004; 114:465–74.

[94] Lewis T. The blood vessels of the human skin and their responses. London: Shaw and Sons; 1927.

[95] Schwartz LB. Mast cells and their role in urticaria. J Am Acad Dermatol 1991;25:190–204.

[96] Sabroe RA, Greaves MW. The pathogenesis of chronic idiopathic urticaria. Arch Dermatol 1997;133:1003–8.

[97] Sabroe RA, Poon E, Orchard GE, et al. Cutaneous inflammatory cell infiltrate in chronic idiopathic urticaria: comparison of patients with and without anti-FcεRI or anti-IgE auto-antibodies. J Allergy Clin Immunol 1999;103:484–93.

[98] Guin JD. Treatment of urticaria. Med Clin North Am 1982;66:831–49.

[99] White MV. The role of histamine in allergic diseases. J Allergy Clin Immunol 1990;86: 599–605.

[100] Leznoff A, Josse RG, Denburg J, et al. Association of chronic urticaria and angioedema with thyroid autoimmunity. Arch Dermatol 1983;119:636–40.

[101] Leznoff A, Sussman GL. Syndrome of idiopathic chronic urticaria and angioedema with thyroid autoimmunity: a study of 90 patients. J Allergy Clin Immunol 1989;84:66–71.

[102] Gruber BL, Baeza ML, Marchese MJ, et al. Prevalence and functional role of anti-IgE autoantibodies in urticarial syndromes. J Invest Dermatol 1988;90:213–7.

[103] Hide M, Francis DM, Grattan CE, et al. Autoantibodies against the high-affinity IgE receptor as a cause of histamine release in chronic urticaria. N Engl J Med 1993;328: 1599–604.

[104] Ferrer M, Nakazawa K, Kaplan AP. Complement dependence of histamine release in chronic urticaria. J Allergy Clin Immunol 1999;104:169–72.

[105] Grattan CE, Francis DM, Slater NG, et al. Plasmapheresis for severe, unremitting chronic urticaria. Lancet 1992;339:1078–80.

[106] Kikuchi Y, Kaplan AP. A role for C5a in augmenting IgG-dependent histamine release from basophils in chronic urticaria. J Allergy Clin Immunol 2002;109:114–8.

[107] Fureder W, Agis H, Willheim M, et al. Differential expression of complement receptors on human basophils and mast cells: evidence for mast cell heterogeneity and CD88/C5aR expression on skin mast cells. J Immuno 1995;155:3152–60.

[108] O'Donnell BF, O'Neill CM, Francis DM, et al. Human leucocyte antigen class II associations in chronic idiopathic urticaria. Br J Dermatol 1999;140:853–8.

[109] Oztas P, Onder M, Gonen S, et al. Is there any relationship between human leucocyte antigenic class II and chronic urticaria? (chronic urticaria and HLA class II). Yonsei Med J 2004;45:392–5.

[110] Haas N, Hermes B, Henz BM. Adhesion molecules and cellular infiltrate: histology of urticaria. J Invest Dermatol Symp Proc 2001;6:137–8.

[111] Ferrer M, Luquin E, Sanchez-Ibarrola A, et al. Secretion of cytokines, histamine and leukotrienes in chronic urticaria. Int Arch Allergy Immunol 2002;129:254–60.

[112] Zuberbier T, Greaves MW, Juhlin L, et al. Management of urticaria: a consensus report. J Investig Dermatol Symp Proc 2001;6:128–31.

[113] Kozel MM, Sabroe RA. Chronic urticaria: aetiology, management and current and future treatment options. Drugs 2004;64:2515–36.

[114] Loew ER, MacMillan R, Kaiser ME. The anti-histamine properties of Benadryl, β-dimethylaminoethyl benzhydryl ether hydrochloride. J Pharmacol Exp Ther 1946;86:229–38.

[115] Breneman D, Bronsky EA, Bruce S, et al. Cetirizine and astemizole therapy for chronic idiopathic urticaria: a double-blind, placebo-controlled, comparative trial. J Am Acad Dermatol 1995;33:192–8.

[116] Finn AF, Kaplan AP, Fretwell R, et al. A double-blind, placebo-controlled trial of fexofenadine HCl in the treatment of chronic idiopathic urticaria. J Allergy Clin Immunol 1999; 103:1071–8.

[117] Nelson HS, Reynolds R, Mason J. Fexofenadine HCl is safe and effective for treatment of chronic idiopathic urticaria. Ann Allergy Asthma Immunol 2000;84:517–22.

[118] Lee EE, Maibach HI. Treatment of urticaria: an evidence-based evaluation of antihistamines. Am J Clin Dermatol 2001;2:27–32.

[119] DuBuske LM. Clinical comparison of histamine H1-receptor antagonist drugs. J Allergy Clin Immunol 1996;98(6 Pt 3):S307–18.

[120] Grant JA, Danielson L, Rihoux J-P, et al. A double-blind, single-dose, crossover comparison of cetirizine, ebastine, epinastine, fexofenadine, terfenadine, and loratadine versus placebo: suppression of histamine-induced wheal and flare response for 24h in healthy male subjects. Allergy 1999;54:700–7.

[121] Simons FE. Comparative pharmacology of H1 antihistamines: clinical relevance. Am J Med 2002;9A:38S–46S.

[122] Kennard CD. Evaluation and treatment of urticaria. Immunol Allergy Clin North Am 1995;15:785–801.

[123] Greaves M, Marks R, Robertson I. Receptors for histamine in human skin blood vessels: a review. Br J Dermatol 1977;97:225–8.

[124] Monroe EW, Cohen SH, Kalbfleisch J, et al. Combined H1 and H2 antihistamine therapy in chronic urticaria. Arch Dermatol 1981;117:404–7.

[125] Paul E, Bodeker RH. Treatment of chronic urticaria with terfenadine and ranitidine: a randomized double-blind study in 45 patients. Eur J Clin Pharmacol 1986;31:277–80.

[126] Bleehan SS, Thomas SE, Greaves MW, et al. Cimetidine and chlorpheniramine in the treatment of chronic idiopathic urticaria: a multi-centre randomized double-blind study. Br J Dermatol 1987;117:81–8.

[127] Richelson E. Tricyclic antidepressants and histamine H1 receptors. Mayo Clin Proc 1979; 54:669–74.

[128] Richelson E. Antimuscarinic and other receptor-blocking properties of antidepressants. Mayo Clin Proc 1983;58:40–6.

[129] Greene SL, Reed CE, Schroeter AL. Double-blind crossover study comparing doxepin with diphenhydramine for the treatment of chronic urticaria. J Am Acad Dermatol 1985;12: 669–75.

[130] Goldsobel AB, Rohr AS, Siegel SC, et al. Efficacy of doxepin in the treatment of chronic idiopathic urticaria. J Allergy Clin Immunol 1986;78:867–73.

[131] Leurs R, Church MK, Taglialatela M. H1-antihistamines: inverse agonism, anti-inflammatory actions and cardiac effects. Clin Exp Allergy 2002;32:489–98.

[132] Nettis E, Dambra P, D'Oronzio L, et al. Comparison of montelukast and fexofenadine for chronic idiopathic urticaria. Arch Dermatol 2001;137:99–100.

[133] Erbagci Z. The leukotriene receptor antagonist montelukast in the treatment of chronic idiopathic urticaria: a single-blind, placebo-controlled, crossover clinical study. J Allergy Clin Immunol 2002;110:484–8.

[134] Bagenstose SE, Levin L, Bernstein JA. The addition of zafirlukast to cetirizine improves the treatment of chronic urticaria in patients with positive autologous serum skin test results. J Allergy Clin Immunol 2004;113:134–40.

[135] Bensch G, Borish L. Leukotriene modifiers in chronic urticaria. Ann Allergy Asthma Immunol 1999;83:348.
[136] Nettis E, Colanardi MC, Paradiso MT, et al. Desloratidine in combination with montelukast in the treatment of chronic urticaria: a randomized, double-blind, placebo-controlled study. Clin Exp Allergy 2004;34:1401–7.
[137] DiLorenzo G, Pacor ML, Mansueto P, et al. Randomized placebo-controlled trial comparing desloratidine and montelukast in monotherapy and desloratidine plus montelukast in combined therapy for chronic idiopathic urticaria. J Allergy Clin Immunol 2004;114: 619–25.
[138] Ellis M. Successful treatment of chronic urticaria with leukotriene antagonists. J Allergy Clin Immunol 1998;102:876–7.
[139] Spector S, Tan RA. Antileukotrienes in chronic urticaria. J Allergy Clin Immunol 1998; 101:572.
[140] Elliott GR, Lauwen AP, Bonta IL. Prostaglandin E2 inhibits and indomethacin and aspirin enhance, A23187-stimulated leukotriene B4 synthesis by rat peritoneal macrophages. Br J Pharmacol 1989;96:265–70.
[141] Soberman RJ, Christmas P. The organization and consequences of eicosanoid signaling. J Clin Invest 2003;111:1107–13.
[142] Anand MK, Nelson HS, Dreskin SC. A possible role for cyclooxygenase 2 inhibitors in the treatment of chronic urticaria. J Allergy Clin Immunol 2003;111:1133–6.
[143] Boehncke WH, Ludwig RJ, Zollner TM, et al. The selective cyclooxygenase-2 inhibitor rofecoxib may improve the treatment of chronic idiopathic urticaria. Br J Dermatol 2003;148:604–6.
[144] Mukherjee D, Nissen SE, Topol EJ. Risk of cardiovascular events associated with selective COX-2 inhibitors. JAMA 2001;286:954–9.
[145] FitzGerald GA. Coxibs and cardiovascular disease. N Engl J Med 2004;351:1709–11.
[146] FitzGerald GA, Patrono C. The coxibs, selective inhibitors of cyclooxygenase-2. N Engl J Med 2001;345:433–42.
[147] Leval X, Julemont F, Delarge J, et al. New trends in dual 5-LOX/COX inhibition. Curr Med Chem 2002;9:941–62.
[148] Celotti F, Durand T. The metabolic effects of inhibitors of 5-lipoxygenase and of cyclooxygenase 1 and 2 are an advancement in the efficacy and safety of anti-inflammatory therapy. Prostaglandins Other Lipid Mediat 2003;71:147–62.
[149] Kennes B, DeMaubeuge J, Delespesse G. Treatment of chronic urticaria with a beta2-adrenergic stimulant. Clin Allergy 1977;7:35–9.
[150] Dunsky EH, Zweiman B, Fischler E, et al. Early effects of corticosteroids on basophils, leukocyte histamine, and tissue histamine. J Allergy Clin Immunol 1979;63:426–32.
[151] Henderson RL, Fleischer AB, Feldman SR. Allergists and dermatologists have far more expertise in caring for patients with urticaria than other specialists. J Am Acad Dermatol 2000;43:1084–91.
[152] Fradin MS, Ellis CN, Goldfarb MT, et al. Oral cyclosporine for severe chronic idiopathic urticaria and angioedema. J Am Acad Dermatol 1991;25:1065–7.
[153] Toubi E, Blant A, Kessel A, et al. Low-dose cyclosporin A in the treatment of severe chronic idiopathic urticaria. Allergy 1997;52:312–6.
[154] Grattan CE, O'Donnell BF, Francis DM, et al. Randomized double-blind study of cyclosporin in chronic idiopathic urticaria. Br J Dermatol 2000;143:365–72.
[155] Stellato C, dePaulis A, Ciccarelli A, et al. Anti-inflammatory effect of cyclosporine A on human skin mast cells. J Invest Dermatol 1992;98:800–4.
[156] Cohan VL, Undem BJ, Fox CC, et al. Dexamethasone does not inhibit the release of mediators from human mast cells residing in airway, intestine, or skin. Am Rev Respir Dis 1989; 140:951–4.
[157] Zackheim HS. The FDA guidelines for the treatment of psoriasis using cyclosporine A: are they adequate? Cutis 2002;70:288–90.

[158] Kessel A, Bamberger E, Toubi E. Tacrolimus in the treatment of severe chronic idiopathic urticaria: an open-label prospective study. J Am Acad Dermatol 2005;52:145–8.

[159] Stanaland BE. Treatment of patients with chronic idiopathic urticaria. Clin Rev Allergy Immunol 2002;23:233–41.

[160] Tedeschi A, Airaghi L, Lorini M, et al. Chronic urticaria: a role for newer immunomodulatory drugs? Am J Clin Dermatol 2003;4:297–305.

[161] Sheikh J. Advances in the treatment of chronic urticaria. Immunol Allergy Clin North Am 2004;24:317–34.

[162] Saini SS, MacGlashan DW, Sterbinsky SA, et al. Down-regulation of human basophil IgE and FC epsilon RI alpha surface densities and mediator release by anti-IgE-infusions is reversible in vitro and in vivo. J Immunol 1999;162:5624–30.

[163] Greaves MW. Autoimmune urticaria. Clin Rev Allergy Immunol 2002;23:171–83.

[164] Van der Valk PG, Moret G, Klemeney LA. The natural history of chronic urticaria and angioedema in patients visiting a tertiary referral center. Br J Dermatol 2002;146:110–3.

[165] Sabroe RA, Seed PT, Francis DM, et al. Chronic idiopathic urticaria: comparison of the clinical features of patients with and without anti-FcepsilonRI or anti-IgE autoantibodies. J Am Acad Dermatol 1999;40:443–50.

[166] Sabroe RA, Fiebinger E, Francis DM, et al. Classification of anti-FcεRI and anti-IgE autoantibodies in chronic idiopathic urticaria and correlation with disease severity. J Allergy Clin Immunol 2002;110:492–9.

[167] Caproni M, Volpi W, Giomi B, et al. Chronic idiopathic and chronic autoimmune urticaria: clinical and immunopathological features of 68 subjects. Acta Derm Venereol 2004;84: 288–90.

[168] Kozel MM, Mekkes JR, Bossuyt PM, et al. Natural course of physical and chronic urticaria and angioedema in 220 patients. J Am Acad Dermatol 2001;45:387–91.

[169] O'Donnell BF, Lawlor F, Simpson J, et al. The impact of chronic urticaria on the quality of life. Br J Dermatol 1997;136:197–201.

[170] Baiardini I, Giardini A, Pasquali M, et al. Quality of life and patients' satisfaction in chronic urticaria and respiratory allergy. Allergy 2003;58:621–3.

ELSEVIER
SAUNDERS

Med Clin N Am 90 (2006) 211–232

THE MEDICAL
CLINICS
OF NORTH AMERICA

# Insect Sting Allergy

## David F. Graft, MD[a,b],*

[a]Asthma and Allergic Diseases, Park Nicollet Clinic, Minneapolis, MN, USA
[b]Department of Pediatrics, University of Minnesota Medical School, Minneapolis, MN, USA

The study of allergy to insect stings holds a unique position in the field of allergy, and because of the usually singular and notable times of exposure, it serves as a model for the development, natural history, and treatment of allergic phenomena. The death of King Menes of Egypt shortly after a wasp sting is often cited as one of the earliest historical examples of anaphylaxis [1]. Soon after the concepts of anaphylaxis were defined by Portier and Richert in 1902 [2], generalized reactions to insect stings were recognized as hypersensitivity phenomena [3]. Ten years later, Braun [4] described a typical patient with insect sting sensitivity and his use of insect venom for diagnosis and treatment. Although this initial treatment used the posterior one eighth inch of the insect to increase the yield of venom, that stipulation was later ignored and for decades, immunotherapy with whole-body extract was used for the treatment of patients with insect sting reaction [5]. In the 1950s and 1960s, events occurred that eventually led to the development of venom immunotherapy (VIT). Loveless and Fackler [6] reported the successful diagnostic and therapeutic use of extracts of venom sacs. Bernton and Brown [7] and Schwartz [8] independently found that whole-body extract skin tests did not discriminate insect allergic patients from subjects with no history of generalized reactions. Methods for collecting large quantities of honeybee venom were developed and the venom contents were characterized [9]. Vespid venom collection was more difficult requiring venom sac extirpation in a tedious one-insect-at-a-time process. In the 1970s, a few case reports of successful VIT appeared [10,11] and then, in 1978, Hunt and coworkers [12] from Johns Hopkins reported a challenge sting trial in which the superiority of VIT was demonstrated when compared with whole-body extract and placebo injections. The immunotherapy protocol with venom is the most effective treatment in the field of allergy. About 97% of venom-treated

* Asthma and Allergic Diseases, Park Nicollet Clinic, 3800 Park Nicollet Boulevard, Minneapolis, MN 55416.
E-mail address: graftd@parknicollet.com

0025-7125/06/$ - see front matter © 2005 Elsevier Inc. All rights reserved.
doi:10.1016/j.mcna.2005.08.006

patients have no reaction when stung [13–15]. The few remaining patients are more appropriately considered partial successes rather than treatment failures because they tend to have reactions that are much less severe than those they have previously experienced.

Insect venoms for immunotherapy became commercially available in 1979. Since then, thousands of patients have received VIT. Venom injections greatly reduce the likelihood of serious allergic reactions and consequently improve the patient's quality of life by reducing anxiety and allowing patients to participate in the outdoor activities that they prefer. Guidelines have been published regarding the selection of patients and the method of VIT and for the discontinuation of VIT [16,17]. Venom injections have proved very safe, with a low occurrence of injection-induced systemic reactions and no reports of fatal reactions. Unfortunately, even after 25 years of use, many patients who should initiate VIT are not referred to allergists for evaluation despite data that demonstrate the lack of effectiveness of single or multiple doses of epinephrine [12,18]. It is hoped that this pattern of underutilization will diminish in the future.

### Epidemiology

Systemic allergic reactions are reported by 0.4% to 3% of individuals [19–21]. There is a 2:1 male/female ratio that is probably a reflection of relative exposure. About one third of those experiencing allergic sting reactions are atopic [22]. Annually, about 45 deaths are attributed to insect stings in the United States (Table 1) [23]. Other data on fatal stings include the following: 20 in Ontario, Canada, from 1986 to 2000 [24]; four per year in the United Kingdom [25]; three per year in Switzerland [26]; and 11 per year in West Germany [27]. About one half of the fatal reactions occur in individuals with no prior history of allergic reactions to stings [28,29]. Many more men (about 3.5-fold) than women die from insect sting reactions, and greater than 80% of the deaths from insect stings occur in persons over 40 years of age [23]. The coexistence of coronary heart disease, atherosclerosis, or emphysema may determine a more severe outcome. The true number of deaths attributed to insect stings is undoubtedly higher because sudden deaths on a golf course or while working outside may be falsely labeled as heart attacks or strokes. In studies of postmortem sera from individuals dying from unknown causes, a significant number had clinically relevant levels of IgE antibodies to one or more Hymenoptera venom or elevated tryptase levels [30,31]. There are many more near-fatal episodes. In the initial controlled trial of VIT, 3 of the 14 patients in the placebo- and whole-body extract–treated groups who sustained challenge sting-induced systemic reactions had significant hypotension; in two of these patients the hypotension persisted despite multiple doses of epinephrine; one patient required intubation [18].

Table 1
Insect sting deaths in the United States

| | No. of deaths | | | | | | | | Total for | |
|---|---|---|---|---|---|---|---|---|---|---|
| Year | 0–9 | 10–19 | 20–29 | 30–39 | 40–49 | 50–59 | 60–69 | 70+ | the year | Sex (M/F) |
| 1980 | 0 | 0 | 1 | 1 | 7 | 13 | 13 | 3 | 38 | 25/13 |
| 1981 | 0 | 1 | 2 | 7 | 6 | 12 | 6 | 5 | 39 | 35/4 |
| 1982 | 0 | 1 | 2 | 4 | 16 | 13 | 10 | 8 | 54 | 45/9 |
| 1983 | 2 | 0 | 3 | 8 | 9 | 9 | 10 | 8 | 49 | 43/6 |
| 1984 | 4 | 0 | 2 | 5 | 11 | 8 | 14 | 4 | 48 | 39/9 |
| 1985 | 1 | 1 | 4 | 4 | 8 | 10 | 9 | 4 | 41 | 32/9 |
| 1986 | 0 | 0 | 2 | 8 | 7 | 7 | 11 | 7 | 42 | 31/11 |
| 1987 | 1 | 0 | 0 | 5 | 9 | 15 | 12 | 11 | 53 | 42/11 |
| 1988 | 0 | 0 | 1 | 3 | 7 | 8 | 9 | 6 | 34 | 27/7 |
| 1989 | 0 | 0 | 2 | 6 | 9 | 13 | 15 | 8 | 53 | 40/13 |
| 1990 | 0 | 1 | 3 | 4 | 6 | 11 | 10 | 3 | 38 | 33/5 |
| 1991 | 1 | 1 | 4 | 11 | 11 | 13 | 14 | 9 | 64 | 48/16 |
| 1992 | 0 | 0 | 2 | 10 | 13 | 10 | 8 | 5 | 48 | 38/10 |
| 1993 | 0 | 2 | 1 | 6 | 8 | 5 | 11 | 6 | 39 | 31/8 |
| 1994 | 0 | 1 | 2 | 7 | 12 | 6 | 13 | 8 | 49 | 37/12 |
| 1995 | 0 | 1 | 0 | 7 | 12 | 13 | 11 | 15 | 59 | 46/13 |
| 1996 | 0 | 1 | 1 | 2 | 9 | 14 | 12 | 6 | 45 | 27/18 |
| 1997 | 0 | 1 | 5 | 5 | 10 | 10 | 10 | 2 | 43 | 40/3 |
| 1998 | 1 | 0 | 4 | 4 | 13 | 12 | 4 | 8 | 46 | 33/13 |
| 1999 | 0 | 0 | 0 | 5 | 13 | 15 | 5 | 5 | 43 | 31/12 |
| **Total** | **10** | **11** | **41** | **112** | **196** | **217** | **207** | **131** | **925** | **723/202** |

Data from Graft DF. Venom immunotherapy for stinging insect allergy. Clin Rev Allergy 1987;5:149–59.

The rate of venom sensitivity is higher than the rate of systemic reactions. In a stratified random sample of 320 adults in a light industrial setting, 3.3% had a history of systemic reaction to insect sting, but 17% had positive venom skin test (VST) and 26% had venom-specific IgE antibodies by radioallergosorbent testing (RAST) [21]. Evidence of venom sensitivity was more likely if the subject had been stung in the last 3 years. Interestingly, these history-negative positive VST subjects had a 17% risk of reaction to field sting [32]. Ludolph-Hauser and coworkers [33] reported a more frequent occurrence of elevated basal serum tryptase in patients with a history of severe systemic reactions to insect stings. Others have also reported severe reactions to insect stings in patients with systemic mastocytosis and often little evidence of venom sensitization is found [34].

## The insects

The stinging insects belong to the order Hymenoptera. A sting is an injection of venom by the female of each species through a modified ovipositor. The most conspicuous members of the superfamily Apidae are the honeybee (*Apis mellifera*) and bumblebees (*Bombus* spp). Honeybees are small, fuzzy insects with alternating tan and black stripes. They are often seen pollinating clover and flowering plants, are relatively nonaggressive, and generally sting only when caught underfoot. The barbs along the shaft of the honeybee stinger cause it to remain embedded at the sting site (autonomy). As it flies away, the honeybee dies through evisceration.

The honeybees in the United States were at one time only of European ancestry. Africanized honeybees were brought to Brazil in 1956 to improve honey production. One year later multiple colonies escaped and began interbreeding with the resident colonies. The Africanized honeybees have expanded northward and by 2002 were present in most of Texas and Arizona and southern areas of Nevada, California, and New Mexico. Africanized honeybees are often referred to as "killer bees" not because of increased venom potency or allergenicity but rather of their tendency to attack en masse; fortunately, even massive stinging incidents of 50 to 100 stings are not usually fatal. Nevertheless, there were at least 70 deaths attributed to Africanized honeybees in Venezuela from 1978 to 1981 [35] and 42 deaths in Mexico from 1987 to 1991 [36]. McKenna [36] recently accounted the 13 deaths in the United States until 2002.

Bumblebees are large, slow-moving, noisy bees with hairy bodies of alternating yellow and black stripes. They are also nonaggressive and account for only a small fraction of stings. Bumblebee stings have become more common, however, because they have been used in confined settings, such as greenhouses, to pollinate tomato plants [37].

The family Vespidae includes the yellow jackets, hornets, and wasps, which make papier-mâché–like nests of wood fiber. The more than 10 species of yellow jackets (*Vespula* spp) are identified by alternating yellow and black body stripes. They usually nest in the ground or in decaying logs near human dwellings and scavenge for food. Closely related are the yellow and white (bald-faced) hornets (also *Vespula* spp), which build teardrop-shaped nests that hang in trees or bushes. Both yellow jackets and hornets are extremely aggressive, especially in the late summer when crowded conditions develop in the nests.

Not quite as aggressive as the other vespids, the thin-bodied paper wasps (*Polistes* spp) build nests in the eaves of buildings in which the development cells are not enclosed by a paper envelope. Allergic reactions resulting from wasp stings account for less than 5% of the cases in the northeast; however, in the southern regions of the United States, they are much more prevalent. Vespids rarely leave a stinger at the sting site, a feature that can be a clue in culprit identification.

Interestingly, common names for these insects are different in the United States and Europe and this must be kept in mind when reviewing the literature [38]. The yellow jacket, yellow hornet, and paper wasp are all called wasps in Europe. The term "hornet" is reserved in Europe for the *Vespa crabro* (European hornet), a large insect that builds its nests in tree hollows and wall cavities. Fortunately, still relatively uncommon in the United States, they account only for a small fraction of stings.

The imported fire ant (*Solenopsis invicta*) is found in the southeastern and south central United States. Its range continues to increase and allergic reactions to fire ants are becoming more common [39]. The fire ant grasps the victim with its jaws, then pivots around, stinging repetitively in a semicircular pattern. The hallmark of their sting is the development of a sterile pustule at each sting site 24 hours later.

## Venoms

The dried weight of the venom deposited by a honeybee, induced to sting a plastic film, is approximately 50 μg. A single sting from a yellow jacket is thought to deliver between 10 and 100 μg. Hymenoptera venoms contain a number of interesting constituents [40]. Most of the venoms contain histamine, dopamine, acetylcholine, and kinins, which cause the characteristic burning and pain and may allow for access to the systemic circulation. The allergens in the venoms are mostly proteins with enzyme activity. Although honeybees and have both phospholipase and hyaluronidase activities in their venom, the proteins bearing the same enzymatic functions in vespid venoms are immunochemically different. Antibody inhibition studies on sera from mice immunized with purified venom allergens show that extensive cross-reactivity exists between white-faced hornet, yellow hornet, and yellow jacket for hyaluronidase and antigen 5, but not phospholipase [41,42]. There is some cross-sensitization between *Polistes* wasp and yellow jacket for antigen 5 and there is limited cross-reactivity between honeybee, vespid, and fire ant venoms.

## Spectrum of reactions

Following a Hymenoptera sting, most individuals experience a small urticarial area that is slightly raised with surrounding redness, pruritus, and pain that starts shortly after the sting and usually resolves in 2 to 3 hours. About 10% of the population develop large local reactions, which has been variably defined as swelling contiguous with the sting site larger than a 2-in diameter [43] or more than a 4-in diameter [44] lasting over 24 hours. Occasionally, these are large enough to involve an entire extremity and may last for as long as a week. Often, these are misdiagnosed as cellulitis and patients receive antibiotics, especially if there is a lymphatic streak toward the axilla or groin.

Systemic allergic reactions (anaphylaxis) may be mild with only cutaneous symptoms (pruritus; urticaria; angioedema of the eyes, lips, hands; and so forth) or severe with potentially life-threatening symptoms of laryngeal edema, bronchospasm, hypotension manifested by an uncomfortable feeling in the throat, gagging, difficulty swallowing, voice change, inspiratory stridor, chest tightness, wheezing, cough, dizziness, tunnel vision, or loss of consciousness. Adults often describe a metallic taste in their mouth or an aura of impending doom, as if they are going to die. Nausea is common in large local and systemic reactions.

Systemic allergic reactions are, in general, less severe in children than adults. Of the approximately 45 deaths per year in the United States attributed to insect stings, only one or two occur in children [23]. Whereas 85% of adults with sting-induced systemic reactions report potentially life-threatening symptoms, such as laryngeal edema, bronchospasm, or hypotension, only 40% of children develop reactions of this level of severity [45]. Diagnosis of anaphylaxis is sometimes complicated by the absence of the more easily recognized cutaneous symptoms of an allergic reaction, such as urticaria. A patient may complain of light-headedness or a brief period of unconsciousness, be found to have hypotension, and the diagnosis of vasovagal reaction may be made. A vasovagal reaction is usually accompanied by bradycardia, however, whereas anaphylaxis often includes compensatory tachycardia in response to vasodilation and leakage of fluid from the blood vessels. An elevated serum tryptase, which signals mast cell degranulation, provides additional evidence for anaphylaxis [46].

Solley [47] recently reported his 17-year experience with insect stings and bites from Queensland, Australia. Of 1194 patients with anaphylaxis, 775 had urticaria with dyspnea, 425 had facial angioedema, and 457 had asthma. Additionally, 454 (38%) reported dizziness and 179 (15%) more patients manifested unconsciousness. Of particular note, 82 patients (7%) experienced dizziness, faintness, weakness, or coma as their sole expression of anaphylaxis; 48 (4%) had airways obstruction only; and an additional 79 (7%) had a combination of these two only.

A variety of atypical reactions have been described after insect stings [48,49]. When the syndrome of urticaria, fever, proteinuria, lymphadenopathy, and arthropathy has occurred, it has been termed "serum sickness" despite the imperfect analogy to classic serum sickness. Although one might worry that symptoms of serum sickness might recur when VIT is used, that has not been reported. Other uncommon outcomes after insect stings including renal disease and neurologic manifestations have been described, but they have not been shown to be IgE-mediated, and the mechanism of these events is unclear.

## Treatment of acute sting reactions

Minor local swelling and pruritus are expected and can be treated with ice and antihistamines. If present, the imbedded stinger should be flicked off with a scraping motion. Some authorities believe that one should not grasp the fleshy venom sac to extract the stinger because more venom might then be injected through the stinger. Schumacher and colleagues [50], however, showed that essentially the entire honeybee venom load is injected in less than 20 seconds; one should quickly remove the stinger.

If a generalized reaction occurs, epinephrine is the keystone of management. Epinephrine halts the further release of mediators and reverses many of the effects of released mediators. An intramuscular (preferred) [51] or subcutaneous injection of epinephrine usually produces prompt resolution of symptoms. The dose of epinephrine is 0.3 to 0.5 mg (0.3 to 0.5 mL of a 1:1000 solution) for adults, and 0.01 mg/kg for children. This may be repeated in 10 to 15 minutes if necessary. An oral or parenteral antihistamine, such as diphenhydramine, 6.25 to 50 mg, is also usually given. It may lessen urticaria, but in more severe or progressive reactions, its use should not delay the administration of epinephrine.

Epinephrine may be ineffective in profound anaphylactic shock unless the functional hypovolemia of this state is corrected with intravenous fluids [18]. Severe reactions often require treatment with oxygen, $H_2$-antihistamines, and pressor agents. Corticosteroids are often used but they have a delayed onset of action. Intubation or tracheostomy is indicated for severe upper airway edema not responding to therapy. Close observation is essential. Overnight hospitalization is suggested for patients who have experienced severe reactions or who have complicated medical problems.

## Decreasing future reactions

### Preventing stings

Future stings can be avoided by taking common sense precautions to significantly reduce exposure. Shoes should always be worn outside. Hives and nests around the home should be exterminated. Good sanitation should be practiced because garbage and outdoor food, especially canned drinks, attract yellow jackets. Unfortunately, insect repellents have little or no effect. Avoidance of attractants, such as fragrances and brightly colored clothes, may be helpful.

### Emergency epinephrine

To encourage prompt treatment, epinephrine is available in emergency kits for self-administration. These are used by insect sting–allergic individuals immediately after the sting to "buy time" to get to a medical facility. A practice self-injection with saline helps to allay such fears. The EpiPen (0.3 mg epinephrine) and EpiPen Jr. (0.15 mg epinephrine) offer a concealed needle and a pressure-sensitive spring-loaded injection device that make them suited for patients and families who are uncomfortable with the injection process. Epinephrine by inhalation may also be used to achieve a therapeutic plasma level and may be especially helpful for laryngeal edema and bronchospasm. Many patients in urgent care settings do not receive a prescription for self-administered epinephrine or referrals to allergists for consideration of VIT [52]. Patients who are receiving maintenance injections of

VIT are advised that emergency self-treatment will probably not be required; however, they should have the kit available if they are distant from medical facilities. A Medic-Alert bracelet is also advised.

## How to initiate venom immunotherapy

### Patient selection

VIT is a safe, highly effective method of preventing future sting reactions in insect-allergic patients. The selection of patients for VIT is determined by the likelihood that a future sting will cause an allergic reaction (Table 2), which is based on the clinical history and the results of venom skin tests (VSTs) (and occasionally RASTs). The risk of recurrence is higher for adults than for children, higher for those allergic to honeybee rather than vespid venom, and higher for patients whose previous reactions were more severe [53–55]. A careful history discloses the type, degree, and time course of symptoms, and often identifies the culprit insect. An individual who has experienced a sting-induced systemic reaction should be referred to an allergist who will perform skin tests with dilute solutions of honeybee, yellow jacket, yellow hornet, white-faced hornet, and *Polistes* wasp venoms and, if indicated, imported fire ant whole-body extract [56,57]. RAST cannot replace VST but may provide additional information [58]. The value of venom RAST is discussed in a subsequent section on the VST-negative patient. To date, fire ant venom has only been available in small research quantities; fortunately, the fire ant whole-body extract material contains a significant amount of venom and has been successfully used for skin testing and treatment. Table 3 lists the indications for VIT. At particularly low risk are children who have had reactions limited to the skin in which there is only a 10% rate of subsequent systemic reactions involving respiratory or cardiovascular symptoms [53]. Children who have had moderate or severe reactions should start VIT; those who do not start VIT have a significantly higher risk of

Table 2
Risk of systemic reaction in untreated patients with a history of sting anaphylaxis and positive venom skin tests

| Original sting reaction | | Risk of systemic reaction (%) | |
|---|---|---|---|
| Severity | Age | 1–9 y | 10–20 y |
| No reaction | Adult | 17 | — |
| Large local | All | 10 | 10 |
| Cutaneous | Child | 10 | 5 |
| Systemic | Adult | 20 | 10 |
| Anaphylaxis | Child | 40 | 30 |
| | Adult | 60 | 40 |

*From* Golden DBK. Insect allergy. In: Adkinson NF, Middleton E, editors. Middleton's allergy: principles and practice. 6th edition. Philadelphia: Mosby; 2003. p. 1475–86.

Table 3
Selection of patients for immunotherapy

| Reaction to sting | Result of skin test or RAST | Venom immunotherapy? |
|---|---|---|
| *Child* | | |
| Systemic, non–life-threatening, immediate, generalized urticaria, angiodema, erythema, pruritus[a] | + or − | No |
| Systemic, life-threatening, possible cutaneous symptoms, but also respiratory symptoms (laryngeal edema or bronchospasm) or cardiovascular symptoms (hypotension, shock) | + | Yes |
| *Adult* | | |
| Systemic | + | Yes |
| Systemic | − | No |
| *Child or adult* | | |
| Large local (>2 in diameter, >24-h duration) | + or − | No |
| Normal (<2 in, <24-h duration) | + or − | No |

[a] It is unknown whether this rule applies to imported fire ant hypersensitivity in children.

reaction as adults, estimated to be 30% [59]. Some clinicians recommend VIT for an adult who experienced any degree of systemic reaction. Most individuals, however, have a stereotypic response to a sting with the symptoms on subsequent stings closely resembling the first episode [60]. When only a mild reaction has occurred, the physician and patient may jointly decide whether to embark on a course of VIT [61]; some experts advise treatment of adults with only cutaneous symptoms [62]. Individuals who have had severe allergic reactions should be advised not to depend only on avoidance and availability of epinephrine but also to receive venom injections. Patients with a history of systemic reactions have a reduced quality of life [63]; this is not improved by having self-administered epinephrine but is with VIT [64].

Individuals with large local reactions or negative skin tests are not candidates for venom therapy. The risk of anaphylaxis to future stings is about 5% to 10% in patients who have had large local reactions to insect stings; many, however, develop large local reactions again [43,44,65]. Many patients with large local reactions have evidence of a high level of venom sensitivity. Because it is also true that some patients with severe anaphylaxis have low levels of venom sensitivity, the level of skin test reactivity (and venom-specific IgE) is poorly correlated with the risk of systemic reactions [56]. A positive VST or RAST in the absence of a sting-induced systemic reaction is not an indication for therapy. Approximately 25% of the general population may have such evidence of sensitization to venom antigens, apparently resulting from past stings. This is usually transient, disappearing in 1 to 3 years [21].

Other factors may influence the decision concerning the need for VIT. Those with an increased risk of being stung, such as landscapers or other individuals who engage in outdoor activities, especially those that take them far away from available medical care, dispose the physician toward initiating venom treatment. Part of the morbidity associated with stinging insect allergy includes psychologic effects of anxiety in the victim and family because of the threat of a sudden "unpreventable" systemic reaction. This high level of anxiety has frequently been exacerbated by a physician warning that "the next sting may be your last." Actually, most victims exhibit an individual pattern of anaphylaxis that varies only slightly in severity from one sting to another. Some investigators have proposed that a diagnostic sting challenge be used to select patients for VIT [60]. Patients who did not react would not be placed on VIT. Other reports, however, have described individuals who tolerated one sting challenge, but reacted later to a second challenge [66,67]. In the United States, the use of sting challenges to determine VIT candidates is impractical and most physicians believe that a challenge sting presents too great a risk [68], especially for patients with life-threatening reactions (ie, hypotension). Indeed, in one study life-threatening reaction recurred in 15% of subjects with histories of severe reactions [60].

*The venom skin test–negative patient (never say never)*

The patient with a history of a sting-induced systemic reaction and negative VSTs presents a unique challenge. It has been commonly assumed that negative VST responses indicate that there is no risk of systemic reaction to a sting. Golden and coworkers [69] recently reported, however, that of 307 subjects with a history of a sting-induced systemic reaction who underwent VST, 99 (32%) had negative VST. Of these, negative RAST was present in 56 patients; 36 had low (1–3 ng/mL) RAST; and 7 had high positive RAST (4–243 ng/mL). Sting challenges in 14 of 56 patients with negative VST and negative RAST resulted in two (14%) systemic reactions. Sting challenges in 37 of 43 patients with negative VST and positive RAST caused nine (24%) systemic reactions. Combined, the negative VST group had a systemic reaction rate of 22%, which was similar to the rate of 21% found in those with positive VST studied at the same time. It is now recommended that a patient with a convincing history of a sting-induced systemic reaction should have VST. If these are negative and the reaction was severe, venom-specific IgE should be measured and VIT initiated if positive. If negative RASTs are obtained, the VST should be repeated 3 to 6 months later [70,71]. Regardless of the VST and venom-specific IgE determinations, the patient should practice usual precautions of insect sting avoidance and should carry antihistamines and injectable epinephrine.

*Venom selection*

The venoms used for immunotherapy are the same as those used for skin testing (honeybee, yellow jacket, yellow hornet, white-faced hornet, wasp, and fire ant whole-body extract if applicable). The regimen begins with an injection of 0.01 μg and advances weekly to 100 μg (0.5 of 1:100 wt/vol for fire ant whole-body extract). The maintenance dose of 100 μg is given every 4 weeks for a year, after which the interval is lengthened to 6 to 8 weeks.

The choice of venoms is based primarily on VST results, and to a lesser extent on clinical history and patterns of venom cross-reactivity. It is currently recommended that immunotherapy include all venoms giving a positive skin test, the aim being to give the maximum security to the patient [62]. Even a patient who has reacted to only one type of insect should not be left with lingering doubts about future stings by other insects to which he or she shows skin test sensitivity. The most common culprit in North America is the yellow jacket, except for some areas of the south central and southwestern states, where wasps and honeybees, respectively, are predominant. In some cases, the skin tests are positive to only one or two venoms. Most yellow jacket–allergic patients also have positive skin tests to yellow hornet and white-faced hornet venoms, however, and consequently require treatment with mixed vespid venom containing the full dose of each venom (yellow jacket, yellow hornet, and white-faced hornet). Half of these patients are also positive to *Polistes* wasp venom and receive this in addition. RAST inhibition studies can disclose whether patients are sensitive to a cross-reacting allergen or multiple unique allergens. The allergenic cross-reactivity of the four vespid venoms has been demonstrated, as has the fact that most patients with multiple vespid venom sensitivity can be fully protected by immunotherapy with yellow jacket venom alone [72,73]. Honeybee venom is administered as indicated.

The 100-µg maintenance dose of venom was initially chosen because it represented approximately twice the venom content of a honeybee sting. One investigator has reported his 10-year experience with a maintenance venom dose of 50 µg [73]. The question of whether or not a lesser dose would suffice was examined in a group of patients who received a 50-µg maintenance dose. It was found that with the reduced venom dose, only 79% of subjects were protected from challenge sting-induced systemic reactions [74].

Yunginger and coworkers [75] reported on a very rapid 1-day rush regimen that had some success but caused many systemic reactions and had to be performed in a hospital. Bernstein and colleagues [76] described a 2- to 5-hour regimen of rush VIT in which 10 gradually increasing doses were administered every 10 to 15 minutes to achieve a total dose on day 1 of about 55 µg per venom followed by doses of 70, 80, 90, and 100 µg on days 3, 7, 14, and 21, respectively. Only 4 of 33 patients had reactions on day 1, and all were mild. These patients subsequently tolerated natural stings without incident.

## How does venom immunotherapy work?

The mechanism of action of immunotherapy is only partially understood. The development of allergic sensitization to venom requires the sting-induced production of venom-specific IgE antibodies that are bound to tissue mast cells and circulating basophils. A subsequent sting may then result in the binding of venom antigens to the IgE molecules followed by the release of mast cell and basophil mediators of anaphylaxis (histamine, leukotrienes, and so forth). It should be remembered that venom vaccines used to immunize patients with insect sting hypersensitivity are not clinically or immunologically identical to the venom injected by live stings. In the initial controlled trial of VIT, some patients tolerated injections of 100 μg of venom administered subcutaneously immediately before challenge stings that caused severe anaphylaxis to challenge stings [12,18]. Successful VIT is associated with many humoral and cellular immunologic changes that are summarized in a recent review [77].

VIT results in significant changes in venom-specific IgE and IgG antibody levels. IgE rises first, peaking at 8 to 12 weeks, before declining slowly over 3 to 5 years to pretreatment levels. The IgG level reaches its mean peak value of 15 μg/mL at 2 to 4 months, and then is fairly constant over 5 to 6 years of treatment in children. Adults have an average peak of 9 μg/mL and then decline to about 6 μg/mL. A few adult patients experience even more extreme declines for reasons that are presently unclear. The cause of the more vigorous IgG response in children is also not known. Analysis of venom-specific IgG levels in children and patient age, body weight, or surface area fails to show any correlation [78].

The production of antigen-specific IgG (blocking) antibodies has been considered the possible means of immunotherapeutic improvement. Lessof and coworkers [79] demonstrated that honeybee-allergic patients could tolerate challenge stings after passive immunization with the gamma globulin fraction of pooled beekeeper's serum that contained a high blocking antibody titer. The serum level of venom-specific IgG has been inversely correlated with the likelihood of challenge sting-induced systemic reactions in patients on VIT [80]. After 4 years of VIT, however, that correlation no longer held true. Other immunologic changes occur that could also influence the development of protection to insect stings. VIT seems to influence the T-cell phenotype away from the Th2-type, which produces interleukin-4 and interleukin-5, and toward the Th-1 type, which produces interferon-$\gamma$ [81,82], or a regulatory type with expression of interleukin-10 and the production of IgG4 [83].

## Management of venom immunotherapy

### Safety of venom immunotherapy

VIT generally is well tolerated. Most patients receive their injections in an allergist's office until the maintenance dose is reached. Patients should remain for 30 minutes after each injection in a setting equipped to handle a systemic reaction. About 3% to 12% of patients have treatment-induced systemic reactions that generally are mild and occur in the early phases of VIT [15,84]. The reaction rate is no higher than that seen in conventional pollen immunotherapy when effective immunizing doses are used [85]. If a systemic reaction occurs, the regimen is interrupted. One half of the dose that resulted in a systemic reaction is given the next week and, if tolerated, the schedule is resumed. Pretreatment with antihistamines reduces VIT reactions and may improve the efficacy of VIT [86,87]. A less serious, but more frequent, problem with VIT is the large local reactions that occur in 25% of children and 50% of adults, usually at doses about 20 to 30 µg. Although bothersome, they do not predict an increased risk of future systemic reactions to treatment and usually the best way to avoid them is to reach higher doses by proceeding with the injections regimen. Further advice in dealing with difficult cases can be found in the literature [88].

All new forms of treatment provoke concern of possible long-term complications. Yunginger and coworkers [89] provided some information regarding venom safety by studying beekeepers and their families who may experience as many as 50 or more stings per year. Although this population showed some minor urine or blood chemistry abnormalities, these did not show a correlation with sting frequency. Also, beekeepers do not have an increased risk of cancer. It should be noted, however, that parallel studies for vespid venoms are not available. No long-term toxicity or side effects have been associated with VIT thus far. Graft and coworkers [14] noted that 3 to 6 years of VIT in children was not associated with abnormalities in histories; physical examinations; or laboratory analyses (hematologic and chemical surveys, and urinalyses).

Few reports of VIT use during pregnancy have been published. Schwartz and coworkers [90] discussed 22 pregnancies in 15 women that resulted in 19 normal children, 1 first-trimester miscarriage, 1 miscarriage secondary to placenta previa, and 1 child with multiple congenital abnormalities of unknown cause. This rate of less than optimal outcome for pregnancy was not higher than expected with pregnancy in normal populations. In one closely studied case, VIT during pregnancy did not result in allergic sensitization to venom in the child [91].

*Interval between venom injections*

The maintenance dose of 100 µg is given every 4 weeks for a year; the interval is usually lengthened to 6 weeks during the second year and to 8 weeks during the third year of treatment [16]. Investigators from Israel described 160 individuals who had the maintenance interval lengthened to 3 months [92]. A subgroup of 47 reached the 3-month maintenance interval only 4.5 months after the maintenance dose was reached. Ninety-three stings in 80 patients on 3-month maintenance interval VIT resulted in four skin reactions (one occurred in one of the few patients on a 50-µg maintenance dose). After VIT was stopped in these patients, 65 stings in 46 patients resulted in four reactions (6.2% per sting, 8.7% per patient). Extending the interval between injections reduces the cost of VIT [93,94].

*Monitoring of venom immunotherapy*

Most patients begin therapy with IgG levels less than 1 µg/mL (usually undetectable), but occasionally they may be elevated because of the previous sting. IgG levels induced by the first 4 to 6 months of therapy are usually between 5 µg/mL and 20 µg/mL, with higher levels observed in children and when multiple venoms are administered [80]. Among immunized patients, those who continue to react to stings generally have exceptionally small increases in their venom-specific IgG antibodies. Patients who are not adequately protected by the 100 µg per venom dose are often protected with higher doses [95]. Because there are so few treatment failures with VIT, it may not be cost-effective to perform venom IgG antibody assays on all immunized patients [96].

At follow-up visits, usually annually, the patient's VIT schedule should be reviewed, noting dose and frequency of injections; local or systemic reactions to injections; and any stings (and their outcome) that may have occurred since the last visit. VSTs may be repeated every several years. Over time, VSTs tend to decline and become negative in a significant proportion of patients. In children, Graft and coworkers [97] found that 45% of those who had received 3 to 6 years of VIT developed negative VSTs to one or more venoms, whereas in adults, Golden and coworkers [98] reported that 20% had negative VSTs after 5 years and 50% to 60% after 7 to 10 years.

*Honeybee allergy versus vespid allergy*

Honeybee sensitivity is generally a more difficult problem than vespid venom sensitivity. Researchers in The Netherlands stung 324 patients and found that patients with history of honeybee sting reactions were twice as likely to react to challenge stings (52% versus 25%) [60]. Once VIT is commenced, Müller reported that honeybee-sensitive patients have more reactions to VIT (41% versus 25%) than those on vespid VIT [54]. Of concern, honeybee VIT is less effective in preventing future sting-induced systemic reactions (77% versus 91%) [54]. Finally, even after VIT is stopped, patients who received honeybee VIT are more than twice as likely to react to challenge stings (17% versus 4%–8%) delivered 1 to 2 years after VIT discontinuation [99].

**Discontinuation of venom immunotherapy**

In 1998, the American Academy of Allergy Asthma and Immunology published a position statement on the discontinuation of hymenoptera VIT [17]. This reviewed data that had been published on outcomes of patients who stopped VIT without a physician's recommendation; those who were able to stop VIT because they developed negative VSTs or significantly lower levels of venom-specific IgE; and those who had completed a specific duration of VIT, such as 3 or 5 years. Most have used challenge stings;

others have reported on the outcome of natural field stings. Importantly, the lack of certainty of identification of the insect clouds the interpretation of studies that used field stings.

When VIT was first used, many thought that it would need to be continued indefinitely. Early on, however, reports began to appear that chronicled the relatively good outcomes of patients who chose to stop their venom injections. Reisman and coworkers [13] reported from Buffalo on 88 patients, ages 10 to 76 years, who stopped VIT after 1 to 78 months without a physician's recommendation. Of these, 61 field stings in 41 patients occurred 1 to 72 months after VIT was terminated and there were 11 (18%) systemic reactions. In Baltimore, Golden and coworkers [100] noted a 22% reaction rate in patients who stopped treatment after 2 to 44 months of venom injections. These rates were much lower than the approximately 60% risk for untreated patients with histories of sting-induced systemic reactions and positive VST.

Next, studies were designed in which VIT was discontinued if the venom allergy had significantly diminished as measured by the fall in venom-specific IgE to low levels. Studies in which the VST became negative reported low numbers of entrants [33,97]. Urbanek and coworkers [101] studied the discontinuation of VIT in 31 honeybee-sensitive children and adolescents in whom venom-specific IgE had fallen to low or unmeasurable levels. One year after stopping VIT, a challenge honeybee sting resulted in a systemic reaction in only 1 (3%) of 29 patients; at 2 years after stopping VIT, 2 (14%) of 14 patients reacted. Randolph and Reisman [102] reported an 8% reaction rate to stings in patients who stopped VIT because of a two-log decline in venom-specific IgE levels. Studies using serum venom-specific IgE levels have been criticized because of potential for variance in assay methods and scoring systems between investigators. Reisman [103] retrospectively reviewed the outcome of 217 field re-stings in 113 patients after discontinuation of VIT and reported a relationship between the severity of the pre-VIT insect sting reaction and the likelihood and severity of sting reactions after a course of VIT was stopped. Systemic reactions occurred in 1 (4%) of 25 patients with initial mild reactions; 2 (5%) of 41 patients with initial moderate reactions; and 7 (15%) of 47 patients with initial severe reactions. In the latter group, five of the seven reactions were again of a severe nature. Furthermore, in Minneapolis a retrospective study found that 148 stings in 117 patients (most were intentional challenge stings) who had discontinued VIT resulted in only two reactions, both of which occurred in patients with initial severe sting reactions [104].

Most recently, studies have been designed in which VIT is administered for a specific duration of time. Haugaard and coworkers [105] of Denmark reported the outcome of sting challenges in 25 adults (mean age, 42.9 years) who had moderate to severe systemic reactions; were primarily yellow jacket sensitive; and had been on VIT for 36 to 83 months (mean, 42.8 months). Twenty-eight sting challenges with the relevant insects 12 to 36 months (mean 25.2 months) after VIT was stopped resulted in no systemic reactions. In Switzerland, Müller and coworkers [99] studied 86 children and adults who had received honeybee venom for a mean period of 56.4 months (range, 32–119 months). All patients had tolerated a honeybee sting in the field or in a hospital challenge setting while receiving VIT. About 13 months (range, 10–24 months) after VIT was discontinued, patients returned for deliberate honeybee sting challenges, and 15 patients (17%) experienced mild systemic reactions.

Keating and coworkers [106] studied 51 patients in Minnesota after cessation of VIT for 2 to 10 years (mean, 5.2 years). Vespid VIT was administered to 46 patients, with 15 patients receiving honeybee venom injections. All patients tolerated stings by the relevant insects at the time VIT was discontinued. One year after stopping VIT, two patients reacted to intentional challenge stings; these patients resumed VIT. Further sting challenges (N = 31) resulted in no reactions. Two of 15 patients with initial severe reactions had reactions to challenge stings compared with none of the 36 patients with milder reactions. Also, the risk of reaction was higher in the 13 patients who received VIT for less than 5 years (2 of 20) than in the patients who received VIT for more than 5 years (0 of 31).

At Johns Hopkins in Baltimore, Golden and coworkers [98,107,108] performed the most comprehensive trial of discontinuation of VIT. They reported the results of challenge stings in 74 adults allergic to insect venom who had stopped treatment after 5 or more years of VIT. Eighty percent of these patients had a history of respiratory or vascular symptoms of anaphylaxis after a pre-VIT sting. VST responses were negative in 28% when VIT was discontinued (VIT duration: mean, 5.95 years; range, 5–9 years). One group of 29 patients was stung annually for 5 years; in year 4 they had two stings, 1 month apart. A second group of 25 patients had sting challenges every 2 years; in year 4 off VIT they received two sting challenges, 1 month apart. A third group of 20 patients had two stings 1 month apart after 2 years off VIT. Systemic reactions followed 8 (3%) of 270 stings in 7 (10%) of 74 patients [98]; only two reactions were clinically significant. By the end of the study, skin test responses were negative in 67% of the subjects.

Subsequently, Golden and coworkers [107] reported on their extended follow-up for these and other patients. Of the original 74 patients in their challenge sting study, 11 sustained field stings after 3 to 7 years off VIT and one developed a systemic reaction involving dyspnea. Of an additional 51 patients, 4 of 15 stings results in systemic reactions. In total, 12 (13.5%) of 89 patients had 14 (4.5%) reactions to 309 stings. Patients who had a systemic reaction to a venom injection or insect sting during VIT had a 46% rate of systemic reaction to stings after VIT was discontinued as compared with only 8% rate in those who had no reactions during VIT. Patients with more severe pre-VIT reactions did not have a higher frequency of reactions to stings but did tend to have more severe reactions. A follow-up paper noted that insect stings had caused systemic reactions in 16 (14%) of 113 patients who were stung after discontinuing 5 or more years of VIT [108]. It seems that patients with more severe reactions before VIT, patients who reacted to stings or venom injections while receiving VIT, and patients with honeybee-venom sensitivity tend to react to stings more frequently when VIT is stopped. No two situations are identical. For some patients, a decision to continue venom injections indefinitely, regardless of other factors, may be in order. Fortunately, most venom-treated patients can extend the interval between maintenance injections to 6 to 8 or even 12 weeks after 2 to 4 years of therapy.

The American Academy of Allergy Asthma and Immunology Position Statement [17] recommendations regarding discontinuation of VIT include the following: (1) the decision should be made on the basis of a thorough discussion of the issues by the physician and patient (individual patient variables, such as vocation or leisure activities, medications, and coexistent diseases, should be considered); (2) the conversion to a negative skin test is one criterion for stopping VIT; (3) patients with mild or moderate sting reactions before VIT was initiated may discontinue VIT after 3 to 5 years; and (4) in patients with severe (hypotension, laryngeal edema, or bronchospasm) sting reactions the physician may wish to continue venom injections for more than 5 years and perhaps indefinitely (because most of even these most-at-risk patients tolerate discontinuation of VIT after 5 years of treatment, stopping treatment is an option).

## Summary

Insect sting allergy has served as an excellent model for the allergic process over the past century. In particular, during the last 30 years, a new form of diagnostic testing and treatment with venom has been one of the great success stories in the entire field of allergy. VIT reduces the risk of recurrent life-threatening reactions from about 60% to less than 2%. Progress and further questions continue with a search for a definitive diagnostic test that more accurately predicts which patients are at risk for future reactions, and defines which patients can stop VIT and which ones need to continue treatment.

## Acknowledgments

I thank Robert N. Anderson, PhD, of the National Center for Health Statistics for his efforts in providing the most current insect sting mortality data and Ms. Penny Marsala for librarian services.

## References

[1] Cohen SG, Samter M, editors. Excerpts from classics in allergy. 2nd edition. Carlsbad (CA): Symposia Foundation; 1993.

[2] Portier P, Richert C. De l'action anaphylactic de certain venins [The anaphylactic action of some venoms]. C R Soc Biol (Paris) 1902;54:170–2 [in French].

[3] Waterhouse AT. Bee sting and anaphylaxis. Lancet 1914;2:946.

[4] Braun LIB. Notes of desensitization of a patient hypersensitive to bee stings. S Afr Med Rec 1925;23:408.

[5] Benson RL, Semenov H. Allergy in its relation to the bee sting. J Allergy 1930;1:105–16.

[6] Loveless MH, Fackler WR. Wasp venom allergy and immunity. Ann Allergy 1956;14: 347–85.

[7] Bernton HS, Brown H. Studies on the Hymenoptera. I. Skin reactions of normal persons to honeybee (*Apis mellifera*) extract. J Allergy 1965;36:315–20.

[8] Schwartz HJ. Skin sensitivity in insect allergy. JAMA 1965;194:703–5.

[9] Benton AW, Morse RA, Stewart JD. Venom collection from honeybees. Science 1963;142: 228–30.

[10] Lichtenstein LM, Valentine MD, Sobotka AK. A case for venom therapy treatment in anaphylactic sensitivity to Hymenoptera sting. N Engl J Med 1974;290:1223–7.

[11] Busse WW, Reed CE, Lichtenstein LM, et al. Immunotherapy in bee-sting anaphylaxis: use of honeybee venom. JAMA 1975;231:1154–6.

[12] Hunt KJ, Valentine MD, Sobotka AK, et al. A controlled trial of immunotherapy in insect hypersensitivity. N Engl J Med 1978;299:157–61.

[13] Reisman RE, Dvorin DJ, Randolph CC, et al. Stinging insect allergy: natural history and modification with venom immunotherapy. J Allergy Clin Immunol 1985;75:735–40.

[14] Graft DF, Schuberth KC, Kagey-Sobotka A, et al. Assessment of prolonged venom immunotherapy in children. J Allergy Clin Immunol 1987;80:162–9.

[15] Golden DBK, Valentine MD, Kagey-Sobotka A, et al. Regimens of Hymenoptera venom immunotherapy. Ann Intern Med 1980;92:620–4.

[16] Moffitt JE, Golden DBK, Reisman RE, et al. Stinging insect hypersensitivity: a practice parameter update. J Allergy Clin Immunol 2004;114:869–86.

[17] Graft DF, Golden DB, Reisman RE, et al. The discontinuation of Hymenoptera venom immunotherapy. Position statement. The American Academy of Allergy Asthma and Immunology. J Allergy Clin Immunol 1998;101:573–5.

[18] Smith PL, Kagey-Sobotka A, Bleecker ER, et al. Physiologic manifestations of human anaphylaxis. J Clin Invest 1980;66:1072–80.

[19] Chafee FH. The prevalence of bee sting allergy in an allergic population. Acta Allergol 1970;25:292–3.

[20] Settipane GA, Boyd GK. Prevalence of bee sting allergy in 4,992 Boy Scouts. Acta Allergol 1970;25:286–91.

[21] Golden DBK, Marsh DG, Kagey-Sobotka A, et al. Epidemiology of insect venom sensitivity. JAMA 1989;262:240–4.

[22] Lockey RF, Turkelstaub PC, Baird-Warren IA, et al. The Hymenoptera venom study I, 1979–1982: demographics and history sting data. J Allergy Clin Immunol 1988;82:370–81.

[23] Deaths from each cause by 5-year age groups, race, and sex: United States, 1980–1999. Hyattsville (MD): National Center for Health Statistics. Available at: http://wonder.cdc.gov.

[24] Salter J, Mehra S, Cairns J, et al. Insect sting-related deaths in Ontario: 1986–2000, a retrospective review [abstract]. J Allergy Clin Immunol 2002;109:5268.

[25] Ewan PW. ABC of allergies: venom allergy. BMJ 1998;316:1365–8.

[26] Müller U. Prophylaxe und therapie der in: insektenstichallergie. Pharma-Kritik 1985;7: 25–8.

[27] Przybilla B, Ring J. Diagnostik und therapie der allergie vom sofort-typ gegenüber bienen-und wespengift. Allergologie 1985;8:31–9.

[28] Barnard JH. Studies of 400 Hymenoptera sting deaths in the United States. J Allergy Clin Immunol 1973;52:259–64.

[29] Mosbech H. Death caused by wasp and bee stings in Denmark 1960–1980. Allergy 1983;38: 195–200.

[30] Schwartz HJ, Squillace DL, Sher TH, et al. Studies in stinging insect hypersensitivity: post-mortem demonstration of antivenom IgE antibody in possible sting-related sudden death. Am J Clin Pathol 1986;85:607–10.

[31] Yunginger JW, Nelson DR, Squillace DL, et al. Laboratory investigation of deaths due to anaphylaxis. J Forensic Sci 1991;36:857–65.

[32] Golden DB, Marsh DG, Freidhoff LR, et al. Natural history of Hymenoptera venom sensitivity in adults. J Allergy Clin Immunol 1997;100:760–6.

[33] Ludolph-Hauser D, Rueff F, Fries C, et al. Constitutively raised serum concentrations of mast-cell tryptase and severe anaphylactic reactions to Hymenoptera stings. Lancet 2001; 357:361–2.

[34] Fricker M, Helblind A, Schwartz L, et al. Hymenoptera sting anaphylaxis and urticaria pigmentosa: clinical findings and results of venom immunotherapy in ten patients. J Allergy Clin Immunol 1997;100:11–5.

[35] Tayler OR. Health problems associated with African bees. Ann Intern Med 1986;104: 267–8.

[36] McKenna WR. Africanized honey bees. In: Levine MI, Locket RF, editors. Monograph on insect allergy. 4th edition. Milwaukee (WI): American Academy of Allergy, Asthma and Immunology; 2003. p. 27–36.

[37] Kochuyt AM, Van Hoeyveld E, Stevens EA. Occupational allergy to bumble bee venom. Clin Exp Allergy 1993;23:190–5.

[38] Mueller UR, Reimers A, Haeberli G. The European experience in Hymenoptera venom allergy. In: Levine MI, Lockey RF, editors. Monograph on insect allergy. 4th edition. Milwaukee (WI): American Academy of Allergy Asthma and Immunology; 2003. p. 243–58.

[39] Kemp SF, deShazo RD, Moffitt JE, et al. Expanding habitat of the imported fire ant (Solenopsis invicta): a public health concern. J Allergy Clin Immunol 2000;105:683–91.

[40] Hoffman DR. Hymenoptera venoms: composition, standardization, stability. In: Levine MI, Lockey RF, editors. Monograph on insect allergy. 4th edition. Milwaukee (WI): American Academy of Allergy Asthma and Immunology; 2003. p. 37–53.

[41] King TP, Valentine MD. Allergens of hymenoptera venoms. Clin Rev Allergy 1987;5: 137–48.

[42] Lu G, Kochoumian L, King TP. Sequence identity and antigenic cross-reactivity of white face hornet venom allergen, also a hyaluronidase, with other proteins. J Biol Chem 1995; 270:4457–65.

[43] Graft DF, Schuberth KC, Kagey-Sobotka A, et al. A prospective study of the natural history of large local reactions after Hymenoptera stings in children. J Pediatr 1984;104:664–8.

[44] Mueller UR. Insect sting allergy. Stuttgart (Germany): Gustav Fischer Verlag; 1990. p. 61–2.

[45] Schuberth KC, Valentine MD, Kagey-Sobotka A, et al. An epidemiologic study of insect allergy in children: characteristics of the disease. J Pediatr 1982;100:546–51.

[46] Schwartz LB, Yunginger JW, Miller J, et al. Time course of appearance and disappearance of human mast cell tryptase in the circulation after anaphylaxis. J Clin Invest 1989;83: 1551–5.

[47] Solley GO. Stinging and biting insect allergy: an Australian experience. Ann Allergy Asthma Immunol 2004;93:532–7.

[48] Light WC, Reisman RE, Shimizu M, et al. Unusual reactions following insect stings: clinical features and immunologic analysis. J Allergy Clin Immunol 1977;59:391–7.

[49] Reisman RE, Livingston A. Late-onset allergic reactions, including serum sickness, after insect stings. J Allergy Clin Immunol 1989;84:331–7.

[50] Schumacher MJ, Tveten MS, Egen NB. Rate and quantity of delivery of venom from honeybee stings. J Allergy Clin Immunol 1994;93:831–5.

[51] Simons FER, Gu X, Simons KJ. Epinephrine absorption in adults: intramuscular versus subcutaneous injection. J Allergy Clin Immunol 2001;108:871–3.

[52] Hutcheson PS, Slavin RG. Lack of preventative measures given to patients with stinging insect anaphylaxis in hospital emergency rooms. Ann Allergy 1990;64:306–7.

[53] Valentine MD, Schuberth KC, Kagey-Sobotka A, et al. The value of immunotherapy with venom in children with allergy to insect stings. N Engl J Med 1990;323:1601–3.

[54] Müller U, Helbling A, Berchtold E. Immunotherapy with honeybee venom and yellow jacket venom is different regarding efficacy and safety. J Allergy Clin Immunol 1992;89: 529–35.

[55] Reisman RE. Natural history of insect sting allergy: relationship of severity of symptoms of initial sting anaphylaxis to re-sting reactions. J Allergy Clin Immunol 1992;90:335–9.

[56] Hunt KJ, Valentine MD, Sobotka AK, et al. Diagnosis of allergy to stinging insects by skin testing with Hymenoptera venoms. Ann Intern Med 1976;85:56–9.

[57] Rhoades RB. Skin test reactivity to imported fire ant whole body extract: comparison of three commercial sources. J Allergy Clin Immunol 1993;91:282.

[58] Sobotka AK, Adkinson NF Jr, Valentine MD, et al. Allergy to insect stings: IV. Diagnosis by radioallergosorbent tests (RAST). J Immunol 1978;121:2477–84.

[59] Golden DBK, Kagey-Sobotka A, Norman PS, et al. Outcomes of allergy to insect stings in children, with and without venom immunotherapy. N Engl J Med 2004;351:668–74.

[60] Van der Linden PG, Hack CE, Struyvenberg A, et al. Insect-sting challenge in 324 subjects with a previous anaphylactic reaction: current criteria for insect-venom hypersensitivity do not predict the occurrence and the severity of anaphylaxis. J Allergy Clin Immunol 1994;94: 151–9.

[61] Reisman RE. Insect stings. N Engl J Med 1994;331:523–7.

[62] Golden DBK. Insect allergy. In: Adkinson NF, Middleton E, editors. Middleton's allergy: principles and practice. 6th edition. Philadelphia: Mosby; 2003. p. 1475–86.

[63] Oude-Elberink JN, deMonchy JG, Golden DB, et al. Quality of life in yellow jacket allergic patients: I. Development and validation of a health-related quality of life questionnaire in yellow jacket patients. J Allergy Clin Immunol 2002;109:162–70.

[64] Oude-Elberink JN, deMonchy JG, Van Der Heide S, et al. Venom immunotherapy improves health-related quality of life in yellow jacket allergic patients. J Allergy Clin Immunol 2002;110:174–82.

[65] Mauriello PM, Barde SH, Georgitis JW, et al. Natural history of large local reactions from stinging insects. J Allergy Clin Immunol 1984;74:494–8.

[66] Franken HH, Debois AEJ, Minkena ITJ, et al. Lack of reproducibility of a single negative sting challenge response in the assessment of anaphylactic risk in patients with suspected yellow jacket sensitivity. J Allergy Clin Immunol 1994;93:431–6.

[67] Golden DB, Kagey-Sobotka A, Norman PS, et al. Sting Challenge Trial I: spectrum of a population with insect sting allergy. J Allergy Clin Immunol 1998;101: S159.

[68] Reisman RE. Insect sting challenges: do no harm. J Allergy Clin Immunol 1995;96:702–3.

[69] Golden DB, Kagey-Sobotka A, Norman PS, et al. Insect sting allergy with negative venom skin test responses. J Allergy Clin Immunol 2001;107:897–901.

[70] Reisman RE. Insect sting allergy: the dilemma of the negative skin test reactor [editorial]. J Allergy Clin Immunol 2001;107:781–2.

[71] Graft DF. Never say never: exchange of comments on negative VST responses [correspondence]. J Allergy Clin Immunol 2001;108:875–6.

[72] Golden DB, Valentine MD, Kagey-Sobotka A, et al. Cross-reactivity of vespid venoms [abstract]. J Allergy Clin Immunol 1981;67:57.

[73] Reisman RE, Livingston A. Venom immunotherapy: 10 years of experience with administration of single venoms and 50 micrograms maintenance dose. J Allergy Clin Immunol 1992;89:1189–95.

[74] Golden DB, Kagey-Sobotka A, Valentine MD, et al. Dose dependence of Hymenoptera venom immunotherapy. J Allergy Clin Immunol 1981;67:370–4.

[75] Yunginger JW, Paull BR, Jones RT, et al. Rush venom immunotherapy program for honeybee venom sensitivity. J Allergy Clin Immunol 1979;63:340–7.

[76] Bernstein DI, Mittman RJ, Kagen SL, et al. Clinical and immunologic studies of rapid venom immunotherapy in Hymenoptera-sensitive patients. J Allergy Clin Immunol 1989; 84:951–9.

[77] Mosbech H, Frew AJ. The immunologic response to Hymenoptera venoms. In: Levine MI, Lockey RF, editors. Monograph on insect allergy. 4th edition. Milwaukee (WI): American Academy of Allergy Asthma and Immunology; 2003. p. 75–81.

[78] Graft DF. Venom immunotherapy for stinging insect allergy. Clin Rev Allergy 1987;5:149–59.

[79] Lessof MH, Sobotka AK, Lichtenstein LM. Effects of passive antibody in bee venom anaphylaxis. Johns Hopkins Med J 1978;142:1–7.

[80] Golden DB, Lawrence ID, Hamilton RG, et al. Clinical correlation of the venom-specific IgG antibody level during maintenance venom. J Allergy Clin Immunol 1992;90:386–93.

[81] McHugh SM, Deighton J, Stewart AG, et al. Bee venom immunotherapy induces a shift in cytokine responses from a TH2 to a TH1 dominant pattern: comparison of rush and conventional immunotherapy. Clin Exp Allergy 1995;25:828–38.

[82] Jutel M, Pichler WJ, Skrbic D, et al. Bee venom immunotherapy results in decrease of IL-4 and IL-5 and increase in IFN-γ secretion in specific allergen stimulated T cell cultures. J Immunol 1995;154:4187–94.

[83] Nasser SM, Ying S, Meng Q, et al. Interleukin-10 levels increase in cutaneous biopsies of patients undergoing wasp venom immunotherapy. Eur J Immunol 2001;31:3704–13.

[84] Lockey RF, Turkeltaub PC, Olive ES, et al. The Hymenoptera venom study III: safety of venom immunotherapy. J Allergy Clin Immunol 1990;86:775–80.

[85] Van Metre TE Jr, Adkinson NF Jr, Amodio FJ, et al. A comparison of immunotherapy schedules for injection treatment of ragweed pollen hay fever. J Allergy Clin Immunol 1982;69:181–93.

[86] Brockow K, Kiehn M, Rietmuller C, et al. Efficacy of antihistamine pretreatment in the prevention of adverse reactions to Hymenoptera immunotherapy: a prospective, randomized, placebo-controlled trial. J Allergy Clin Immunol 1997;100:458–63.

[87] Müller U, Han Y, Berchtold E. Premedication with antihistamines may enhance efficacy of specific allergen immunotherapy. J Allergy Clin Immunol 2001;107:81–6.

[88] Golden DBK. Insect sting allergy in adults. In: Lichtenstein LM, Fauci AS, editors. Current therapy in allergy and immunology 1983–1984. Philadelphia: BC Decker; 1983. p. 70–5.

[89] Yunginger JW, Jones RT, Leiferman KM, et al. Immunological studies in beekeepers and their family members. J Allergy Clin Immunol 1978;61:93–101.

[90] Schwartz HJ, Golden DBK, Lockey RF. Venom immunotherapy in the Hymenoptera-allergic pregnant patient. J Allergy Clin Immunol 1990;85:709–12.

[91] Graft DF. Venom immunotherapy during pregnancy. Allergy Proc 1988;9:563–5.

[92] Goldberg A, Confino-Cohen R. Maintenance venom immunotherapy at 3-month intervals is both safe and efficacious. J Allergy Clin Immunol 2001;107:902–6.

[93] Kochuyt AM, Stevens EA. Safety and efficacy of a 12 week maintenance interval in patients treated with Hymenoptera venom immunotherapy. Clin Exp Allergy 1994;24:35–41.

[94] Golden DBK, Kelly D, Hamilton RG. Extended maintenance intervals during long-term venom immunotherapy (VIT) [abstract]. J Allergy Clin Immunol 2005;115: S108.

[95] Rueff F, Wenderoth A, Przybilla B. Patients still reacting to a sting challenge while receiving conventional Hymenoptera venom immunotherapy are protected by increased venom doses. J Allergy Clin Immunol 2001;108:1027–32.

[96] Reisman RE. Should routine measurements of serum venom-specific IgG be a standard of practice in patients receiving venom immunotherapy? J Allergy Clin Immunol 1992;90: 282–4.

[97] Graft DF, Schuberth KC, Kagey-Sobotka A, et al. The development of negative venom skin tests in children treated with venom immunotherapy. J Allergy Clin Immunol 1984; 73:61–8.

[98] Golden DBK, Kwiterovich KA, Kagey-Sobotka A, et al. Discontinuing venom immunotherapy: outcome after five years. J Allergy Clin Immunol 1996;97:579–87.

[99] Müller U, Berchtold E, Helbling A. Honeybee venom allergy: results of a sting challenge 1 year after stopping successful venom immunotherapy in 86 patients. J Allergy Clin Immunol 1991;87:702–9.

[100] Golden DBK, Johnson K, Addison BI, et al. Clinical and immunologic observations in patients who discontinue venom immunotherapy. J Allergy Clin Immunol 1986;77:435–42.

[101] Urbanek R, Forster J, Kuhn W, et al. Discontinuation of bee venom immunotherapy in children and adolescents. J Pediatr 1985;107:367–71.

[102] Randolph CC, Reisman RE. Evaluation of decline in serum venom-specific IgE as a criterion for stopping venom immunotherapy. J Allergy Clin Immunol 1986;77:823–7.

[103] Reisman RE. Duration of venom immunotherapy: relationship to the severity of symptoms of initial insect sting anaphylaxis. J Allergy Clin Immunol 1993;92:831–6.

[104] Graft DF, Schoenwetter WF. Insect sting allergy: analysis of a cohort of patients who initiated venom immunotherapy from 1978 to 1986. Ann Allergy 1994;73:481–5.

[105] Haugaard L, Norregaard OF, Dahl R. In-hospital sting challenge in insect venom-allergic patients after stopping venom immunotherapy. J Allergy Clin Immunol 1991;87:699–702.

[106] Keating MV, Kagey-Sobotka A, Hamilton RG, et al. Clinical and immunologic follow-up of patients who stop venom immunotherapy. J Allergy Clin Immunol 1991;88:339–48.

[107] Golden DBK, Kwiterovich KA, Kagey-Sobotka A, et al. Discontinuing venom immunotherapy: extended observations. J Allergy Clin Immunol 1998;101:298–305.

[108] Golden DB, Kagey-Sobotka A, Lichtenstein LM. Survey of patients after discontinuing venom immunotherapy. J Allergy Clin Immunol 2000;105:385.

ELSEVIER
SAUNDERS

THE MEDICAL
CLINICS
OF NORTH AMERICA

Med Clin N Am 90 (2006) 233–260

# Drug Hypersensitivity

## Roland Solensky, MD*

*Division of Allergy and Immunology, The Corvallis Clinic, Corvallis, OR, USA*

Adverse drug reactions (ADRs) are everyday occurrences in both in- and outpatient practice settings. Based on a recent meta-analysis, the overall incidence of ADRs in hospitalized patients was 15.1%, with nearly half of these reactions being serious in nature [1]. The incidence of fatal ADRs was found to be 0.32%, a figure that the authors estimated translates to 106,000 deaths annually in United States hospitals [1]. Although there are less data on the incidence of ADRs in the outpatient setting, two recent studies found that between 17% and 25% of ambulatory primary care clinic patients reported ADRs, and more than half of these were considered serious [2,3].

Allergic drug reactions are ADRs that are known (or presumed) to be mediated by an immunologic mechanism. They are thought to account for approximately 6% to 10% of all ADRs [4]. Because of space limitations, this review does not address the entire spectrum of drug hypersensitivity disorders (Box 1). Instead, the discussion focuses on the most clinically relevant reactions: to penicillins and other beta-lactam antibiotics, sulfonamides, aspirin/nonsteroidal anti-inflammatory drugs (NSAIDs), and local anesthetics. For a more comprehensive review of drug hypersensitivity, the reader is referred to two recent texts [5,6].

## Definitions and mechanisms

An ADR is defined as any noxious, unintended, and undesired effect of a drug that occurs at doses used in humans for prevention, diagnosis, or treatment [7]. ADRs are divided into two broad categories: predictable (also called type A) reactions and unpredictable (or type B) reactions (Table 1) [8]. Predictable reactions are usually dose-dependent, are related to the

---

* Division of Allergy and Immunology, The Corvallis Clinic, 3680 NW Samaritan Drive, Corvallis, OR 97330.

*E-mail address:* roland.solensky@corvallis-clinic.com

0025-7125/06/$ - see front matter © 2005 Elsevier Inc. All rights reserved.
doi:10.1016/j.mcna.2005.08.010

**Box 1. Partial list of drug hypersensitivity disorders**

*Multisystem*
  Anaphylaxis
  Serum-sickness and serum sickness–like reactions
  Drug fever
  Hypersensitivity syndrome
  Vasculitis
  Lupus erythematosus–like syndrome
  Generalized lymphadenopathy

*Skin*
  Urticaria/angioedema
  Stevens-Johnson syndrome
  Toxic epidermal necrolysis
  Fixed drug eruption
  Maculopapular or morbilliform rashes
  Contact dermatitis
  Photosensitivity
  Erythema nodosum

*Bone marrow*
  Hemolytic anemia
  Thrombocytopenia
  Neutropenia
  Aplastic anemia
  Eosinophilia

*Lung*
  Bronchospasm
  Pneumonitis
  Pulmonary edema
  Pulmonary infiltrates with eosinophilia

*Kidney*
  Interstitial nephritis
  Nephrotic syndrome

*Liver*
  Hepatitis
  Cholestasis

*Heart*
  Myocarditis

Table 1
Classification of adverse drug reactions

| Reactions | Example Drug | Result |
|---|---|---|
| Predictable[a] | | |
| Overdosage | Acetaminophen | Hepatic necrosis |
| Side effect | Albuterol | Tremor |
| Secondary effect | Clindamycin | *Clostridium difficile* pseudomembranous colitis |
| Drug–drug interaction | Terfenadine/erythromycin | Torsade de pointes arrhythmia |
| Unpredictable[b] | | |
| Intolerance | Aspirin | Tinnitus (at usual doses) |
| Idiosyncratic | Chloroquine | Hemolytic anemia in G6PD-deficient patient |
| Allergic | Penicillin | Anaphylaxis |
| Pseudoallergic | Radiocontrast material | Anaphylactiod reaction |

[a] Predictable, or type A, reactions occur in otherwise normal patients, are generally dose-dependent, and related to the known pharmacologic actions of the drug.

[b] Unpredictable, or type B, reactions occur only in susceptible individuals, are dose-independent, and not related to the pharmacologic actions of the drug.

known pharmacologic actions of the drug, and occur in otherwise normal patients. Unpredictable reactions are usually dose-independent, are unrelated to the pharmacologic actions of the drug, and occur only in susceptible individuals. Although predictable reactions make up approximately 80% of all ADRs, most serious and life-threatening reactions fall into the unpredictable category.

Allergic (ie, hypersensitivity) drug reactions are distinguished from other unpredictable reactions in that they are mediated by a specific immune mechanism. No single classification scheme is able to account for all allergic drug reactions. The widely used Gell and Coombs classification scheme of type 1 to type 4 hypersensitivity reactions [9] may be applied to some drug-induced allergic reactions (Table 2). Certain reactions cannot be categorized into any classification scheme despite our insight into their

Table 2
Gell and Coombs classification scheme for allergic reactions

| Reaction Type | Mechansim | Drug | Result |
|---|---|---|---|
| I | IgE antibodies leading to mast-cell/basophil degranulation | Penicillin | Anaphylaxis |
| II | IgG/IgM-mediated cytotoxic reaction against cell surface | Quinidine | Hemolytic anemia |
| III | Immune complex reaction | Cephalexin | Serum sickness |
| IV | Delayed T lymphocyte–mediated reaction | Neomycin | Contact dermatitis |

underlying mechanism. In other instances, reactions cannot be classified because the mechanism of their elicitation is not understood.

Most medications, because of their small size, are unable to elicit an immune response independently. Drugs must first covalently bind to larger carrier molecules such as tissue or serum proteins to act as complete multivalent antigens. This process is called haptenation, and the drugs act as haptens [10]. The elicited immune response may be humoral, with the production of specific antibodies, cellular, with the generation of specific T lymphocytes, or both.

Most drugs are chemically inert in their native state and must be enzymatically metabolized to chemically reactive intermediates to form covalent bonds with macromolecules [10]. A notable exception is penicillin, which spontaneously degrades under physiologic conditions to reactive intermediates capable of binding to proteins [11]. Although the immunochemistry of the intermediates is well characterized in the case of penicillin, frequently, the identity of the metabolites is unknown, making it impossible to develop accurate diagnostic tests for drug allergy.

## Drug allergy history

A thorough history is an essential component of the evaluation of patients with suspected drug allergies. The history helps guide the clinician in the choice of diagnostic tests and the decision whether it is safe to reintroduce the medication. If possible, the original medical record that describes the drug reaction should be reviewed. Typically, years or decades have passed since reactions occurred, and, as a result, these records are usually unavailable at the time of consultation. However, for inpatients who experienced recent reactions while hospitalized, the chart notes should be available. The most important components of a drug allergy history are as follows:

- What is the name of the medication? Although it may be obvious that a drug allergy history starts with the name of the implicated medication, frequently patients are unable to give this basic piece of information. This problem may be due to the reaction's being distant in time, to the similar-sounding names of many medications, or, in the case of patients with a history of multiple drug reactions, to the inability to say with certainty which drug caused which reaction.
- How long ago did the reaction occur? The time elapsed since the reaction is important, because some allergies, such as penicillin allergy, are known to wane over time.
- Which systems (eg, cutaneous, respiratory, gastrointestinal) were involved in the reaction, and what were the exact characteristics? If a cutaneous eruption occurred, what kind was it? Urticarial, morbilliform, bullous, exfoliative? Showing the patient pictures of different types of rashes may be helpful.

- When during the course did the reaction occur? Alternatively, did the onset of symptoms follow completion of the course? Occasionally, patients blame a medication for symptoms that began days after a course was completed, which are highly unlikely to be drug related.
- Why was the medication prescribed? The indication is important because symptoms of the underlying disease may be misattributed to the medication. For example, a truncal rash related to strep pharyngitis may be blamed on penicillin. Similarly, some patients claim an allergy to oral diphenhydramine because it exacerbated their urticaria, or to sulfonamide ocular drops because the medication worsened their ocular discharge.
- Was the patient taking concurrent medications at the time of the reaction? Antibiotics are usually first to be blamed for a reaction, but other medications, such as narcotics or NSAIDs, are frequently coadministered and may be responsible.
- What was the therapeutic management required secondary to the reaction? Self-discontinuation of a medication by a patient suggests a reaction of different severity from a patient's requiring hospitalization. Interestingly, some patients recall treatment they received more readily than the characteristics of the reaction itself, and this can give the clinician a clue as to the type of reaction.
- Had the patient taken the same or a cross-reacting medication before the reaction? Truly allergic reactions require a period of sensitization, typically during a previous course that was tolerated.
- Has the patient been exposed to the same or similar medication since the reaction? For instance, some patients who report a penicillin allergy later tolerate a course of amoxicillin clavulanate, not realizing the latter is a penicillin-class compound.
- Has the patient experienced symptoms similar to his or her reaction in the absence of drug treatment? The most common such situation is chronic recurrent idiopathic urticaria, which may be confused with drug allergy.
- Does the patient have an underlying condition that favors reactions to certain medications? Examples of such conditions include ampicillin-induced morbilliform rash in patients with mononucleosis and trimethoprim/sulfamethoxazole reactions in patients infected with HIV.

**Evaluation and management**

*Antibiotics*

*Penicillins*

Penicillin is the most prevalent medication allergy, with approximately 10% of patients reporting being penicillin-allergic [11]. However, when patients with a history of penicillin allergy are evaluated, more than 90% of them are found not to be allergic and are able to tolerate the drug [12,13]. The discrepancy between *claimed* and *real* penicillin allergies probably results from several factors. The reaction may have been predictable or due to the underlying illness and hence may have been mislabeled as allergic from the onset. Another contributor to the discrepancy is the tendency of patients with a type 1 penicillin allergy to lose penicillin-specific IgE antibodies over time. Patients labeled penicillin-allergic are more likely to be treated with more expensive and broad-spectrum antibiotics [14,15], a practice that leads to the development and spread of multiple drug-resistant bacteria and higher direct and indirect health care costs.

Under physiologic conditions, penicillin spontaneously degrades to a number of reactive intermediates that act as haptens and covalently bind to self-proteins, which then may elicit an immune response [16–18]. Approximately 95% of penicillin degrades to the penicilloyl moiety, which is referred to as the major antigenic determinant (Fig. 1). The remaining portion of penicillin degrades to several derivatives; of these, penicilloate and penilloate are the most important in inducing allergic responses. These two compounds, along with penicillin itself, are collectively known as the minor antigenic determinants, and they cover all clinically relevant allergenic determinants not covered by penicilloyl. Less commonly, the R-group side chain, which distinguishes different penicillin compounds, may also serve as an allergenic determinant (see Fig. 1). Descriptions exist of patients who selectively react to a particular semisynthetic penicillin yet are able to tolerate other penicillins [19,20]. These individuals presumably form IgE antibodies directed against the R-group side chain, rather than the core beta-lactam portion of the molecule.

Insight into the immunochemistry of penicillin has allowed for the development of validated skin-test reagents to detect penicillin-specific IgE

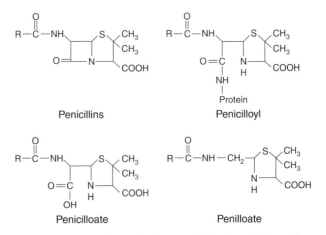

Fig. 1. Structures of major and minor penicillin allergenic determinants.

antibodies (Table 3). The major determinant, penicilloyl-polylysine, became commercially available in the United States as Pre-Pen in 1974, but its production was discontinued in the fall of 2004. It is highly probable that Pre-Pen will become commercially available from a different manufacturer at some time in 2005 or 2006; therefore, this discussion assumes that clinicians have access to this important reagent. Without Pre-Pen, accurate diagnosis of type 1 penicillin allergy is impossible, because the vast majority of penicillin-allergic patients react to the major determinant. Of the minor determinants, only penicillin G is commercially available. Penicilloate and penilloate are synthesized by some medical centers for local use, and allergists may have access to them. It is hoped that all penicillin minor determinants will become commercially available, along with Pre-Pen, in the near future. For patients who have reacted to a semisynthetic penicillin, the skin testing panel should also include a nonirritating concentration of that compound, in addition to the major and minor penicillin determinants.

The penicillin skin test procedure is analogous to other immediate-type allergy skin testing [21]. Appropriate positive and negative controls should be used. Tests are read 15 to 20 minutes after application, and a positive response is defined by the size of the wheal, which should be 3 mm or greater than that of the negative control [22]. Penicillin skin testing should only be performed by trained personnel in a setting prepared to treat possible allergic reactions. Epicutaneous testing should be performed first, and, if it is negative, intradermal tests should follow. When a standard protocol is followed, the safety of penicillin skin testing is comparable to that of other types of allergy testing, and it only rarely results in systemic reactions [13,23–25].

Because an accurate diagnosis of penicillin allergy cannot be made clinically, any patient with a history of a possible IgE-mediated reaction to penicillin is a candidate for skin testing. One cannot rely on the history to make the diagnosis, because approximately one third of patients with positive skin tests have vague reaction histories [26]. Additionally, patients with an unequivocal history of penicillin-induced anaphylaxis may be able to tolerate penicillin, because approximately 80% of such individuals lose their sensitivity over a period of 10 years [11]. Patients with a clear history of serious

Table 3
Commonly used penicillin skin test reagents

| Reagent | Concentration |
| --- | --- |
| Penicilloyl-polylysine (Pre-Pen)[a] | $6 \times 10^{-5}$ mol/L |
| Penicillin G | 10,000 U/mL |
| Penicilloate[a] | 0.01 mol/L |
| Penilloate[a] | 0.01 mol/L |
| Ampicillin/amoxicillin | 1–20 mg/mL |

[a] At the time or this writing, Pre-Pen, penicilloate, and penilloate were commercially unavailable. It is, however, anticipated they will become available in the near future.

non–IgE-mediated penicillin reactions, such as Stevens-Johnson syndrome, toxic epidermal necrolysis, or interstitial nephritis, should not undergo skin testing.

Ideally, patients should undergo penicillin skin testing electively, when they are well and not in immediate need of antibiotic treatment. Patients need not have an absolute need to be treated with a penicillin-class compound to undergo skin testing. In present-day medical practice, situations in which penicillin is the drug of choice and no acceptable alternatives exist are rare. However, a negative result on penicillin skin testing in 90% of patients with a history of penicillin allergy allows these patients to avoid treatment with broad-spectrum, and typically more expensive and toxic, antibiotics. Efforts to implement penicillin skin testing have demonstrated decreased use of broad-spectrum antibiotics and were found to be cost-effective [27–30]. A notable example is the use of vancomycin in hospitalized patients, which is associated with development of drug-resistant bacteria [31,32] and has a less favorable side effect profile than do beta-lactam antibiotics. Surveys have shown that between one third and one half of inpatients are treated with vancomycin solely because of a history of penicillin allergy [15,33,34]. At the Mayo Clinic, when penicillin skin testing was incorporated into the preoperative evaluation of surgical patients with a history of penicillin allergy, there was a 10-fold decrease in the use of vancomycin in these patients [29,35].

The negative predictive value of penicillin skin testing is extremely high. When appropriate major and minor determinants are used, a negative skin test essentially rules out the potential for a serious immediate-type reaction. In large-scale studies, 1% to 3% of skin test–negative patients developed mild and self-limiting reactions on being challenged with the drug [12,13,23,36]. As mentioned previously, until recently, commercial availability was limited to Pre-Pen and penicillin G, excluding other minor determinants (penicilloate and penilloate). Controversy exists as to how many truly allergic patients are missed when one tests only with Pre-Pen and penicillin G, but this value is probably at most 1% to 2% of all comers who present with a history of penicillin allergy [11]. Therefore, in cases where patients test negative to Pre-Pen and penicillin G (and other minor determinants are unavailable), some experts recommend a cautious initial administration of penicillin (ie, 0.01 of the therapeutic dose followed by the full dose, assuming no reaction occurs during a brief observation period) [22].

Although penicillin skin testing has excellent negative predictive value, in the real world practice setting, many skin test–negative patients still do not receive treatment with penicillins [37,38]. In some cases, patients are unwilling to trust a negative skin test result. Additionally, prescribing physicians may be unaware of the high negative predictive value of penicillin skin testing, or they may be fearful of legal consequences if the patient has a reaction. To alleviate everyone's apprehension and prove the medication's safety unequivocally, most experts (including this author) recommend that, following a negative skin test, an elective oral challenge (with the same antibiotic implicated in the previous reaction) be performed.

Penicillin resensitization is defined as redevelopment of penicillin allergy in patients who have lost their sensitivity. When penicillin skin testing first came into clinical use 3 decades ago, it was assumed (without supporting data) that the risk of resensitization was high. As a result, penicillin skin testing was routinely repeated before each course of the antibiotic in patients with a history of penicillin allergy [39]. Also, because of a presumed risk of resensitization, elective penicillin skin testing was discouraged [39]. Studies of penicillin resensitization after oral penicillin have shown resensitization rates of 0% to 3% [36,40–42], which is comparable to the rate of sensitization. Typically, the resensitization rate in these studies was based on the number of patients who converted their skin tests from negative (before the challenge) to positive (after the challenge). The study by Solensky and colleagues [42] is the only one to evaluate resensitization after repeated courses of penicillin. Patients with a convincing history of penicillin allergy and initially negative penicillin skin tests were challenged with three separate courses of penicillin and underwent three repeat penicillin skin tests; none converted to a positive skin test [42]. Based on these data, it is not necessary routinely to re–skin test patients with a history of penicillin allergy whose results are found to be negative on penicillin skin testing. Resensitization following parenteral administration of penicillin appears to be more likely—rates of 0% to 20% have been reported—but these data are from smaller-scale studies [43–45]. Pending additional research, patients with a history of penicillin allergy who have tolerated a parenteral course of penicillin should have skin testing repeated before receiving the drug again.

*Cephalosporins*

Cephalosporins share a common four-member beta-lactam ring with penicillin, whereas the five-member thiazolidine ring is replaced by a six-member dihydrothiazine ring (Fig. 2). Cephalosporins appear to be less allergenic than penicillins, particularly in causing IgE-mediated reactions. The incidence of anaphylaxis as a reaction to cephalosporins [46] is about an order of magnitude lower than it is to penicillin [47–49]. Diagnosis of IgE-mediated allergy to cephalosporins is limited by a lack of insight into the relevant immunogenic determinants that are produced by the process of degradation. Unlike penicillin, cephalosporin has no validated diagnostic skin test reagents available. Skin testing using nonirritating concentrations of native cephalosporins has been performed, but its predictive value is unknown. A positive skin test response using a nonirritating concentration of native cephalosporins is suggestive of IgE-mediated allergy, but, importantly, a negative result does not rule out sensitivity. A recent study of nonallergic subjects found that intravenous formulations of cephalosporins were nonirritating for intradermal skin testing at 10-fold dilution from full strength [50].

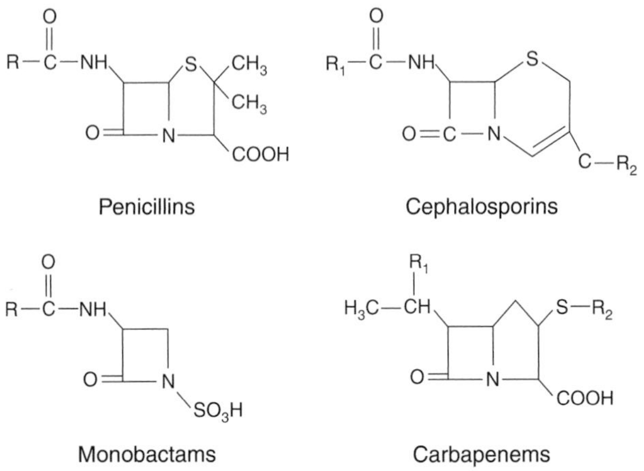

Fig. 2. Structures of beta-lactam antibiotics.

Although cephalosporin allergenic determinants are unknown, it is believed that immune responses to these drugs are directed toward R-group side chains rather than the core portion of the molecule (see Fig. 2). Case reports exist of patients who are proved by challenge to be allergic to a particular cephalosporin and are able to tolerate others [51–54]. Based on these data and clinical experience, it is generally believed that patients with a history of cephalosporin allergy may safely receive other cephalosporins that have dissimilar side chains [22]. Because this recommendation is not based on extensive clinical trials of cephalosporin-allergic patients, this author suggests that the cephalosporin initially be given cautiously by means of graded challenge (to be discussed later in this article).

*Penicillin/cephalosporin cross-reactivity*

Penicillins and cephalosporins have a potential for allergic cross-reactivity due to the common beta-lactam ring or, possibly, to identical R-group side chains. In vitro studies in both animals and humans have shown a high degree (ie, up to 50%) of immunologic cross-reactivity between these compounds [55,56]. Although clinical cross-reactivity occurs much less frequently, the exact incidence is still a topic of controversy. After cephalosporins were introduced to clinical use in the 1960s, a number of case reports of reactions to them in patients with a history of penicillin allergy appeared in the literature [57–60]. These publications, however, are subject to several limitations and confounders. The patients were not proved to be penicillin-allergic at the time of their cephalosporin reactions, either by penicillin skin testing or by oral challenge. Initial cephalosporin preparations contained trace amounts of penicillin [61], which could have been the actual cause of the patients' reactions. Most first-generation cephalosporins implicated in these reactions have similar (although not identical) R-group side chains to benzylpenicillin, and this factor (rather than the beta-lactam portion) may have led to the cross-reactivity. Finally, it is known that patients who are allergic to one medication are more likely to react to other non–cross-reacting drugs; this is a condition called multiple drug allergy syndrome [62,63]. Hence, the cephalosporin reactions may have been due to de novo cephalosporin hypersensitivity in patients who are generally prone to react to drugs, rather than to cross-reactivity.

According to retrospective studies performed in the 1970s, cephalosporin reaction rates in patients with a history of penicillin allergy were approximately 8%, compared with 1% to 2% in patients without a history of penicillin allergy [64,65]. The authors did not describe the types of reactions the patients experienced. Two recent publications employing similar retrospective protocols did not confirm these findings [66,67]. Collectively, out of 1089 patients with a history of penicillin allergy, only two developed mild reactions while being treated with mostly parenteral cephalosporins [66,67]. The major weakness of retrospective studies is a lack of confirmation of penicillin allergy by skin testing, because it is likely that the vast majority of these patients lack penicillin-specific IgE antibodies. This author has reviewed the published literature and found reports of more than 300 penicillin skin test–positive patients who have been challenged with a variety of cephalosporins [11]. The overall reaction rate is approximately 3%, which is comparable to the rate observed in patients without a history of penicillin allergy. Moreover, in virtually all reported positive cephalosporin challenges, the implicated cephalosporin shares a similar R-group side chain with benzylpenicillin. These findings suggest that the occasional observed cross-reactivity may be due to the side chain rather than to the core beta-lactam portion of the molecules. In fact, there are case reports of patients who react to amoxicillin and cefadroxil (which share an identical side chain) but not to other beta-lactams [68,69].

Although it is not clear why a small proportion of patients with a history of penicillin allergy react to cephalosporins, the drug allergy practice parameter recognizes this phenomenon and recommends penicillin skin testing in patients with a history of penicillin allergy who require treatment with cephalosporins [22]. Fig. 3 summarizes the approach to patients who have a history of penicillin allergy and are to be treated with cephalosporins.

*Monobactams*

Monobactams are a newer family of beta-lactam antibiotics that contain a monocyclic ring structure, in contrast to the other, bicyclic core beta-lactams (see Fig. 2). Aztreonam is the only clinically available monobactam antibiotic. Aztreonam is less immunogenic than penicillin and cephalosporins [70], and clinical experience confirms that allergic reactions to aztreonam are uncommon. Evaluation of possible type 1 allergy to aztreonam is analogous to that of cephalosporins, in that relevant allergenic degradation products are unknown; hence no standardized skin test reagents are available. Skin

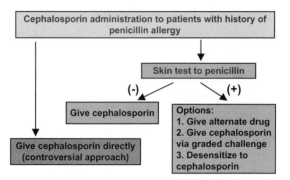

Fig. 3. Algorithm for administration of cephalosporins to patients with a history of penicillin allergy. (*Adapted from* Bernstein IL, Gruchalla RS, Lee RE, et al. Disease management of drug hypersensitivity: a practice parameter. Ann Allergy Asthma Immunol 1999;83:687; with permission.)

testing with a nonirritating concentration of native aztreonam has the same limitation and questionable predictive value as in the case of cephalosporins.

Fortunately, the allergic cross-reactivity between aztreonam and other beta-lactams has been determined. In vitro, skin test, and patient challenge studies have consistently shown no cross-reactivity between penicillin and aztreonam [71–76]. Likewise, no cross-reactivity has been demonstrated between cephalosporins and aztreonam, except in the case of ceftazidime, which shares an identical R-group side chain with aztreonam [70,73,77]. Therefore, penicillin- and cephalosporin-allergic patients may safely receive aztreonam, with the exception of patients who are allergic to ceftazidime. Conversely, aztreonam-allergic patients may be treated with all beta-lactams except for ceftazidime [78].

*Carbapenems*

Imipenem is the prototype agent in this newest class of beta-lactams that contain a bicyclic nucleus similar to penicillin (see Fig. 2). As in the case of other nonpenicillin beta-lactams, lack of knowledge of the relevant immunogenic breakdown products limits evaluation of possible carbapenem-induced type 1 allergy to skin testing with the native antibiotic. Limited data exist on potential allergic cross-reactivity between carbapenems and other beta-lactams. Retrospective chart review–type studies of inpatients with a history of penicillin allergy who received carbapenems show that 6% to 8% experienced allergic reactions [79,80]; however, no patients underwent penicillin skin testing. Among skin test–proven penicillin-allergic patients, 50% also showed skin test reactivity to imipenem, but none was challenged with the drug [81]. No published reports exist of carbapenem challenges of penicillin skin test–positive patients.

Ideally, the approach to a patient who requires treatment with a carbapenem-class antibiotic should include penicillin skin testing. Skin test–negative patients may be safely treated with carbapenems as well as with all other beta-lactams. Skin test–positive patients should receive carbapenems by means of desensitization. If penicillin skin testing is not available, patients with a history of penicillin allergy should receive carbapenems by means of graded challenge or desensitization, depending on the type of reaction history.

*Sulfonamides*

Sulfonamides are defined as compounds that contain an $SO_2NH_2$ moiety. Sulfonamide antibiotics differ from other sulfonamides in that they also contain an aromatic amine (arylamine) group at the N4 position and a substituted ring at the N1 position (Fig. 4). This difference is important when considering the potential cross-reactivity between sulfonamide antibiotics and nonantibiotic sulfonamides. The presence of the N4 arylamine group and particular types of substituted ring at the N1 position has been found to be critical for the development of various types of sulfonamide allergic reaction [82–84]. Therefore, on theoretic grounds, one would not expect allergic cross-reactivity between sulfonamide antibiotics and other sulfonamides. Recent data support an absence of clinical cross-reactivity in patients allergic to sulfonamide antibiotics who are treated with nonantimicrobial sulfonamides [85–88].

Although sulfonamide antibiotics (referred to as sulfonamides from here on) have been associated with virtually every drug hypersensitivity disorder listed in Box 1, by far the most common reactions are delayed maculopapular and morbilliform eruptions [84]. Patients who are infected with HIV are at greatly increased risk for cutaneous reactions with sulfonamides [89]. For instance, although the incidence of skin rash reactions to trimethoprim/sulfamethoxazole (TMP-SMX) in normal individuals is 3.3% [90], reaction rates of 40% to 80% have been reported in patients who have HIV [89].

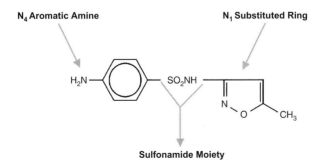

Fig. 4. Structure of sulfamethoxazole—the prototype sulfonamide antibiotic. Nonantibiotic sulfonamides lack an N4 aromatic amine group and N1 substituted ring, which are important for allergic reactions to sulfonamide antibiotics.

The remainder of this section focuses on the pathogenesis, evaluation, and management of TMP-SMX reactions in HIV-positive patients.

The typical reaction to TMP-SMX in HIV-positive patients consists of a generalized maculopapular eruption that occurs during the second week of treatment and is usually accompanied by pruritus and fever. These reactions are not caused by TMP-SMX–specific IgE or IgG antibodies [91]. Rather, the delayed onset is suggestive of a T-cell–mediated mechanism, although this has not been established definitively. Several possible explanations exist for the increased risk of HIV-positive patients reacting to sulfonamides. First, slow acetylation may cause more of the parent drug to be shunted toward the oxidative cytochrome P450 pathway, with subsequent formation of reactive hydroxylamine and nitroso metabolites (Fig. 5); these are responsible for most adverse reactions to sulfonamides. Second, a relative deficiency of glutathione or other scavengers would have a similar effect, resulting in an excess of reactive intermediates. Third, viral or other opportunistic infections may stimulate the activity of cytochrome P450 enzymes and lead to an increased rate of oxidation and production of reactive metabolites. Finally, viral infections are known to stimulate production of interferon-γ, which leads to increased expression of major histocompatibility complex (MHC) class I and class II cell surface molecules, including those on keratinocytes. This process would result in a condition favorable

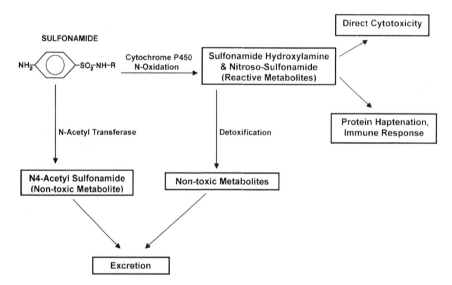

Fig. 5. Sulfonamide metabolic pathways. N-acetylation yields nontoxic metabolites that are excreted. N-oxidation forms reactive intermediates that may cause direct cytotoxicity or haptenate proteins and lead to an immunologic response. Glutathione reduces reactive metabolites to nontoxic products that are excreted. (*From* Solensky R. Drug desensitization. Immunol Allergy Clin N Am 2004;24:438; with permission.)

for the presentation of processed drug antigens on MHC molecules to drug-specific $CD4^+$ and $CD8^+$ T cells, resulting in delayed skin rashes. The pathogenesis of TMP-SMX reactions in HIV-positive patients is probably multifactorial, and limited data suggest that all these elements play some role in the process [84,89,91,92].

Clinicians are frequently confronted with HIV-positive patients who require treatment with TMP-SMX, because it is the drug of choice for prophylaxis and treatment of *Pneumocystis carinii* pneumonia and other potentially life-threatening opportunistic infections [93]. Over the last 2 decades, numerous protocols have been devised in an attempt to administer TMP-SMX safely to HIV-positive patients who have a history of previous reactions to the antibiotic [94]. The term *desensitization* is commonly used to describe these procedures, but it is imprecise, because IgE antibodies are not implicated in these reactions. All the protocols start with a low, subtherapeutic dose of TMP-SMX, which is incrementally increased until the full dose is reached. However, the study designs vary greatly in such aspects as the starting dose, the time interval between doses, the extent of increase between doses, and the total duration of the desensitization. The reported desensitization success rates range from 60% to 100%, but the lack of consistency among the protocols regarding premedication and the question of whether to treat through reactions makes comparison impossible [94]. Without any comparative trials, it appears that clinicians may employ a number of different TMP-SMX desensitization protocols with similar hopes for success and safety [94]. Importantly, these protocols should only be used in HIV-positive patients with a history of the typical delayed reactions described earlier. They are not intended for patients with a history of other delayed serious reactions, such as Stevens-Johnson syndrome or toxic epidermal necrolysis, or for patients with type 1 reactions (these individuals should undergo rapid desensitization, as discussed later in this article).

## Other drugs

### Aspirin and nonsteroidal anti-inflammatory drugs

Unpredictable adverse reactions to aspirin (ASA) and NSAIDs fall into several major categories (Table 4). Respiratory reactions occur in patients with underlying asthma, nonallergic rhinitis, and, frequently, nasal polyposis. The preferred term for this disorder is aspirin-exacerbated respiratory disease (AERD) [95]. The reactions typically involve the entire respiratory tract, with symptoms of rhinitis, conjunctivitis, and bronchospasm, but some patients experience solely upper or solely lower respiratory tract reactions. It is estimated that approximately 5% to 10% of adult asthmatics have AERD, whereas the prevalence increases to about a third in adult patients who have asthma and nasal polyposis [96]. AERD is rare in prepubescent children. The pathogenesis of AERD is partially understood and involves aberrant arachidonic acid metabolism, in that patients are

Table 4
Unpredictable adverse reactions to aspirin, nonsteroidal anti-inflammatory drugs, and selective cyclo-oxygenase-2 inhibitors

| Reaction type | Underlying disease | Drugs involved | Cross-reaction | Mechanism |
|---|---|---|---|---|
| Respiratory | Rhinitis, polyps, asthma | ASA, NSAIDs | All except COX-2 | COX-1 inhibition |
| Multiple-drug urticaria/ andioedema | Chronic urticaria | ASA, NSAIDs | All except COX-2 | COX-1 inhibition |
| Single-drug urticaria/ andioedema | None | ASA, NSAIDs, COX-2 | None | IgE (probable) |
| Anaphylaxis | None | ASA, NSAIDs, COX-2 | None | IgE (probable) |
| Aseptic meningitis | None | NSAIDs | None | T cell (probable) |
| Hypersensitivity pneumonitis | None | NSAIDs | None | T cell (probable) |

*Modified from* Stevenson DD. Adverse reactions to nonsteroidal anti-inflammatory drugs. Immunol Allergy Clin North Am 1998;18:775.

exquisitely susceptible to inhibition of cyclo-oxygenase by ASA. Patients who have AERD exhibit cross-reactivity with all NSAIDs, but they can tolerate cyclo-oxygenase 2 enzyme (COX-2) selective inhibitors [97,98]. No in vitro tests to detect ASA sensitivity exist, and oral challenge remains the gold standard diagnostic test for AERD [96].

ASA desensitization refers to the induction of a state of tolerance in which patients who have AERD are able to take ASA and other NSAIDs without experiencing adverse sequelae. This procedure is not intended for patients with other types of reactions to ASA and NSAIDs. It is another example of imprecise use of the term *desensitization*, because IgE antibodies are not involved in AERD. The goal of ASA desensitization is cautiously to induce a reaction following which the patient becomes refractory to the deleterious effects of ASA/NSAIDs for 2 to 5 days [99,100]. To maintain the patient in a refractory state indefinitely, ASA must be continually administered on a daily basis. ASA desensitization should be performed only by clinicians familiar with the procedure, in a controlled clinical setting with intravenous access and readiness to treat potentially severe bronchospastic reactions. For further details of the ASA desensitization procedure, the reader is referred to recent reviews of this topic [99,100].

Patients selected for ASA desensitization fall into two categories. First, there are patients with AERD whose respiratory disease is well controlled but who require ASA or NSAIDs for other indications, such as cardiac prophylaxis or treatment of arthritis. Because of the introduction of newer platelet inhibitors (such as clopidogrel) and COX-2 inhibitors, which patients who have AERD are able to tolerate, this indication is not encountered as frequently as it was in the past. Second, ASA desensitization should be considered for patients with AERD who have poor control of their disease despite use of topical corticosteroids and leukotriene-modifying drugs and for patients who require chronic treatment with systemic corticosteroids. Several long-term studies of patients maintained on chronic ASA desensitization demonstrated improved clinical courses [101–103]. For upper respiratory disease, long-term ASA desensitization was associated with significant improvements in nasal symptom scores, frequency of sinusitis, need for polypectomies or sinus surgeries, sense of smell, and dose of intranasal corticosteroids [101–103]. For lower respiratory disease, improved clinical outcomes included reductions in asthma symptom scores, hospitalizations, emergency room visits, and dose of inhaled corticosteroids [101–103]. ASA desensitization also resulted in a reduction in the number of bursts of oral corticosteroids and allowed patients on chronic corticosteroids to decrease their dose [101–103].

Other unpredictable reactions to ASA/NSAIDs are summarized in Table 4. Approximately one third of patients who have chronic idiopathic urticaria experience an exacerbation of their disease with ingestion of ASA/NSAIDs [100]. The reactions are thought to be related to COX-1 inhibition, and therefore cross-reactivity occurs among all NSAIDs. As one would expect, COX-2 selective inhibitors have been found to be safe in these patients [100].

Urticarial and anaphylactic reactions due to ASA/NSAIDs in patients without underlying chronic urticaria may be IgE-mediated [100]. This connection is sometimes difficult to prove, because the relevant metabolites to which IgE antibodies are formed are unknown. However, the clinical presentation is consistent with a type 1 mechanism in that there is generally a period of sensitization, during which patients tolerate the NSAID, before a reaction occurs. Because the mechanism is not COX-related, and NSAIDs vary greatly in their chemical structure, these reactions are medication-specific rather than class-specific [100]. Additionally, COX-2 selective inhibitors, as well as ASA and NSAIDs, have the potential to cause anaphylactic reactions [104–106]. Retrospective reviews of patients with drug-induced anaphylaxis have found that, aside from penicillin, ASA/NSAIDs are the most commonly implicated medications [107,108].

## Local anesthetics

True hypersensitivity reactions to local anesthetics are uncommon and usually consist of delayed contact dermatitis; anaphylaxis from local anesthetics occurs rarely if ever [109]. Most adverse reactions are vasovagal, psychogenic, toxic, or predictable side effects of the epinephrine that is often used in combination with local anesthetics. Another possible but rare cause of immediate-type reactions is preservatives, such as methylparaben, that are present in multidose vials [109]. Large-scale studies have found that, following full evaluation, virtually all patients with a history of allergy to local anesthetics are able to tolerate these drugs [110–112].

Unfortunately, patients who experience any adverse reaction to local anesthetics are frequently labeled *allergic* and told to avoid all "-caines" in the future. Because evaluation of these patients invariably finds them able to receive a local anesthetic, such evaluation prevents them from being subjected to the increased risk of general anesthesia or, alternatively, to pain from the absence of anesthesia. Evaluation of patients with a supposed allergy to local anesthetics is also important because it serves to alleviate dentists' or physicians' legal (ie, malpractice-related) concerns regarding use of a drug to which a patient is listed as being allergic. Fig. 6 summarizes the approach to patients with previous reactions to local anesthetics. It involves skin testing followed by an incremental dose challenge with the local anesthetic. Data from patch testing suggest that there is cross-reactivity among the benzoate esters but not among the amides (Table 5). Although these findings may have no significance for immediate-type reactions, it is generally recommended that, when a patient has previously reacted to an ester, an amide should be used in evaluation for readministration. If the identity of the previous local anesthetic is unknown, or if it was an amide, another amide may be used. During skin testing and challenge, one should attempt to employ the same agent that will subsequently be used by the dentist or physician.

## Rapid desensitization

Rapid desensitization to a drug should be considered in patients who have an IgE-mediated allergy to a medication when no acceptable

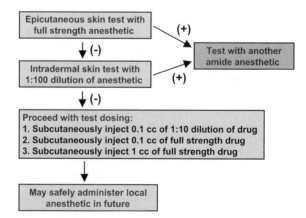

Fig. 6. Management of patients with previous reactions to local anesthetics. Intervals between steps are 15 minutes. (*Data from* Patterson R, DeSwarte RD, Greenberger PA, et al. Drug allergy and protocols for management of drug allergies. Allergy Proc 1994;15:239–64.)

Table 5
Benzoate esters and amides that comprise the two major classes of local anesthetics

| Generic name | Available forms | Examples of trade names |
| --- | --- | --- |
| Benzoate esters | | |
| Benzocaine | Topical | Orajel, Hurricane, Lanacaine, etc |
| Butamben picrate | Topical | Butesin |
| Chloroprocaine | Injectable | Nesacaine |
| Cocaine | Topical | Cocaine |
| Procaine | Injectable | Novocain |
| Proparacaine | Ophthalmic | Alcaine, Optheaine, Opthetic |
| Tetracaine | Injectable, topical, ophthalmic | Pontocaine |
| Amides | | |
| Bupivacaine | Injectable | Marcaine, Sensorcaine |
| Dibucaine | Topical | Nupercaine |
| Etidocaine | Injectable | Duranest, Durnest MPF |
| Lidocaine | Injectable, topical | Xylocaine, Dilocaine, Nervocaine, etc |
| Mepivacaine | Injectable | Carbocaine, Polocaine, Isocaine |
| Prilocaine | Injectable | Citanest |
| Ropivacaine | Injectable | Naropin |
| Combination | | |
| Lidocaine/Prilocaine | Topical | EMLA |

Patch testing data indicate there is cross-reactivity among the esters but not the amides.

alternative treatment is available. The aim of desensitization is to convert a patient who is highly allergic to a drug to a state in which he or she can tolerate treatment with the medication. Although most published desensitization protocols involve penicillin, the principle has been applied successfully to virtually all other classes of antibiotics, as well as to some chemotherapeutic agents [113–118]. Rapid desensitization somehow renders mast cells unresponsive to the drug used in the procedure, but the exact immunologic mechanism is not known [94]. Desensitization can be performed by oral, intravenous, or subcutaneous routes; when possible, the oral route is preferred, because it is thought to be safer than parenteral administration. Tables 6–8 list representative protocols for penicillin desensitization; these may be modified and used for other medications.

Several principles of management have been derived from studies of penicillin desensitization [119–122]; these are presumed to hold true for other drugs. First, the amount of the drug the patient tolerated during skin testing determines a safe initial dose for desensitization, which generally translates to 0.0001 or less of the full therapeutic dose. Second, doubling the dose every 15 minutes until the recommended dose is reached is effective in nearly all instances. Mild reactions occur in approximately a third of patients (typically during treatment after desensitization is completed), but no fatal or life-threatening reactions have been reported. Third, desensitization does not prevent the occurrence of non-IgE reactions, such as serum sickness,

Table 6
Penicillin oral desensitization protocol

| Step[a] | Penicillin (mg/mL) | Amount (mL) | Dose given (mg) | Cumulative dose (mg) |
|---|---|---|---|---|
| 1 | 0.5 | 0.1 | 0.05 | 0.05 |
| 2 | 0.5 | 0.2 | 0.1 | 0.15 |
| 3 | 0.5 | 0.4 | 0.2 | 0.35 |
| 4 | 0.5 | 0.8 | 0.4 | 0.75 |
| 5 | 0.5 | 1.6 | 0.8 | 1.55 |
| 6 | 0.5 | 3.2 | 1.6 | 3.15 |
| 7 | 0.5 | 6.4 | 3.2 | 6.35 |
| 8 | 5 | 1.2 | 6 | 12.35 |
| 9 | 5 | 2.4 | 12 | 24.35 |
| 10 | 5 | 5 | 25 | 49.35 |
| 11 | 50 | 1 | 50 | 100 |
| 12 | 50 | 2 | 100 | 200 |
| 13 | 50 | 4 | 200 | 400 |
| 14 | 50 | 8 | 400 | 800 |

Observe patient for 30 minutes, then give full therapeutic dose by the desired route.
[a] Interval between doses is 15 minutes.
*From* Sullivan TJ. Drug allergy. In: Middleton E, Reed CE, Ellis EF, et al, editors. Allergy: principles and practice. 4th edition. St. Louis (MO): Mosby; 1993. p. 1740.

hemolytic anemia, or interstitial nephritis. Fourth, in order for the patient to remain desensitized, it is necessary continually to administer the medication. In the case of penicillin, if treatment is discontinued for more than 48 hours, the patient is again at risk for developing anaphylaxis, and desensitization needs to be repeated.

Rapid desensitization should only be performed by a physician experienced in the procedure, in a hospital setting, with intravenous access and necessary medications and equipment to treat anaphylaxis. The hospital pharmacy staff may be consulted before the procedure to assist with preparation of the required drug dilutions. Patients should not be pretreated with corticosteroids or antihistamines, because they may mask early signs of an allergic reaction. If mild reactions do occur, they should be treated, and the dose should not be advanced until they have resolved.

## Graded challenge

Graded challenge, also known as test dosing, refers to cautious administration of a medication to a patient who is unlikely to be truly allergic to it. Unlike desensitization, graded challenge does not modify or attempt to fool the immune system into accepting a medication to which an allergy exists. Graded challenges are most commonly used in situations where diagnostic testing cannot sufficiently rule out an allergy, and the clinician has reason to believe the patient has a low likelihood of being allergic. One

Table 7
Penicillin intravenous desensitization protocol with drug added by piggyback infusion

| Step[a] | Penicillin (mg/mL) | Amount (mL) | Dose given (mg) | Cumulative dose (mg) |
|---|---|---|---|---|
| 1 | 0.1 | 0.1 | 0.01 | 0.01 |
| 2 | 0.1 | 0.2 | 0.02 | 0.03 |
| 3 | 0.1 | 0.4 | 0.04 | 0.07 |
| 4 | 0.1 | 0.8 | 0.08 | 0.15 |
| 5 | 0.1 | 1.6 | 0.16 | 0.31 |
| 6 | 1 | 0.32 | 0.32 | 0.63 |
| 7 | 1 | 0.64 | 0.64 | 1.27 |
| 8 | 1 | 1.2 | 1.2 | 2.47 |
| 9 | 10 | 0.24 | 2.4 | 4.87 |
| 10 | 10 | 0.48 | 4.8 | 10 |
| 11 | 10 | 1 | 10 | 20 |
| 12 | 10 | 2 | 20 | 40 |
| 13 | 100 | 0.4 | 40 | 80 |
| 14 | 100 | 0.8 | 80 | 160 |
| 15 | 100 | 1.6 | 160 | 320 |
| 16 | 1000 | 0.32 | 320 | 640 |
| 17 | 1000 | 0.64 | 640 | 1280 |

Observe patient for 30 minutes, then give full therapeutic dose by the desired route.
[a] Interval between doses is 15 minutes.
*From* Sullivan TJ. Drug allergy. In: Middleton E, Reed CE, Ellis EF, et al, editors. Allergy: principles and practice. 4th edition. St. Louis (MO): Mosby; 1993. p. 1741.

such example is that of patients who are positive on penicillin skin testing yet require treatment with cephalosporins. As outlined earlier, only about 3% of such patients react to cephalosporins; therefore, a reasonable approach is to administer the cephalosporin by means of graded challenge (Table 9). Another example is administration of a cephalosporin to a patient who previously reacted to another cephalosporin. Assuming the two cephalosporins do not contain identical R-group side chains, the cephalosporin may be given by graded challenge (Table 10). Patients with histories of severe non–IgE-mediated reactions (such as Stevens-Johnson syndrome, toxic epidermal necrolysis, and so on) are not candidates for graded challenge, because even small doses of the drug may induce severe progressive reactions.

Most graded challenges may be safely conducted in an office without intravenous access but with preparation to treat potential allergic reactions, including anaphylaxis. The pace of the challenge and the degree of caution exercised depend on the likelihood that the patient is allergic and on the physician's experience and comfort level with the procedure. Generally, the starting dose is 0.1 to 0.01 of the full dose, and approximately five-fold increasing doses are administered every 30 to 60 minutes until the full therapeutic dose is reached. At the first sign of any allergic reaction, the procedure should be abandoned, and the patient should be treated

Table 8
Penicillin intravenous desensitization protocol using a continuous infusion pump

| Step[a] | Penicillin (mg/mL) | Flow rate (mL/h) | Dose (mg) | Cumulative dose (mg) |
|---|---|---|---|---|
| 1 | 0.01 | 6 | 0.015 | 0.015 |
| 2 | 0.01 | 12 | 0.03 | 0.045 |
| 3 | 0.01 | 24 | 0.06 | 0.105 |
| 4 | 0.1 | 5 | 0.125 | 0.23 |
| 5 | 0.1 | 10 | 0.25 | 0.48 |
| 6 | 0.1 | 20 | 0.5 | 1 |
| 7 | 0.1 | 40 | 1 | 2 |
| 8 | 0.1 | 80 | 2 | 4 |
| 9 | 0.1 | 160 | 4 | 8 |
| 10 | 10 | 3 | 7.5 | 15 |
| 11 | 10 | 6 | 15 | 30 |
| 12 | 10 | 12 | 30 | 60 |
| 13 | 10 | 25 | 62.5 | 123 |
| 14 | 10 | 50 | 125 | 250 |
| 15 | 10 | 100 | 250 | 500 |
| 16 | 10 | 200 | 500 | 1000 |

Observe patient for 30 minutes, then give full therapeutic dose by the desired route.
[a] Interval between doses is 15 minutes.

appropriately. If the patient requires the medication at a later point, it should only be administered by means of formal desensitization.

## Summary

Allergic drug reactions compose a small percentage of ADRs, yet they are commonly encountered in clinical practice, and physicians are taught routinely to question patients about these reactions during history taking. Among antibiotics, the immunochemistry of penicillins has been elucidated, leading to the development of validated skin test reagents to diagnose type 1 allergy. Currently, the temporary commercial unavailability of Pre-Pen makes accurate penicillin skin testing impossible; however, this important skin test reagent is expected to become available sometime in 2006. Type 1 allergies to most other drugs lack comparable diagnostic tests, and their diagnosis is therefore driven by the patient's history. When readministration

Table 9
Example of graded challenge with oral cefuroxime using a commercially-available liquid suspension in penicillin skin test–positive patient

| Step[a] | Cefuroxime (mg/mL) | Amount (mL) | Dose (mg) |
|---|---|---|---|
| 1 | 25 | 0.2 | 5 |
| 2 | 50 | 5 | 250 |

[a] Interval between doses is 30 minutes. If an allergic reaction occurs, rapid desensitization should be performed.

Table 10
Example of graded challenge with oral cefdinir in patient with history of previous type-1 allergic reaction to cephalexin

| Step[a] | Cefdinir (mg/mL) | Amount (mL) | Dose (mg) |
|---|---|---|---|
| 1 | 25 | 0.1 | 2.5 |
| 2 | 25 | 1 | 25 |
| 3 | 25 | 10 | 250 |

[a] Interval between doses is 30 minutes. If an allergic reaction occurs, rapid desensitization should be performed.

of medications to which patients report previous reactions is indicated, it may be almost always successfully accomplished by means of either graded challenge or desensitization.

## References

[1] Lazarou J, Pomeranz BH, Corey PN. Incidence of adverse drug reactions in hospitalized patients: a meta-analysis of prospective studies. JAMA 1998;279:1200–5.
[2] Gandhi TK, Burstin HR, Cook EF, et al. Drug complications in outpatients. J Gen Intern Med 2000;15:149–54.
[3] Gandhi TK, Weingart SN, Borus J, et al. Adverse drug events in ambulatory care. N Engl J Med 2003;348:1556–64.
[4] DeSchazo RD, Kemp SF. Allergic reactions to drugs and biologic agents. JAMA 1997;278: 1895–906.
[5] Ditto AM, Greenberger PA, Grammer LC. Drug allergy. In: Grammer LC, Greenberger PA, editors. Patterson's allergic diseases. 6th edition. Philadelphia: Lippincott Williams & Wilkins; 2002. p. 295–387.
[6] Volcheck GW, Hagan JB, Li JT, editors. Drug hypersensitivity. Immunol Allergy Clin N Am 2004;24(3):345–549.
[7] World Health Organization. International drug monitoring: the role of the hospital. Geneva (Switzerland): World Health Organization; 1966.
[8] Rawlins MD, Thompson W. Mechanisms of adverse drug reactions. In: Davies DM, editor. Textbook of adverse drug reactions. New York: Oxford University Press; 1991. p. 18–45.
[9] Coombs RRA, Gell PGH. Classification of allergic reactions responsible for clinical hypersensitivity and disease. In: Gell PGH, Coombs RRA, Lachman PJ, editors. Clinical aspects of immunology. Oxford (UK): Blackwell Scientific; 1975. p. 761–81.
[10] Park BK, Coleman JW, Kitteringham NR. Drug disposition and drug hypersensitivity. Biochem Pharmacol 1987;36:581–90.
[11] Solensky R. Hypersensitivity reactions to beta-lactam antibiotics. Clin Rev Allergy Immunol 2003;24:201–19.
[12] Sogn DD, Evans R, Shepherd GM, et al. Results of the National Institute of Allergy and Infectious Diseases collaborative clinical trial to test the predictive value of skin testing with major and minor penicillin derivatives in hospitalized adults. Arch Intern Med 1992;152:1025–32.
[13] Gadde J, Spence M, Wheeler B, et al. Clinical experience with penicillin skin testing in a large inner-city STD clinic. JAMA 1993;270:2456–63.
[14] Lee CE, Zembower TR, Fotis MA, et al. The incidence of antimicrobial allergies in hospitalized patients: implications regarding prescribing patterns and emerging bacterial resistance. Arch Intern Med 2000;160:2819–22.

[15] Solensky R, Earl HS, Gruchalla RS. Clinical approach to penicillin allergic patients: a survey. Ann Allergy Asthma Immunol 2000;84:329–33.

[16] Parker CW, deWeck AL, Kern M, et al. The preparation and some properties of penicillenic acid derivatives relevant to penicillin hypersensitivity. J Exp Med 1962;115:803–19.

[17] Levine BB, Ovary Z. Studies on the mechanism of the formation of the penicillin antigen. III. The N-(D-alpha-benzyl-penicilloyl) group as an antigenic determinant responsible for hypersensitivity to penicillin G. J Exp Med 1961;114:875–904.

[18] Levine BB, Redmond AP. Minor haptenic determinant–specific reagins of penicillin hypersensitivity in man. Int Arch Allergy Appl Immunol 1969;35:445–55.

[19] Blanca M, Vega JM, Garcia J, et al. Allergy to penicillin with good tolerance to other penicillins: study of the incidence in subjects allergic to betalactams. Clin Exp Allergy 1990;20: 475–81.

[20] Vega JM, Blanca M, Garcia JJ, et al. Immediate allergic reactions to amoxicillin. Allergy 1994;49:317–22.

[21] Bernstein IL, Storms WW. Practice parameters for allergy diagnostic testing. Ann Allergy Asthma Immunol 1995;75:543–625.

[22] Bernstein IL, Gruchalla RS, Lee RE, et al. Disease management of drug hypersensitivity: a practice parameter. Ann Allergy Asthma Immunol 1999;83:665–700.

[23] Sullivan TJ, Wedner HJ, Shatz GS, et al. Skin testing to detect penicillin allergy. J Allergy Clin Immunol 1981;68:171–80.

[24] Valyasevi MA, VanDellen RG. Frequency of systematic reactions to penicillin skin tests. Ann Allergy Asthma Immunol 2000;85:363–5.

[25] Green GR, Rosenblum AH, Sweet LC. Evaluation of penicillin hypersensitivity: value of clinical history and skin testing with penicilloyl-polylysine and penicillin G. J Allergy Clin Immunol 1977;60:339–45.

[26] Solensky R, Earl HS, Gruchalla RS. Penicillin allergy: prevalence of vague history in skin test–positive patients. Ann Allergy Asthma Immunol 2000;85:195–9.

[27] Harris AD, Sauberman L, Kabbash L, et al. Penicillin skin testing: a way to optimize antibiotic utilization. Am J Med 1999;107:166–8.

[28] Forrest DM, Schellenberg RR, Thien VV, et al. Introduction of a practice guideline for penicillin skin testing improves the appropriateness of antibiotic therapy. Clin Infect Dis 2001; 32:1685–90.

[29] Li JT, Markus PJ, Osmon DR, et al. Reduction of vancomycin use in orthopedic patients with a history of antibiotic allergy. Mayo Clin Proc 2000;75:902–6.

[30] Arroliga ME, Radojicic C, Gordon SM, et al. A prospective observational study of the effect of penicillin skin testing on antibiotic use in the intensive care unit. Infect Control Hosp Epidemiol 2003;24:347–50.

[31] Fridkin SK, Edwards JR, Courval JM, et al. The effect of vancomycin and third-generation cephalosporins on prevalence of vancomycin-resistant enterococci in 126 US adult intensive care units. Ann Intern Med 2001;135:175–83.

[32] Martinez JA, Ruthazer R, Hansjosten K, et al. Role of environmental contamination as a risk factor for acquisition of vancomycin-resistant enterococci in patients treated in a medical intensive care unit. Arch Intern Med 2003;163:1905–12.

[33] Kwan T, Lin F, Ngai B, et al. Vancomycin use in 2 Ontario tertiary care hospitals: a survey. Clin Invest Med 1999;22:256–64.

[34] Cieslak PR, Strausbaugh LJ, Fleming DW, et al. Vancomycin in Oregon: who's using it and why. Infect Control Hosp Epidemiol 1999;20:557–60.

[35] Severson RJ, Pongdee T, Markus PJ, et al. Two-year review of clinical outcomes of antibiotic recommendations after consultation and penicillin allergy skin testing prior to orthopedic surgery [abstract]. Ann Allergy Asthma Immunol 2003;90:149.

[36] Mendelson LM, Ressler C, Rosen JP, et al. Routine elective penicillin allergy skin testing in children and adolescents: study of sensitization. J Allergy Clin Immunol 1984;73: 76–81.

[37] Warrington RJ, Burton R, Tsai E. The value of routine penicillin allergy skin testing in an outpatient population. Allergy Asthma Proc 2003;24:199–202.

[38] Warrington RJ, Lee KR, McPhillips S. The value of skin testing for penicillin allergy in an inpatient population: analysis of the subsequent patient management. Allergy Asthma Proc 2000;21:297–9.

[39] Parker CW. Practical aspects of diagnosis and treatment of patients who are hypersensitive to drugs. In: Samter M, Parker CW, editors. Hypersensitivity to drugs. New York: Pergamon Press; 1972. p. 367–94.

[40] Macy E, Mangat R, Burchette RJ. Penicillin skin testing in advance of need: multiyear follow-up in 568 test result–negative subjects exposed to oral penicillins. J Allergy Clin Immunol 2003;111:1111–5.

[41] Macy E. Elective penicillin skin testing and amoxicillin challenge: effect on outpatient use, cost, and clinical outcomes. J Allergy Clin Immunol 1998;102:281–5.

[42] Solensky R, Earl HS, Gruchalla RS. Lack of penicillin resensitization in patients with a history of penicillin allergy after receiving repeated penicillin courses. Arch Intern Med 2002; 162:822–6.

[43] Perencevich EN, Weller PF, Samore MH, et al. Benefits of negative penicillin skin test results persist during subsequent hospital admissions. Clin Infect Dis 2001;32:317–9.

[44] Parker PJ, Parrinello JT, Condemi JJ, et al. Penicillin resensitization among hospitalized patients. J Allergy Clin Immunol 1991;88:213–7.

[45] Lopez-Serrano MC, Caballero MT, Barranco P, et al. Booster responses in the study of allergic reactions to beta-lactam antibiotics. J Investig Allergol Clin Immunol 1996;6: 30–5.

[46] Lin RY. A perspective on penicillin allergy. Arch Intern Med 1992;152:930–7.

[47] International Rheumatic Fever Study Group. Allergic reactions to long-term benzathine penicillin prophylaxis for rheumatic fever. Lancet 1991;337:1308–10.

[48] Napoli DC, Neeno TA. Anaphylaxis to benzathine penicillin G. Pediatr Asthma Allergy Immunol 2000;14:329–32.

[49] Idsoe O, Guthe T, Willcox RR, et al. Nature and extent of penicillin side-reactions, with particular reference to fatalities from anaphylactic shock. Bull World Health Organ 1968;38:159–88.

[50] Empedrad R, Darter AL, Earl HS, et al. Nonirritating intradermal skin test concentrations for commonly prescribed antibiotics. J Allergy Clin Immunol 2003;112:629–30.

[51] Igea JM, Fraj J, Davila I, et al. Allergy to cefazolin: study of in vivo cross reactivity with other betalactams. Ann Allergy 1992;68:515–9.

[52] Marcos Bravo C, Luna Ortiz I, Vazquez Gonzalez R. Hypersensitivity to cefuroxime with good tolerance to other beta-lactams. Allergy 1995;50:359–61.

[53] Romano A, Quaratino D, Venuti A, et al. Selective type-1 hypersensitivity to cefuroxime. J Allergy Clin Immunol 1998;101:564–5.

[54] Romano A, Quaratino D, Venemalm L, et al. A case of IgE-mediated hypersensitivity to ceftriaxone. J Allergy Clin Immunol 1999;104:1113–4.

[55] Batchelor FR, Dewdney JM, Weston RD, et al. The immunogenicity of cephalosporin derivatives and their cross-reaction with penicillin. Immunology 1966;10:21–33.

[56] Abraham GN, Petz LD, Fudenberg HH. Immunohaematological cross-allergenicity between penicillin and cephalothin in humans. Clin Exp Immunol 1968;3:343–57.

[57] Grieco MH. Cross-allergenicity of the penicillins and the cephalosporins. Arch Intern Med 1967;119:141–6.

[58] Kabins SA, Eisenstein B, Cohen S. Anaphylactoid reaction to an initial dose of sodium cephalothin. JAMA 1965;193:165–6.

[59] Rothschild PD, Doty DB. Cephalothin reaction after penicillin sensitization. JAMA 1966; 196:372–3.

[60] Scholand JF, Tennenbaum JI, Cerilli GJ. Anaphylaxis to cephalothin in a patient allergic to penicillin. JAMA 1968;206:130–2.

[61] Pederson-Bjergaard J. Cephalothin in the treatment of penicillin sensitive patients. Acta Allergol 1967;22:299–306.

[62] Asero R. Detection of patients with multiple drug allergy syndrome by elective tolerance tests. Ann Allergy Asthma Immunol 1998;80:185–8.

[63] Moseley EK, Sullivan TJ. Allergic reactions to antimicrobial drugs in patients with a history of prior drug allergy [abstract]. J Allergy Clin Immunol 1991;87:226.

[64] Dash CH. Penicillin allergy and the cephalosporins. J Antimicrob Chemother 1975;1(Suppl 3):107–18.

[65] Petz LD. Immunologic cross-reactivity between penicillins and cephalosporins: a review. J Infect Dis 1978;137(Suppl):S74–9.

[66] Goodman EJ, Morgan MJ, Johnson PA, et al. Cephalosporins can be given to penicillin-allergic patients who do not exhibit an anaphylactic response. J Clin Anesth 2001;13:561–4.

[67] Daulat SB, Solensky R, Earl HS, et al. Safety of cephalosporin administration to patients with histories of penicillin allergy. J Allergy Clin Immunol 2004;113:1220–2.

[68] Sastre J, Quijano LD, Novalbos A, et al. Clinical cross-reactivity between amoxicillin and cephadroxil in patients allergic to amoxicillin and with good tolerance of penicillin. Allergy 1996;51:383–6.

[69] Miranda A, Blanca M, Vega JM, et al. Cross-reactivity between a penicillin and a cephalosporin with the same side chain. J Allergy Clin Immunol 1996;98:671–7.

[70] Adkinson NF, Saxon A, Spence MR, et al. Cross-allergenicity and immunogenicity of aztreonam. Rev Infect Dis 1985;7(Suppl 4):S613–21.

[71] Adkinson NF. Immunogenicity and cross-allergenicity of aztreonam. Am J Med 1990;88(Suppl 3C):S3–S14.

[72] Saxon A, Hassner A, Swabb EA, et al. Lack of cross-reactivity between aztreonam, a monobactam antibiotic, and penicillin in penicillin-allergic subjects. J Infect Dis 1984;149:16–22.

[73] Saxon A, Swabb EA, Adkinson NF. Investigation into the immunologic cross-reactivity of aztreonam with other beta-lactam antibiotics. Am J Med 1985;78(Suppl 2A):19–26.

[74] Vega JM, Blanca M, Garcia JJ, et al. Tolerance to aztreonam in patients allergic to betalactam antibiotics. Allergy 1991;46:196–202.

[75] Moss RB. Sensitization to aztreonam and cross-reactivity with other beta-lactam antibiotics in high-risk patients with cystic fibrosis. J Allergy Clin Immunol 1991;87:78–88.

[76] Graninger W, Pirich K, Schindler I, et al. Aztreonam efficacy in difficult-to-treat infections and tolerance in patients with betalactam hypersensitivity. Chemioterapia 1985;4(Suppl 1):64–6.

[77] Adkinson NF, Swabb EA, Sugerman AA. Immunology of the monobactam aztreonam. Antimicrob Agents Chemother 1984;25:93–7.

[78] Perez Pimiento A, Gomez Martinez M, Minguez Mena A, et al. Aztreonam and ceftazidime: evidence of in vivo cross-allergenicity. Allergy 1997;53:624–5.

[79] Prescott WA, DePestel DD, Ellis JJ, et al. Incidence of carbapenem-associated allergic-type reactions among patients with versus patients without a reported penicillin allergy. Clin Infect Dis 2004;38:1102–7.

[80] McConnell SA, Penzak SR, Warmack TS, et al. Incidence of imipenem hypersensitivity reactions in febrile neutropenic marrow transplant patients with a history of penicillin allergy. Clin Infect Dis 2000;31:1512–4.

[81] Saxon A, Adelman DC, Patel A, et al. Imipenem cross-reactivity with penicillin in humans. J Allergy Clin Immunol 1988;82:213–7.

[82] Harle DG, Baldo BA, Wells JV. Drugs as allergens: detection and combining site specificities of IgE antibodies to sulfamethoxazole. Mol Immunol 1988;25:1347–54.

[83] Naisbitt DJ, Hough SJ, Gill HJ, et al. Cellular disposition of sulphamethoxazole and its metabolites: implications for hypersensitivity. Br J Pharmacol 1999;126:1393–407.

[84] Cribb AE, Lee BL, Trepanier LA, et al. Adverse reactions to sulphonamide and sulphonamide-trimethoprim antimicrobials: clinical syndromes and pathogenesis. Adverse Drug React Toxicol Rev 1996;15:9–50.

[85] Morgan M, Gruchalla RS, Earl HS. Patients with sulfonamide antimicrobial "allergy": are they able to tolerate sulfonamide-containing non-antimicrobial agents? [abstract]. J Allergy Clin Immunol 2004;113:S180.

[86] Strom BL, Schinnar R, Apter AJ, et al. Absence of cross-reactivity between sulfonamide antibiotics and sulfonamide nonantibiotics. N Engl J Med 2003;349:1628–35.

[87] Shapiro LE, Knowles SR, Seber EW, et al. Safety of celecoxib in individuals allergic to sulfonamide: a pilot study. Drug Saf 2003;26:187–95.

[88] Patterson R, Bello AE, Lefkowith F. Immunologic tolerability profile of celecoxib. Clin Ther 1999;21:2065–79.

[89] Koopmans PP, van der Ven AJ, Vree TB, et al. Pathogenesis of hypersensitivity reactions to drugs in patients with HIV infection: allergic or toxic? AIDS 1995;9:217–22.

[90] Jick H. Adverse reactions to trimethoprim-sulfamethoxazole in hospitalized patients. Rev Infect Dis 1982;4:426–8.

[91] Choquet-Kastylevsky G, Vial T, Descotes J. Allergic adverse reactions to sulfonamides. Curr Allergy Asthma Rep 2002;2:16–25.

[92] Solensky R, Gruchalla RS. Non-anaphylactic drug disorders. In: Zweiman B, Schwartz LB, editors. Inflammatory mechanisms in allergic diseases. New York: Marcel Dekker; 2001. p. 411–33.

[93] Centers for Disease Control and Prevention. 1997 USPHS/IDSA guidelines for the prevention of opportunistic infections in persons infected with human immunodeficiency virus. MMWR Morb Mortal Wkly Rep 1997;46:4–6.

[94] Solensky R. Drug desensitization. Immunol Allergy Clin N Am 2004;24:425–43.

[95] Stevenson DD, Sanchez-Borges M, Szczeklik A. Classification of allergic and pseudoallergic reactions to drugs that inhibit cyclooxygenase enzymes. Ann Allergy Asthma Immunol 2001;87:177–80.

[96] Stevenson DD. Adverse reactions to nonsteroidal anti-inflammatory drugs. Immunol Allergy Clin N Am 1998;18:773–98.

[97] Stevenson DD, Simon RA. Lack of cross-reactivity between rofecoxib and aspirin in aspirin-sensitive patients with asthma. J Allergy Clin Immunol 2001;108:47–51.

[98] Woessner K, Simon RA, Stevenson DD. The safety of celecoxib in aspirin exacerbated respiratory disease. Arthritis Rheum 2002;46:2201–6.

[99] Solensky R. Drug allergy: desensitization and treatment of reactions to antibiotics and aspirin. In: Lockey RF, Bukantz SC, Bousquet J, editors. Allergens and allergen immunotherapy for allergic diseases. 3rd edition. New York: Marcel Dekker; 2004. p. 585–606.

[100] Stevenson DD. Aspirin and NSAID sensitivity. Immunol Allergy Clin N Am 2004;24: 491–505.

[101] Berges-Gimeno MP, Simon RA, Stevenson DD. Long-term treatment with aspirin desensitization in asthmatic patients with aspirin-exacerbated respiratory disease. J Allergy Clin Immunol 2003;111:180–6.

[102] Stevenson DD, Hankammer MA, Mathison DA, et al. Aspirin desensitization treatment of aspirin-sensitive patients with rhinosinusitis-asthma: long-term outcomes. J Allergy Clin Immunol 1996;98:751–8.

[103] Sweet JM, Stevenson DD, Simon RA, et al. Long-term effects of aspirin desensitization-treatment for aspirin-sensitive rhinosinusitis-asthma. J Allergy Clin Immunol 1990;85: 59–65.

[104] Levy MB, Fink JN. Anaphylaxis to celecoxib. Ann Allergy Asthma Immunol 2001;87:72–3.

[105] Gagnon R, Marlene J, Gold P. Selective celecoxib-associated anaphylactoid reaction. J Allergy Clin Immunol 2003;111:1404–5.

[106] Grob M, Pichler WJ, Wuthrich B. Anaphylaxis to celecoxib. Allergy 2002;57:264–5.

[107] Cianferoni A, Novembre E, Mugnaini L, et al. Clinical features of acute anaphylaxis in patients admitted to a university hospital: an 11-year retrospective review (1985–1996). Ann Allergy Asthma Immunol 2001;87:27–32.

[108] Brown AFT, McKinnon D, Chu K. Emergency department anaphylaxis: a review of 142 patients in a single year. J Allergy Clin Immunol 2001;108:861–6.

[109] Soto-Aguilar MC, deSchazo RD, Dawson ES. Approach to the patient with suspected local anesthetic sensitivity. Immunol Allergy Clin N Am 1998;18:851–65.

[110] Chandler MJ, Grammer LC, Patterson R. Provocative challenge with local anesthetics in patients with a prior history of reaction. J Allergy Clin Immunol 1985;75:525–7.

[111] Schatz M. Skin testing and incremental challenge in the evaluation of adverse reactions to local anesthetics. J Allergy Clin Immunol 1984;74:606–16.

[112] Gall H, Kaufmann R, Dalveram CM. Adverse reactions to local anesthetics: analysis of 197 cases. J Allergy Clin Immunol 1996;97:933–7.

[113] Turvey SE, Cronin B, Arnold AD, et al. Antibiotic desensitization for the allergic patient: 5 years of experience and practice. Ann Allergy Asthma Immunol 2004;92:426–32.

[114] Lee CW, Matulonis UA, Castells MC. Carboplatin hypersensitivity: a 12-step protocol effective in 35 desensitizations in patients with gynecological malignancies and mast cell/IgE–mediated reactions. Gynecol Oncol 2004;95:370–6.

[115] Earl HS, Sullivan TJ. Acute desensitization of a patient with cystic fibrosis allergic to both beta-lactam and aminoglycoside antibiotics. J Allergy Clin Immunol 1987;79:477–83.

[116] Lantner RR. Ciprofloxacin desensitization in a patient with cystic fibrosis. J Allergy Clin Immunol 1995;96:1001–2.

[117] Wong JT, Ripple RE, MacLean JA, et al. Vancomycin hypersensitivity: synergism with narcotics and "desensitization" by a rapid continuous intravenous protocol. J Allergy Clin Immunol 1994;94:189–94.

[118] Gorman SK, Zed PJ, Dhingra VK, et al. Rapid imipenem/cilastatin desensitization for multidrug-resistant Acinetobacter pneumonia. Ann Pharmacother 2003;37:513–6.

[119] Stark BJ, Earl HS, Gross GN, et al. Acute and chronic desensitization of penicillin-allergic patients using oral penicillin. J Allergy Clin Immunol 1987;79:523–32.

[120] Sullivan TJ, Yecies LD, Shatz GS, et al. Desensitization of patients allergic to penicillin using orally administered beta-lactam antibiotics. J Allergy Clin Immunol 1982;69:275–82.

[121] Sullivan TJ. Antigen-specific desensitization of patients allergic to penicillin. J Allergy Clin Immunol 1982;69:500–8.

[122] Wendel GD, Stark BJ, Jamison RB, et al. Penicillin allergy and desensitization in serious infections during pregnancy. N Engl J Med 1985;312:1229–32.

ELSEVIER
SAUNDERS

THE MEDICAL
CLINICS
OF NORTH AMERICA

Med Clin N Am 90 (2006) 261–262

Erratum

# Toxin-Induced Hyperthermic Syndromes

Daniel Rusyniak, MD[a,b,c,*],
Jon E. Sprague, PhD[d,e]

[a]Division of Medical Toxicology, Department of Emergency Medicine,
Indiana University School of Medicine, Indianapolis, IN, USA
[b]Department of Neurology, Indiana University School of Medicine, Indianapolis, IN, USA
[c]Department of Pharmacology and Toxicology, Indiana University School of Medicine,
Indianapolis, IN, USA
[d]Virginia College of Osteopathic Medicine, Blacksburg, VA, USA
[e]Department of Biomedical Sciences and Pathobiology, Virginia Polytechnic Institute
and State University, Blacksburg, VA, USA

The printer inadvertently published the article without making the following corrections as requested by the author during the publication process (see bold text):

*On page 1278, second full paragraph, the following text,*

Oxidative phosphorylation requires proteins in the mitochondrial inner membrane transport chain to shuttle electrons through a series of oxidation/reduction reactions that ultimately result in oxygen being converted to carbon dioxide, water, and **electrons** being pumped from the cystolic side of the inner membrane into the inner membrane space.

*should have been updated as*

Oxidative phosphorylation requires proteins in the mitochondrial inner membrane transport chain to shuttle electrons through a series of oxidation/reduction reactions that ultimately result in oxygen being converted to carbon dioxide, water, and **protons** being pumped from the cystolic side of the inner membrane into the inner membrane space.

*On page 1284, first full paragraph, the following text,*

In one of these studies, the commonly used antipsychotic olazapine reduced MDMA hyperthermia and cutaneous vasoconstriction; in the other,

* Corresponding author. Division of Medical Toxicology, Department of Emergency Medicine, Indiana University School of Medicine, 1050 Wishard Boulevard, Room 2200, Indianapolis, IN 46202.
*E-mail address:* drusynia@iupui.edu (D. Rusyniak).

0025-7125/06/$ - see front matter © 2005 Elsevier Inc. All rights reserved.
doi:10.1016/j.mcna.2005.11.001

carvedilol reduced MDMA hyperthermia and rhabdomyolysis [65,75]. Olanzapine antagonizes a variety of receptor systems, including 5-HT2a, D-1, and $\alpha_1$ receptors, although which of these is responsible for its effects in MDMA hyperthermia is currently unknown.

*should have been updated as*

In one of these studies, the commonly used antipsychotics olazapine **and clozapine** reduced MDMA hyperthermia and cutaneous vasoconstriction; in the other, carvedilol reduced MDMA hyperthermia and rhabdomyolysis [65,75]. Olanzapine **and clozapine** affect of variety of receptor systems, including 5-HT2a, D-1, **D-2**, and $\alpha_1$ receptors, although which of these is responsible for its effects in MDMA hyperthermia is currently unknown.

*On page 1285, first full paragraph, the following text,*

Of note, the theoretic benefit of benzodiazepines, which hyperpolarize neurons, reducing central mediated catecholamine release [83], and **prevent** serotonin syndrome in rats [56].

*should have been updated as*

Of note, the theoretic benefit of benzodiazepines, which hyperpolarize neurons, reducing central mediated catecholamine release [83], and **decrease** serotonin syndrome in rats [56].

ELSEVIER
SAUNDERS

Med Clin N Am 90 (2006) 263–273

THE MEDICAL
CLINICS
OF NORTH AMERICA

# Index

*Note:* Page numbers of article titles are in **boldface** type.

0025-7125/06/$ - see front matter © 2005 Elsevier Inc. All rights reserved.
doi:10.1016/S0025-7125(05)00124-0 *medical.theclinics.com*

Vocal cord dysfunction
   asthma and, 41, 48–49
   versus asthma, 62, 67–68

**W**

Wasp stings, allergy to. *See* Insect sting
   allergy.

**Y**

Yellow jacket stings, allergy to. *See* Insect
   sting allergy.

**Z**

Zafirlukast, for allergic rhinitis, 31–32

Zileuton, for allergic rhinitis, 31–32

# Elsevier is proud to announce...

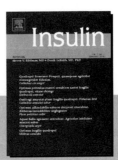

# Insulin

www.insulinjournal.com

## ...the newest addition to its group of premier journals.

*Insulin* is a peer-reviewed clinically oriented journal covering the latest advances in insulin-related disorders. Review articles will focus on the clinical care of patients with diabetes, complications, education, and treatments within special patient populations. The journal will also feature editorials, case studies, and patient handouts. *Insulin* will be of interest to family practitioners, diabetes educators, and other health care professionals.

**Co-Editors-in-Chief:**
Steven V. Edelman, MD, and
Derek LeRoith, MD, PhD
insulin@elsevier.com

**Contact:**
Cindy Jablonowski, Publisher
908.547.2090
c.jablonowski@elsevier.com

---

### Yes! I would like a FREE subscription (4 issues).

| Name | | Degree | Affiliation | | |
| Street | | | | | |
| City | | State | Zip | | Country |
| Telephone | | E-mail | | | |

**Fax to:** Insulin
(908) 547-2204

**Mail to:** Insulin
685 Route 202/206
Bridgewater, NJ 08807, USA

# Changing Your Address?

Make sure your subscription changes too! When you notify us of your new address, you can help make our job easier by including an exact copy of your Clinics label number with your old address (see illustration below.) This number identifies you to our computer system and will speed the processing of your address change. Please be sure this label number accompanies your old address and your corrected address—you can send an old Clinics label with your number on it or just copy it exactly and send it to the address listed below.

We appreciate your help in our attempt to give you continuous coverage. Thank you.

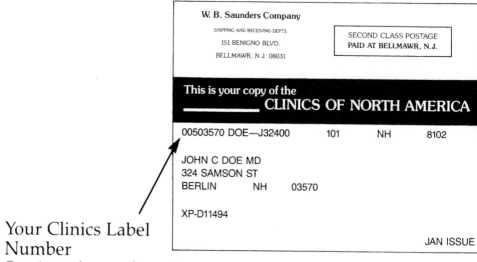

**W. B. Saunders Company**

SHIPPING AND RECEIVING DEPTS.
151 BENIGNO BLVD.
BELLMAWR, N.J. 08031

SECOND CLASS POSTAGE
PAID AT BELLMAWR, N.J.

**This is your copy of the**
_____ **CLINICS OF NORTH AMERICA**

00503570 DOE—J32400          101        NH        8102

JOHN C DOE MD
324 SAMSON ST
BERLIN          NH        03570

XP-D11494

JAN ISSUE

## Your Clinics Label Number

Copy it exactly or send your label along with your address to:
**W.B. Saunders Company, Customer Service**
Orlando, FL 32887-4800
Call Toll Free 1-800-654-2452

Please allow four to six weeks for delivery of new subscriptions and for processing address changes.

Allergy

616.97                                    130005
AL54

GAYLORD S